# Nursing in Critical Care Setting

Irene Comisso • Alberto Lucchini
Stefano Bambi • Gian Domenico Giusti
Matteo Manici

# Nursing in Critical Care Setting

## An Overview from Basic to Sensitive Outcomes

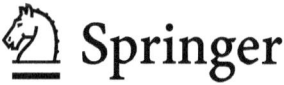 Springer

Irene Comisso
University Anesthesia and
Intensive Care Unit
University Hospital S. Maria della
Misericordia
Udine, Italy

Stefano Bambi
Emergency and Trauma ICU
University Hospital Careggi
Florence, Italy

Matteo Manici
Anesthesia, Intensive Care and
Hub Pain Service
University Hospital of Parma
Parma, Italy

Alberto Lucchini
General Intensive Care Unit - San
Gerardo Hospital – ASST Monza
University of Milano-Bicocca
Milan, Italy

Gian Domenico Giusti
Intensive Care Unit
University Hospital of Perugia
Perugia, Italy

ISBN 978-3-030-09595-6        ISBN 978-3-319-50559-6   (eBook)
https://doi.org/10.1007/978-3-319-50559-6

Printed on acid-free paper

This Springer imprint is published by the registered company Springer
International Publishing AG part of Springer Nature
The registered company address is: Gewerbestrasse 11, 6330 Cham,
Switzerland

# Dedication and Acknowledgements

The Authors wish to dedicate this manuscript to their families and beloved ones, and thank them for the important support given during the editing.

Thanks to all the components of our working groups. They daily collaborate with us , often providing us inspiration and precious suggestions. Also, thanks to the collaborators, who helped us in editing the manuscript.

A special thought is directed to our nursing students. They are the future of our profession, and we wish them to keep working with passion and curiosity lifelong.

Finally, this manuscript originated from our patients and their families. By this publication, we wish to give nurses a tool to improve patients' care, always keeping the person we care for as the main focus of our job.

The Authors' Group

# Preface

In May 2015, me and two co-authors were contacted by Springer's editor, offering to travel this route. We accepted with enthusiasm, but at the same time with several perplexities. We decided to enlarge the group, and started working to define essential concepts to be considered within the manuscript. Day by day, the project gathered consistency, and the path we wanted to offer to readers became clear in our minds.

Nursing care in ICU is complex and requires continuos competences and knowledges update. As in other contexts, both basic and advanced competences can be found in ICU care. The book is directed to students and newly employee ICU nurses, but also to experienced ones. We aimed to underline the importance of basic aspects in ICU nursing, in the past often disregarded in favor of more technical approaches. In our advice, today's ICU nurse is a very complex professional. Technical, assessment, relational, team working competences are all required to face daily challenges. This is what we tried to offer within this book, together with the consciousness that it only constitutes a part of a larger view.

The author's group comes from different ICU experiences around Italy. Trying to get an advantage of it, we networked each other, giving mutual supervision to the forthcoming contents. At the end of this travel, I think we all somehow grew up from the professional point of view, and learned more.

Our wish is to give a similar feeling to our readers.

Irene Comisso and the Authors' Group

# Contents

## Part II   Basic Care in ICU

# Contributors

**Giacomo Alemanno, R.N.** Vascular Surgery, Kent and Canterbury Hospital, East Kent Hospital University Foundation Trust, Canterbury, UK

**Stefano Bambi, R.N., M.S.N., Ph.D.** Emergency & Trauma ICU, University Hospital Careggi, Florence, Italy

**Giovanni Becattini, R.N., M.S.N.** Nursing Service-Siena Urban Area, AUSL South Eastern Tuscany, Italy

**Irene Comisso, R.N., M.S.N.** University Anesthesia and Intensive Care Unit, University Hospital S. Maria della Misericordia, Udine, Italy

**Stefano Elli, R.N.** General Intensive Care Unit, San Gerardo Hospital, ASST Monza, Monza, Italy

**Christian De Felippis, R.N.** Adult Intensive Care Unit, Glenfield Hospital, University Hospital of Leicester-NHS Trust, Leicester, UK

**Francesca Ghillani** Research Fellow, Oxford Institute of Population Ageing, University of Oxford, Oxford, UK

**Gian Domenico Giusti, R.N., M.S.N.** Intensive Care Unit, University Hospital of Perugia, Perugia, Italy

**Alberto Lucchini, R.N.** General Intensive Care Unit, San Gerardo Hospital, ASST Monza, University of Milano-Bicocca, Milan, Italy

**Matteo Manici, R.N., M.S.N.** Anesthesia, Intensive Care and Hub Pain Service, University Hospital of Parma, Parma, Italy

**Giovanni Mistraletti, M.D., Ph.D.** Department of Pathophysiology and Transplantation, University of Milan, Milan, Italy

**Alessandra Negro, R.N.** Vita-Salute San Raffaele University, Milan, Italy

IRCCS San Raffaele Hospital, Milano, Italy

**Margherita I. Nuzzaco, R.N.** Intensive Care Unit, Kent and Canterbury Hospital, East Kent Hospital University Foundation Trust, Canterbury, UK

**Angela Peghetti, R.N., M.S.N.** Nurse Staff. Nurse Department, AOU "S.Orsola Malpighi", Bologna, Italy

**Michele Pirovano, R.N., M.S.N.** AREU Regional Emergency System-IT, Milan, Italy

**Claudio Torbinio, R.N.** Trauma Centre, Emergency Department, Ancona Hospital, Province of Ancona, Italy

# Introduction

ICU caring underwent a constant development during the last 15 years, with the introduction of new standard treatments. At the same time, ongoing problems are challenging healthcare workers, whilst others are announced as decisive ones for future years.

In this process, the importance of technology increased, but at the same time humanising caring and end of life related dilemmas gathered growing consideration.

Nowadays, ICU generally set themselves up as most complex specialistic level of care, mainly belonging to surgical, trauma or respiratory pathways. General ICUs developed within peripheral areas, whilst specialistic ones belong to second or third level hospitals and are characterised for advanced treatments, for which they are considered referral centres (such as for ECMO or solid organs transplants).

Another visible trend in ICU refers to mortality. In the past, ICUs were considered as the last possible step during hospital stay, moving forward the care limit with consequent high mortality rates. Today's ICUs have often lower mortality rates, compared to other hospital facilities, but advancements in diagnosis and organ support claim a structured reflection about limits of care.

At the same time, mean patients- age increased. Elderly, previously screened for ICU eligibility, are now usually assisted in these contexts, and require specific consideration for age-related problems and needs.

ICU stay often occupies an early stage during hospitalisation, followed by less critical and invasive approaches. Therefore, performances-evaluation should overcome traditional measurements, such as mortality and length of stay, and start looking upon specific nursing care outcomes and quality of life indicators, often disregarded because too simple.

Care outcomes, including those related to nursing, became therefore a central issue. In fact, the quality-of-life concept together with life-saving approaches, spread the debate about ethical considerations. At the same time, focus on nursing techniques in critical care settings should be matched with a renewed scientific approach to basic care problems.

"Back to basics" becomes therefore the fil rouge of the entire manuscript, deepening the concepts of basic nursing applicable in the whole critical care (including High dependency Units). This philosophy, together with the ABCDEF bundle, approaches a new tendency in patients care, hopefully early belonging to the whole care pathway during hospitalisation.

Modern nursing deals with such development, claiming for a more specific definition of competences belonging to the profession and for the development of certification systems. Consequently, building a professional portfolio of activities and performances could help to develop and maintain nurses-education and develop standards of care.

Further considerations concern the role of management in ICU. Clinical and technological complexities, together with required knowledge and competences and multidisciplinary approaches, solicit an expert management. Within organisational challenges, the entire set of competences should always be granted. Therefore, a flexible nurse-to-patient ratio could be one of the mail solutions to guarantee specific clinical interventions in a dynamic organizational contex.

This manuscript is mainly oriented towards two main groundings of nursing care: assessment and outcomes. Patients assessment in ICU cannot forget technological-based information collection, that, together with clinical observation, represent the common nursing asset. At the same time, nursing care approaches are moving toward definition and evaluation of outcomes-related problems, thus giving a new dimension and dignity to the nursing diagnosis concept. In these situations, the border between medical and nursing competences becomes sometimes very thin. Nevertheless, the authors defined to approach such topics mainly from nursing point of view, only briefing touching upon medical issues. In this paradigm, we choose to face emerging nursing care aspects, with an evidence based approach.

The wish is to keep alive and strengthen critical thinking, and spread curiosity for a novel approach to nursing problems.

Enjoy reading!

Giovanni Becattini

# Part I
# Assessment and Monitoring in ICU

# Chapter 1
# Monitoring Patients: What's New in Intensive Care Setting?

**Matteo Manici and Claudio Torbinio**

## 1.1 Introduction

Monitoring ("to monitor") is a term that involves the observation, actions, measuring, and understanding of many human activities in time. The origin of the word "monitoring" comes from the Latin *monitor, -oris*, derived from the verb *monēre* (literally, to warn) and means a continuous or repeated observation, measurement, and evaluation of health and/or environmental or technical data for defined purposes, in accordance with predetermined programs in space and time. Monitoring can be implemented using comparable methods for the detection and collection of data [1]. The term originated in industrial environment, to indicate the continuous control of an operating machine, with appropriate instruments which measure some characteristic parameters (speed, consumption, production, etc.). The original meaning was later expanded: from the machine to the whole process, for an operational structure, and also human resources. Monitoring is widespread used in technical and in social sciences, with the general meaning of "data collections" significant for context.

Historically, monitoring started as a physiological measurement problem (Table 1.1) and probably will end up as an overall

© Springer International Publishing AG, part of Springer Nature 2018    3
I. Comisso et al., *Nursing in Critical Care Setting*,
https://doi.org/10.1007/978-3-319-50559-6_1

**Table 1.1** Short history of physiological data measurements [2]

| When | Who | What |
|------|-----|------|
| 1625 | *Santorio* | Measurement of body temperature with spirit thermometer. Timing pulse with pendulum. Principles were established by Galileo. These results were ignored |
| 1707 | *Sir John Foyer* | Published pulse watch |
| 1852 | *Ludwig Taube* | Course of patient's fever measurement. At this time temperature, pulse rate, and respiratory rate had become standard vital signs |
| 1896 | *Scipione Riva-Rocci* | Introduced the sphygmomanometer (blood pressure cuff) |
| 1900 | *Nikolaj Sergeevič Korotkov* | Applied the cuff with the stethoscope (developed by Rene Laennec—French physician) to measure systolic and diastolic blood pressures |
| 1900 | *Harvey Cushing* | Applied routine blood pressure in operating rooms |
| 1903 | *Willem Einthoven* | Devised the string galvanometer to measure ECG (Nobel Prize 1924) |
| 1939–1945 | | World War II: development of transducers |
| 1948–1950 | *George Ludwig, Ian Donald, Douglass Howry, and Joseph Holmes* | Pioneers of ultrasounds in health science |
| 1950 | | The ICU's were established to meet the increasing demands for more acute and intensive care required by patients with complex disorders |
| 1953 | | Danish patients with poliomyelitis received invasive mechanical ventilation |

**Table 1.1** (continued)

| When | Who | What |
|------|-----|------|
| 1963 | Hughes W. Day | Reported that treatment of post-myocardial infarction patients in a coronary care unit reduced mortality by 60% |
| 1968 | Maloney | Suggested that having the nurse record vital signs every few hours was "only to assure regular nurse-patient contact" |
| Early 1970s | | Bedside monitors built around bouncing balls or conventional oscilloscope |
| 1972 | Takuo Aoyagi | Developed a pulse oximeter based on the ratio of red to infrared light absorption in blood. After obtained an US patent, oximetry became clinically feasible |
| 1973 | Jeremy Swan and William Ganz | Pulmonary artery balloon flotation catheter starts advanced hemodynamic study |
| 1990s | | Computer-based patient monitors; systems with database functions, report-generation systems, and some decision-making capabilities |

assessment of intensive care unit (ICU) patient. This chapter has an introductory function for the first section: the concept of generality of instrumental monitoring, the monitoring carried out through applying scales at patient's bed, to propose a new monitoring model for ICU patient.

ICUs are very different, such as medical and surgical wards, because of different staff availability (especially nurses) and expertise, skills, technologies, and environments. Monitoring activity involves the entire ICU staff (nurses, physician, respiratory therapists and rehabilitation therapists, dietitians) and is based on different operational models implemented in several countries around the world. Nurses, wherever present 24 h a day, often act as liaison between the various staff components, ensuring security, continuity, and harmony and coordinating and communicating all aspects of treatment and care the patient needs. Nurses also provide continuous monitoring and caring for patients and equipment and for their interactions [3].

## 1.2 Instrumental Monitoring

Technology is extremely pervasive and is continuously increasing in ICU. It is commonly used in a multitude of tools for monitoring and supporting patient's vital functions: the brain, lung, heart, and kidney. The widespread use of electronic monitoring and support to vital function has probably helped to prevent errors and to improve outcomes [4].

The monitoring tools are able to detect multiple parameters, such as continuous electrocardiogram (ECG), end-tidal carbon dioxide $(EtCO)_2$, various measurements of peripheral oxygen saturation $(SpO_2)$, cardiac output, and intracranial and cerebral perfusion pressure. The supporting devices can affect the respiratory system (noninvasive mechanical ventilation), circulatory (pacemakers, intra-aortic balloon pump, ventricular devices), cardiorespiratory (extracorporeal membrane oxygenation—ECMO), and kidney (continuous renal replacement therapy (CRRT) and slow low-efficiency daily dialysis (SLEDD)). All these supporting systems contextually also provide monitoring parameters (e.g., the ventilator). Understanding the functions of the devices commonly used in ICU can help in caring for patients in critical conditions [5].

The monitoring technique in intensive care has risks and benefits. Intensive monitoring provides a high data value and information, but it can increase some risks of complications.

For example, intensive monitoring could be useful in acute medical interventions aiming to maintain the essential variables within a narrow physiological range and improve the outcome in people with acute stroke [6] (Fig. 1.1).

At the same time, continuous monitoring can increase unnecessary medical interventions and limit patient's mobility, thus increasing the risk of complications related to forced immobility as bedsores, stasis pneumonia, deep vein thrombosis (DVT), thromboembolism (TE), and pain [7].

All recorded data must be evaluated in the clinical context. The value of data must be compared with the accuracy of the instrument, its need for calibration, artifacts, and fictitious events (such

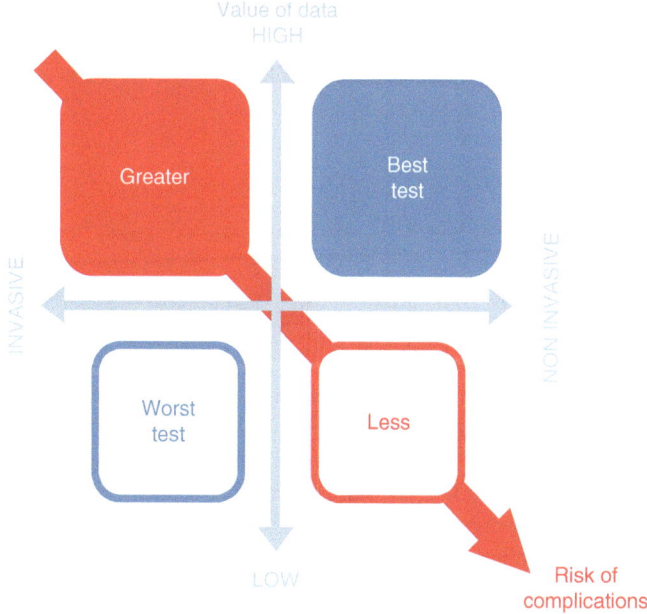

**Fig. 1.1** Conceptual framework-related value of data

as a cough during ventilation). As told it is essential to treat patients and their disease instead of numbers. All monitored parameters must be considered in relation to the disease as the best method to treat the same.

In medical literature there are many studies concerning the false alarm rates in the critical patient monitoring. These studies show more than 90% of ICU alarms are false flags. In many cases, these are caused by measurement errors and by patient's movement. The majority of ICU alarms have no real clinical impact on patient care [8].

A too sensitive monitoring can create "panic" within the team. Staff alarm fatigue can determine inadequate and routine alarm settings. Alarms settings should be tailored on patients individual clinical needs and targets [9]. However, the biggest danger is given by turning off the alarms without understanding events actually occurring to patients. Alarm management is a part of the skills that intensive care staff need to learn at the beginning of their professional careers.

## 1.3   Monitoring and Scales

Through the use of a variety of assessment scales (mono-dimensional or multidimensional, according to the complexity of the construct they want to observe), it is possible to obtain measures of many functional states that cannot be described by any instrumental monitoring systems.

Some aspects have been carefully studied by many authors such as pain, sedation, delirium, and state of consciousness. Other authors made comparisons between tools to determine their adequacy in psychometric characteristics, becoming recommended in international guidelines [10].

An example of the use of scales (and their variations) is represented by functional evaluation. ICU patients frequently experience prolonged immobilization and tend to lose their functional ability. In these patients functional skills assessment during ICU stay and prior ICU discharge becomes crucial to prevent damage from immobility. Many scales have been used for the evaluation of functional abilities, impairments, and/or patients' disabilities. The extent of these outcomes includes different measurement scales. The choice of the right one will depend on the specific cohort of patients, the diagnosis, the stage of rehabilitation, and the available measure sets [11]. These scales are summarized in Table 1.2. Their applicability in ICU environments (including the follow-up period) is indicated in the last column.

## 1.4 Bedside Monitoring: An Overview

The ICU monitoring is a component of critical area skill set, featuring as neurological monitoring, respiratory, hemodynamic, renal, hepatic, and nutritional. Each function can be both assessed using validated tools and/or instrumental monitoring [12–14].

The rating scales are mostly developed in the assessment of psychosocial functions (neurologic evaluation, pain, sedation, and delirium) and the instrumental monitoring for detection of biological parameters (respiration, hemodynamics, temperature, and metabolism).

The main monitoring variables "to read and feel" are summarized in Table 1.3.

A useful example of the effectiveness of the interpretation of monitoring takes us outside the ICU with Early Warning Score (EWS) in the National Early Warning Score (NEWS) variants and Modified Early Warning Score (MEWS) (Table 1.4). The basic

**Table 1.2** Functional assessment scales in the ICUs [11], modified with permission

| Scale | Description | Interpretation | Applicability in ICU setting |
|---|---|---|---|
| Functional Status Score for the ICU (FSS-ICU) | Consists of three preambulation categories (rolling, supine to sit transfer, and unsupported sitting) and two ambulation categories (sit to stand transfers and ambulation) | • Rating: 1 (total dependent assistance) to 7 (complete independence) scale<br>• Score: 0–35 (0 score: unable to perform a task due to physical limitations or medical status) | ++ |
| 4P questionnaire | Evaluates physical and psychosocial problems following ICU recovery | • 4P: patients, physical, psychosocial, and problems<br>• 4P comprises 53 items: 16 physical items, 26 psychosocial items, and 11 follow-up ICU care items, scored on a 5-point Likert scale measuring level of agreement from "strongly agree" to "do not agree at all" | ++ |

| Physical Function ICU Test (PFIT) | Used with critically ill patients who may not be able to mobilize away from the bedside, employing four domains | • Amount of assistance for sit to ++ stand, rated from 0 (no physical assistance required) to 3 (assistance of three people required) |
| | | • Strength for shoulder flexion and knee extension (rated on the Oxford Muscle Test Scale) |
| | | • Marching in place (number of steps taken and the time required to complete these steps) |
| | | • An upper extremity endurance task of arm elevation to 90° shoulder flexion (number of times both upper extremities are lifted above 90° of shoulder flexion) |

(continued)

**Table 1.2** (continued)

| Scale | Description | Interpretation | Applicability in ICU setting |
|---|---|---|---|
| Modified Rankin Scale (mRS) | Quantifies independence and disability, with a scale of 6 grades (0–5) | • 0, no symptoms<br>• 1, no significant disability despite symptoms<br>• 2, slight disability<br>• 3, moderate disability<br>• 4, moderately severe disability<br>• 5, severe disability | + |
| Glasgow Outcome Scale (GOS) | Provides a global assessment of function (see text for modified GOS scales) | • Score 1: good recovery<br>• Score 2: moderate disability<br>• Score 3: severe disability<br>• Score 4 vegetative state<br>• Score 5: death | + |
| Karnofsky Performance Scale Index | A descriptive, ordinal scale that ranges from 100 (good health) to 0 (dead) and emphasizes physical performance and dependency | • Karnofsky index of 70–100: a favorable functional outcome measure | ± |

| | | | ± |
|---|---|---|---|
| Barthel Index (BI) | It measures the capacity to perform ten basic activities of daily living self-care (feeding, grooming, bathing, dressing, bowel and bladder care, and toilet use) and mobility (ambulation, transfers, and stair climbing) | • Scoring ranges from 0 (totally dependent) to 100 (totally independent)<br>• BI index score >90: minimal or no disability<br>• BI index 55–90: moderate disability<br>• BI index <55: severe disability | ± |
| Disability Rating Scale (DRS) | A common outcome measure of impairment, disability, and handicap; the scale is intended to assess accurately general functional changes over the course of recovery | • Impairment ratings: "eye opening," "communication ability," and "motor response"<br>• Level of disability: ability for "feeding," "toileting" and "grooming"<br>• Handicap: "level of functioning" and "employability"<br>• Rating for each functioning area: scale of 0 to either 3 or 5<br>• Maximum score (29): extreme vegetative state<br>• Lowest score (0): a person without disability | ± |

**Table 1.3** Synoptic table of principal monitoring

| Monitoring | Main technological devices | Main assessment scale |
|---|---|---|
| Neurological | • Electroencephalography<br>• ICP (intracranial pressure) and CPP (central perfusion pressure)<br>• Brain tissue oxygen monitoring [15]<br>• Cerebral microdialysis [16] | • GCS (Glasgow coma scale)<br>• FOUR (Full Outline of UnResponsiveness)<br>• Pupillary reactivity [15] |
| Pain | | • NRS (Numerical Rating Scale)<br>• NRS-V (NRS-Visual horizontal)<br>• BPS (Behavioral Pain Scale)<br>• BPS-NI (Behavioral Pain Scale Non-Intubated)<br>CPOT (Critical-Care Pain Observation Tool) [17] |
| Agitation (sedation) | • BIS (bispectral index) [18] | • SAS (Sedation-Agitation Scale)<br>• RASS (Richmond Agitation-Sedation Scale) [17] |
| Delirium | | • CAM-ICU (Confusion Assessment Method-ICU)<br>• ICDSC (Intensive Care Delirium Screening Checklist) [17] |

| | |
|---|---|
| Respiratory and ventilator | • Basic respiratory system mechanics |
| | • Static compliance of the respiratory system |
| | • Resistance of the respiratory system |
| | • Dynamic hyperinflation |
| | • Gas exchange (monitoring oxygenation, arterial oximetry, efficacy of oxygen exchange, monitoring carbon dioxide, assessment of $PaCO_2$, dead space ventilation and $PCO_2$) [19] |
| | • Graphic curve ventilator monitoring [20] |
| Traditional hemodynamic | • Cardiac ECG (HR, HR variability, arrhythmias, ST monitoring) |
| | • IBP (invasive blood pressure) |
| | • NIBP (noninvasive BP) |
| | • CVP (central venous pressure) |
| | • SwGa measurement (PAP, PW, SV, CO, indexed value, etc.) [19] |
| Central hemodynamic monitoring | • Macrocirculation monitoring (pulse contour analysis, Vigileo/FloTrac system, LiDCO, the PiCCO system, esophageal Doppler, thoracic electrical bioimpedance, echocardiography) [19] |

(continued)

**Table 1.3** (continued)

| Monitoring | Main technological devices | Main assessment scale |
|---|---|---|
| Peripheral hemodynamic–tissue perfusion | • Microcirculation monitoring<br>• Gastric tonometry and sublingual capnography<br>• Mixed venous or central venous saturation ($SvO_2$ and oxygen extraction, interpreting $SvO_2$, $ScvO_2$, and perfusion)<br>• Lactate clearance<br>• Venous-to-arterial $CO_2$ gradient ($CO_2$ production and transport physiology, determinants of $P(v–a)CO_2$, $P(v–a)CO_2$ increase, and clinical hypoperfusion) [19]<br>• IAP (intra-abdominal pressure) and APP (abdominal perfusion pressure) | |
| Temperature | • Accurate measurement in the pulmonary artery, distal esophagus, tympanic membrane, bladder, or nasopharynx [19] | |
| Nutritional and metabolic care | • Protein and energy delivery for the prevention of protein-energy deficit<br>• Glycemia and insulin therapy for optimized glycemic control [19] | • NRI (Nutritional Risk Index)<br>• GNRI (Geriatric Nutritional Risk Index)<br>• SGA (Subjective Global Assessment)<br>• MNA-SF (Mini Nutritional Assessment-Screening Form)<br>• MUST (Malnutrition Universal Screening Tool)<br>• NRS 2002 (Nutritional Risk Screening 2002) [21] |

**Table 1.4** NEWS and MEWS comparison

| Physiological parameters | NEWS (National Early Warning System) | | | | | | | MEWS (Modified Early Warning System) | | | | | | |
|---|---|---|---|---|---|---|---|---|---|---|---|---|---|---|
| | 3 | 2 | 1 | 0 | 1 | 2 | 3 | 3 | 2 | 1 | 0 | 1 | 2 | 3 |
| Respiration rate (breath/min) | ≤8 | | 9 11 | 12 20 | | 21 24 | ≥25 | | ≤8 | | 9 14 | 15 20 | 21 29 | ≥30 |
| Oxygen saturation (%) | ≤90 | 91–93 | 94 95 | ≥96 | | | | | | | | | | |
| Supplemental oxygen | | Yes | | No | | | | | | | | | | |
| Temperature (°C) | ≤35.0 | | 35.1 36.0 | 36.1 38.0 | 38.1 39.0 | ≥39.1 | | | ≤35.0 | 35.1 36 | 36.1 38 | 38.1 38.5 | ≥38.6 | |
| Systolic BP (mmHg) | ≤90 | 91 100 | 101 110 | 111 219 | | | ≥220 | ≤70 | 71 80 | 81 100 | 101 199 | | ≥200 | |
| Heart rate (beat/min) | ≤40 | | 41 50 | 51 90 | 91 110 | 111 130 | ≥131 | | ≤40 | 40 50 | 51 100 | 101 110 | 111 129 | ≥129 |
| Level of consciousness (AVPU) | | | | A | | | V, P o U | U | P | V | A | | New Agit. Conf. | |
| Hourly urine for 2 h (mL/h) | | | | | | | | ≤10 | 11 30 | 31 45 | | | | |

0–4—low level of clinical risk: monitoring
5–6—medium level of clinical risk: call physician
≥7 or single item at level 3—high level of clinical risk: call emergency team

principle is the collection of common physical parameters and variables in a score that allows a fast and shared evaluation of clinical status. In hospitalized patients, addressing the deterioration of physiological functions before they precipitate and to define the intensity of required care can be helpful. In the community, the numerical values expressed by NEWS provide a clear indication of the severity level and help to find the limit for referral to the emergency department and urgent.

In general, the NEWS score provides a universal standard for the evaluation of the clinical course, with the sole exception of obstetrical and pediatric cases, and end of life care [22]. The comparison of the two instruments is reported in Table 1.4.

## 1.5   A New Monitoring Model

Which point of view can we provide with the monitoring for an interpretation pace with the expectations of nurses who study, who approach, and who are eventually working in intensive care? What we propose with this text is a more holistic view of the event "monitoring": a nursing activity that concerns first the person as a whole and, then, individual organ parameters and vital signs.

Monitoring can be defined in a conceptual area bounded by the level of invasiveness and objectivity of the systems that we use in the "measurement." Increasing the level of invasiveness and objectivity of the measures will also increase the precision level of the measured variables. Collected information must be sufficient and necessary to determine the diagnosis, the performance of the clinical status, and the response to therapies, but, the collection of unnecessary data (such as the execution of ECG 12 times a day in people without cardiac problems, performing unnecessary blood tests, or even the advanced hemodynamic monitoring in patients with only slightly altered parameters) worsens costs without improving outcomes. In a context of limited resources, the selection of the right level of monitoring should be based on proven systems that maximize the cost-benefit ratio [23].

The concept can be expressed in a diagram (Fig. 1.2) in which the operator is bounded by increasing levels of invasiveness and objectivity of the measures, resulting in three different monitoring levels:

- Level 1: intuitive observational monitoring
- Level 2: discontinuous monitoring
- Level 3: continuous monitoring

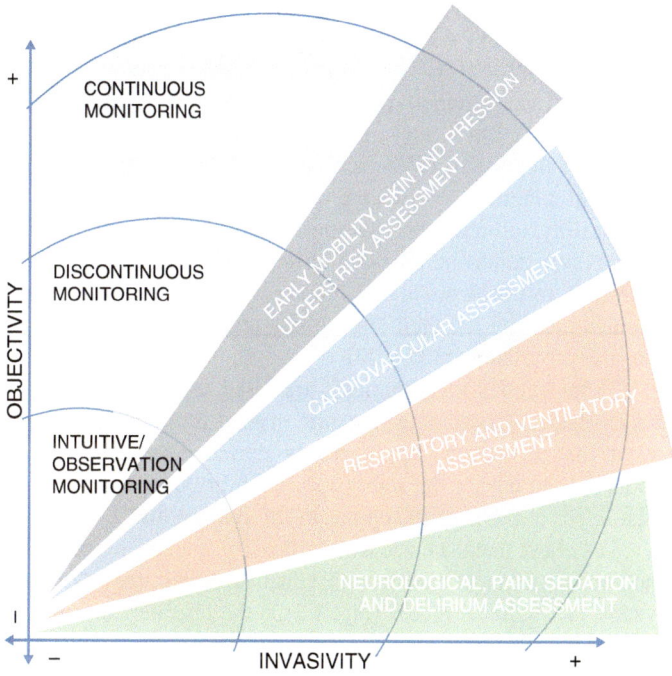

**Fig. 1.2** The MAGIS (acronym of the initials of authors' names) model of intensive care nursing monitoring

The effective observation of hospitalized patients is the first step to identify the patient's concerns and the effectiveness of care management. In all contexts, it is vital for nurses to understand the dataset collected, for a positive impact on outcome of patients through the prevention of problems, which otherwise can drive to acute illness, ICU readmission, or death [24].

Poor technology leads to nurse's feelings play an important role in the perception of patient's deterioration, and vital parameters are used to support the "gut" feelings [25], that is, highly complex and influenced by many factor process, including the experience and preparation of nurses as well as their ability to relate to the medical staff.

There is a lot of difference in the world regarding "ICU numbers": the number of ICU beds for 100 hospital beds or for 100,000 people and technologies and health staff as well as the level of education [26]. But feeling and observation are available for all.

The evaluation of EWS facilitated the early identification of a critical condition. Nurses are called to act professionally and responsibly, to understand the meaning of the observations collected on patients and recorded during time. With a partnership approach to problem-solving, nurses can be effective in communicating with the multidisciplinary team and in bringing the most appropriate care [24, 27].

Discontinuous measurements are often carried out with the rating scales. Continuous ones are instead often obtained with electronic instruments appropriately alerted. These are a lot of tools able to ensure the safety and reliability of the monitoring that arises at the base of support of the ICU quality.

We believe that the nurse who approaches in intensive care cannot think in terms of machine/scale dualism as happened for many years. The MAGIS model (Fig. 1.2) is the operationalization of monitoring construct shown in this text. It suggests a systematic approach to monitoring that begins by insights and observation of clinical variables and appearance of the patient and deepens the clinical trial on rating scales and instrumental monitoring.

Monitoring is a dynamic process, a set of details that, correctly linked and interpreted, describe the entirety of the person in relation to his state of health in the moment of observation and over time, through the evolution of trends. The multimodal monitoring offered by different equipments require high levels of expertise within nursing staff to find answers that are not wasteful and respect the proper use of resources in terms of cost/effectiveness.

In conclusion, the new monitoring technologies are to be built up and have to demonstrate a positive impact on the result before being used. We believe that there is no easy answer to this question. Most hospital administrators require outcome data before purchasing any new and expensive technology. This approach, however, could delay application of useful technologies.

There are few studies that have analyzed the impact of monitoring on results. For example, the oximeter has shown no impact on patients' outcomes [28], and the role of intracranial pressure routine monitoring in comatose patients with acute trauma fails to provide evidence in support of the operation [29]. Despite of these results, those systems are considered essential in monitoring.

A more reflective evaluation of clinical indications and the training of doctors in the area of Swan-Ganz catheter and hemodynamic management would have avoided many patients the unnecessary placement of the cardiac catheter-related damage [30].

Daily challenges will come from deep knowledge of monitoring technologies and appropriate choice according to patient's condition, available resources, and staff expertise.

# References

1. Nič M, Jirát J, Košata B, Jenkins A, McNaught A. IUPAC compendium of chemical terminology—the gold book. Research Triangle Park, NC: International Union of Pure and Applied Chemistry; 2009.
2. Patient Care and Monitoring Systems. 2013. http://www.eng.tau.ac.il/~gannot/MI/file2.ppt. Accessed 12 May 2016.

3. Welch JR, Theaker C. Ruolo infermieristico in terapia intensiva. In: Bersten AD, Soni N, editors. Oh Manuale di terapia intensiva. sesta edizione ed. Milano: Elsevier Health Sciences Italy; 2010. p. 3197–647.
4. Vincent JL, Singer M. Critical care: advances and future perspectives. Lancet. 2010;376(9749):1354–61. https://doi.org/10.1016/S0140-6736(10)60575-2.
5. Schallom M. Monitoring and support devices in the Intensive Care Unit. Support Line. 2014;36(6):20–5. 10.21037/jtd.2016.05.37.
6. Ciccone A, Celani MG, Chiaramonte R, Rossi C, Righetti E. Continuous versus intermittent physiological monitoring for acute stroke. Cochrane Database Syst Rev 2013;(5):CD008444. doi: https://doi.org/10.1002/14651858.CD008444.pub2.
7. Adams HP Jr, del Zoppo G, Alberts MJ, Bhatt DL, Brass L, Furlan A, et al. Guidelines for the early management of adults with ischemic stroke: a guideline from the American Heart Association/American Stroke Association Stroke Council, Clinical Cardiology Council, Cardiovascular Radiology and Intervention Council, and the Atherosclerotic Peripheral Vascular Disease and Quality of Care Outcomes in Research Interdisciplinary Working Groups: The American Academy of Neurology affirms the value of this guideline as an educational tool for neurologists. Circulation. 2007;115(20):e478–534.
8. Imhoff M, Kuhls S. Alarm algorithms in critical care monitoring. Anesth Analg. 2006;102(5):1525–37.
9. ECRI Institute. Top 10 technology hazards for 2012. The risks that should be at the top of your prevention list. Health Devices. 2011;40(11): 358–73.
10. Tomasi CD, Grandi C, Salluh J, Soares M, Giombelli VR, Cascaes S, et al. Comparison of CAM-ICU and ICDSC for the detection of delirium in critically ill patients focusing on relevant clinical outcomes. J Crit Care. 2012;27(2):212–7. https://doi.org/10.1016/j.jcrc.2011.05.015.
11. Christakou A, Papadopoulos E, Patsaki E, Sidiras G, Nanas S. Functional Assessment Scales in a general intensive care unit. Hosp Chron. 2013;8(4):164.
12. Gentili A. Il paziente critico. Clinica e assistenza infermieristica in anestesia e rianimazione. Milano: CEA; 1993.
13. Besso J, Lumb PD, Williams G. Intensive and critical care medicine. WFSICCM World Federation of Societies of Intensive and Critical Care Medicine. Milano: Springer; 2009.
14. Bersten AD, Soni N. Oh Manuale di terapia intensiva. London: Elsevier Health Sciences Italy; 2010.

15. Citerio G, Oddo M, Taccone FS. Recommendations for the use of mul-timodal monitoring in the neurointensive care unit. Curr Opin Crit Care. 2015;21(2):113–9. https://doi.org/10.1097/MCC.0000000000000179.

16. Schomer AC, Hanafy K. Neuromonitoring in the ICU. Int Anesthesiol Clin. 2015;53(1):107–22. https://doi.org/10.1097/AIA.0000000000000042.

17. Barr J, Fraser GL, Puntillo K, Ely EW, Gelinas C, Dasta JF, et al. Clinical practice guidelines for the management of pain, agitation, and delirium in adult patients in the intensive care unit. Crit Care Med. 2013;41(1):263–306. https://doi.org/10.1097/CCM.0b013e3182783b72.

18. Stammet P, Collignon O, Werer C, Sertznig C, Devaux Y. Bispectral index to predict neurological outcome early after cardiac arrest. Resuscitation. 2014;85(12):1674–80. https://doi.org/10.1016/j.resuscitation.2014.09.009.

19. Kipnis E, Ramsingh D, Bhargava M, Dincer E, Cannesson M, Broccard A, Vallet B, Bendjelid K, Thibault R. Monitoring in the intensive care. Crit Care Res Pract. 2012;2012:473507. https://doi.org/10.1155/2012/473507.

20. Bulleri E, Fusi C. Manuale di monitoraggio grafico della ventilazione meccanica. Guida pratica alla rilevazione delle asincronie. FareLibri; 2015.

21. Poulia KA, Yannakoulia M, Karageorgou D, Gamaletsou M, Panagiotakos DB, Sipsas NV, Zampelas A. Evaluation of the efficacy of six nutritional screening tools to predict malnutrition in the elderly. Clin Nutr. 2012;31(3):378–85. https://doi.org/10.1016/j.clnu.2011.11.017.

22. Berni G, Francois C, Tonelli L. National Early Warning Score (NEWS) Misurazione standardizzata della gravità della malattia. 2016. http://www.regione.toscana.it/documents/10180/320308/National+early+warning+score+(NEWS)/072cf23a-213e-4dac-9ad3-4070579417fa. Accessed 16 Jun 2016.

23. Rando K, Niemann CU, Taura P, Klinck J. Optimizing cost-effective-ness in perioperative care for liver transplantation: a model for low- to medium-income countries. Liver Transpl. 2011;17(11):1247–78. https://doi.org/10.1002/lt.22405.

24. Odell M, Victor C, Oliver D. Nurses' role in detecting deterioration in ward patients: systematic literature review. J Adv Nurs. 2009;65(10):1992–2006.

25. Cabrera D, Thomas JF, Wiswell JL, Walston JM, Anderson JR, Hess EP, et al. Accuracy of 'My Gut Feeling:' comparing system 1 to system 2 decision-making for acuity prediction, disposition and diagnosis in an Academic Emergency Department. West J Emerg Med. 2015;16(5):653–7. https://doi.org/10.5811/westjem.2015.5.25301.

26. Adhikari NKJ, Fowler RA, Bhagwanjee S, Rubenfeld GD. Critical care and the global burden of critical illness in adults. Lancet. 2010; 376(9749):1339–46. https://doi.org/10.1016/S0140-6736(10)60446-1.
27. Kisiel M. Nursing observations: knowledge to help prevent critical illness. Br J Nurs. 2006;15(19):1052–6. 10.12968/bjon.2006.15.19.22105.
28. Moller JT, Johannessen NW, Espersen K, Ravlo O, Pedersen BD, Jensen PF, et al. Randomized evaluation of pulse oximetry in 20,802 patients; II. Perioperative events and postoperative complications. J Am Soc Anesthesiol. 1993;78(3):445–53.
29. Forsyth RJ, Raper J, Todhunter E. Routine intracranial pressure monitoring in acute coma. Cochrane Database Syst Rev. 2015;(11):CD002043. doi: https://doi.org/10.1002/14651858. CD002043.pub3.
30. Cannesson M, Broccard A, Vallet B, Bendjelid K. Monitoring in the intensive care unit: its past, present, and future. Crit Care Res Pract. 2012;2012:452769. https://doi.org/10.1155/2012/452769.

# Chapter 2
# Neurological, Pain, Sedation, and Delirium Assessment

**Gian Domenico Giusti and Giovanni Mistraletti**

## 2.1 Introduction

Altered cerebral state can be defined as "any mental state, induced by various pathological, physiological, or pharmacological maneuvers or agents, which can be recognized subjectively by the individual himself (or by an objective observer) as representing a deviation in subjective experience or psychological functioning from certain norms for that individual during alert, waking consciousness"[1].

A proper neurological evaluation is an ICU doctors and nurses' concern [2]. Critically ill patients often show a dysfunction connected to a primary neurological deterioration, or they show a secondary damage related to other vital function's changes; therefore a neurological assessment can help the clinical judgment in treating the primary pathological event [3].

In ICU a proper neurological evaluation can be affected by alteration in cognitive state, agitation, delirium, anxiety, pain, sedation, hypothermia, neuromuscular blockage, intubation and mechanical ventilation, traumatic injuries, and surgical

© Springer International Publishing AG, part of Springer Nature 2018    25
I. Comisso et al., *Nursing in Critical Care Setting*,
https://doi.org/10.1007/978-3-319-50559-6_2

**Table 2.1**  Indications for neurological evaluation in ICU patients [5]

| |
|---|
| • Detect early neurological worsening before irreversible brain damage occurs |
| • Individualize patient care decisions |
| • Guide patient management |
| • Monitor the response to treatment, in order to avoid any adverse effects |
| • Allow clinicians to better understand the physiopathology of complex disorders |
| • Design and implement management protocols |
| • Improve neurological outcome and quality of life in survivors of severe brain injuries |
| • Through understanding disease physiopathology, begin to develop new mechanistically oriented therapies where treatments currently are lacking or are empiric in nature |

interventions [4]. For these reasons and for an accurate and reliable assessment, the ICU staff needs validated tools (Table 2.1).

Furthermore, using a validated evaluation scale both with sedated and nonsedated patients can allow staff members to evaluate patient condition through the assessment of cognitive state, presence of pain or delirium [2].

## 2.2 Neurological Assessment

There isn't a single brain area responsible for consciousness, but its neuro-topical localization can be found in the ascending reticular activating system (ARAS). Whenever this system is functionally impaired bilaterally, one must anticipate disturbances of consciousness ultimately attaining the degree of coma. The ARAS connects the thalamic and subthalamic nuclei with the reticular intermediary gray substance of the spinal cord. The etiology and exact localization of the functional neuronal disturbance in the ARAS are not especially important: reversible metabolic CNS disease in a context of metabolic derangement is just as well possible as structural lesions along the thalamic loop structures.

Coma is a common clinical sign in ICU, and it is defined as a severe disturbance of consciousness, which precludes awakening and the directed movement of limbs. The comatose person shows closed eyes and no purposeful reaction to painful stimuli. The quantitative reduction of wakefulness, or better of arousal function, is the main feature of this condition [6].

Besides these signs we can also detect other cognitive and consciousness disorders before leading to a coma. If both events occur alternatively, or fluctuate, a delirium diagnosis should be considered. Following several brain damage, some patients can be *awaken* (the patient opens and moves its eyes), but still *unresponsive* (showing no voluntary movement) [7]; this syndrome is called *vegetative/unresponsive state*. A patient in this state has an alternated sleep-wake cycle, can swallow and breathe, and shows a response to pain stimuli and nonfinalized movement. However he is not able to voluntarily move his eyes to visual stimuli and verbal response nor finalize movements. If this state continues for more than a month, this clinical syndrome, initially termed "apallic syndrome" or "vigil coma," will be defined as "persistent vegetative state" (PVS), although many neuroscientists prefer to describe this state of consciousness as "unresponsive wakefulness syndrome" (UWS). This choice is due to ethical questions about whether a patient can be called "vegetative" or not [8].

The minimally conscious state (MCS) is an impairment of consciousness; the patient shows awareness of self and/or the environment. Both actions and awareness are unstable during the day. If this condition is detected in acute stage, its outcome seems to improve.

Patients with MCS open their eyes spontaneously and show a response to visual stimuli, are able to show aware response to simple orders or imitate actions, and usually don't speak and pronounce unmeaning sounds instead. Patients are able to show finalized movement or emotional behaviors, and they usually swallow properly [8].

ICU nurses are skilled to assess patient's consciousness; they evaluate and detect changes of neurological state and report them to medical staff in case early interventions are needed to improve the outcome and reduce the long-term sequelae [9].

Nursing care focuses on:

- Evaluation of awaken state using a score tool to define the level of consciousness and the stimuli needed to achieve a response from the patient
- Evaluation of the patient awareness of self and environment (testing orientation, ability to concentrate and speak) and performing test to assess presence of delirium

The most common scoring scale to assess the consciousness is the Glasgow Coma Scale (GCS) introduced in the 1970s [10]. An updated tool, the Full Outline of UnResponsiveness (FOUR), is also available (Table 2.2).

The GCS remains the most widely used in critical care settings. The assessment of motor, verbal, and eye responses of the GCS characterizes the level of consciousness. The picture provided by these responses enables comparison both between patients and changes in patients over the time that crucially guides management. The three components can be scored separately or combined in a sum score, ranging from 3 to 15 [11].

This value must be associated to pupil diameter and reactivity evaluation, arterial blood pressure, heart rate, body temperature, breathing pattern and, when prescribed, $CO_2$ ($EtCO_2$) measurement, intracranial pressure (ICP), and cerebral perfusion pressure (CPP).

Its main limitations are that verbal responses are not assessable in mechanically ventilated patients and that brainstem examination is not directly considered. The total GCS on ED arrival is a strong predictor of in-hospital mortality (area under

**Table 2.2** Glasgow Coma Scale (GCS) and Full Outline of UnResponsiveness (FOUR) score

|  | Glasgow Coma Scale (GCS) | Full Outline of UnResponsiveness (FOUR) |
|---|---|---|
| Eye response | 4 = eyes open spontaneously<br>3 = eyes opening to verbal command<br>2 = eyes opening to pain<br>1 = no eyes opening | 4 = eyelids open or opened, tracking, or blinking to command<br>3 = eyelids open but not tracking<br>2 = eyelids closed but open to loud voice<br>1 = eyelids closed but open to pain<br>0 = eyelids remain closed with pain |
| Motor response | 6 = obeys commands<br>5 = localizing pain<br>4 = withdrawal from pain<br>3 = flexion response to pain<br>2 = extension response to pain<br>1 = no motor response | 4 = thumbs-up, fist, or peace sign<br>3 = localizing to pain<br>2 = flexion response to pain<br>1 = extension response to pain<br>0 = no response to pain or generalized myoclonus status |
| Verbal response | 5 = oriented<br>4 = confused<br>3 = inappropriate words<br>2 = incomprehensible sounds<br>1 = no verbal response | |
| Brainstem reflexes | | 4 = pupil and corneal reflexes present<br>3 = one pupil wide and fixed<br>2 = pupil or corneal reflexes absent<br>1 = pupil and corneal reflexes absent<br>0 = absent pupil, corneal and cough reflex |

(continued)

**Table 2.2** (continued)

|  | Glasgow Coma Scale (GCS) | Full Outline of UnResponsiveness (FOUR) |
| --- | --- | --- |
| Respiration |  | 4 = not intubated, regular breathing pattern |
|  |  | 3 = not intubated, Cheyne-Stokes breathing pattern |
|  |  | 2 = not intubated, irregular breathing |
|  |  | 1 = breathes above ventilator rate |
|  |  | 0 = breathes at ventilator rate or apnea |
| Max–min | 15–3 | 16–0 |

the ROC curve (AUC) of 0.91) and need for neurosurgical intervention (AUC of 0.87), with the eye score as the weakest predictor and sum score the best. An initial GCS sum score of 3 is associated with poor clinical outcomes in traumatic brain injury (TBI) (mortality 50–76%) [12].

The FOUR score, introduced in 2005, provides additional information not captured by the GCS including details about brainstem reflexes and respiratory drive and an opportunity to recognize the locked-in syndrome [13].

It assesses eye response, motor response, brainstem reflexes, and respiratory pattern. The FOUR score has been tested in a range of clinical settings and in different countries; moreover it has been further validated in the medical ICU, in the ED, and among ICU nurses well experienced in neurological care [12].

Patients with the lowest GCS score can be further differentiated using the FOUR score: among patients with GCS3, only 25% have FOUR = 0, while the others show scores from 1 to 8 [13].

The FOUR score showed good interrater reliability and prognostic content in a range of neurological conditions and may help to differentiate between several conditions when a patient is unresponsive [14]. However, experience with this instrument is still limited when compared to the GCS. Current evidence suggests that both the GCS and FOUR score provide useful and reproducible measures of neurological state and can be routinely used to chart trends in clinical progress [5].

Sedation, major analgesics (e.g., opioids), and neuromuscular blockage remain a problem for any clinical scale of consciousness.

## 2.3  Pain Assessment

Pain remains a common symptom among ICU patients [15]; the gold standard to assess pain remains the patient reports, because it's well known that pain attributed from the staff could easily be underestimated. A good application of an evaluation tool is very important, so as proper illustration of its working principles, in order to understand and evaluate the patient's response. Nurses should choose pain assessment scales according to patient's conditions and their own confidence level in using each tool:

- Self-reported:
    - (a) One dimensional (acute and chronic pain—to monitor and verify the efficacy in pain-relieving treatment)
    - (b) Multidimensional (chronic pain—long-term evaluation or for research purpose)
- Behavioral assessment tool (children or adult with compromised cognitive status).
- Information given by the caregiver.
- Alterations in vital signs (breathing rate, blood pressure, and heart rate) are not valid indicators to assess the presence and intensity of pain, but they are useful combined with other informations [16].

With cooperative patients both one- and multidimensional scales can be applied (Table 2.3).

**Table 2.3** Pain evaluation scales

| Scale | Method | Validated for | Comments |
|---|---|---|---|
| *One dimensional* | | | |
| Visual Analogue Scale, VAS | Visual | • Acute and chronic pain<br>• Rheumatic disease<br>• Children >5 y.o. | It's the most reliable and solid tool, but not easy to use<br>It's not reliable in patients with cognitive impairment (after surgery, dementia). Some patients are not able to understand how to represent graphically the intensity of pain<br>Up to 7–11% of adult patients and more than 25% of elderly are not able to fill in VAS |
| Numeric Rating Scale, NRS | Visual and/or verbal | • Rheumatic disease<br>• Acute and chronic pain<br>• Oncological pain<br>• Pain post trauma<br>• Illiterates | Verbal numeric scale is an easy tool to assess pain, similar to VAS, which has a good concordance with<br>NRS is easily understood because the patient has to choose a number between 0 and 10 to explain its pain level<br>NRS doesn't need the visual and motor coordination required for VAS, for this reason can be easily performed<br>It's indicated to assess the pain after surgery<br>Failure to complete this scale is 2%. It's a very reliable tool to assess the efficacy in pain relief treatment<br>Less reliable in case of older age and visual, hearing, or cognitive impairment |

**Table 2.3** (continued)

| Scale | Method | Validated for | Comments |
|---|---|---|---|
| Verbal Rating Scale, VRS | Visual and/or verbal | • Chronic pain | VRS needs a description of the level of pain through adjectives<br>Even if these scales are easy and quick to use, they aren't able to assess the intensity of pain since adjectives used in this scale could have different meaning to different people<br>Furthermore, these adjectives could not describe exactly the level of pain<br>VRS scales aren't enough representative in showing modification in pain level in case of too few items<br>Best results could be achieved if the scale has at least six different items |
| Facial Pain Scale, FPS | | • Bieri: children and adults<br>• Wong-Baker: children | Facial Pain Scale is a graphic tool which represents different face expressions hypothetically connected to the absence or presence of pain<br>It's been used with children not able to understand an analogue scale before 5 years old<br>The main weakness of this tool is that facial expressions could have a correlation with different variables as anxiety, depression, anger, and satisfaction<br>It's not affected by cultural or ethnic differences |

(continued)

**Table 2.3** (continued)

| Scale | Method | Validated for | Comments |
|---|---|---|---|
| *Multidimensional* | | | |
| Brief Pain Inventory (BPI) | Verbal | • Oncological pain<br>• Rheumatic disease | This scale assesses location, intensity and feature of pain, relief of pain, associated feelings, affected quality of life |
| McGill Pain Questionnaire | Verbal | • Chronic pain | It's a complex tool requiring 30 min, there is a short form too requiring only 2–3 min<br><br>It assesses location, intensity and features of pain provide also an affective score |

For patients unable to self-report, either the Behavioral Pain Scale (BPS) [17] or the Critical-Care Pain Observation Tool (CPOT) can be used [18].

The BPS is validated for both intubated and non-intubated ICU patients and it's recommended in the new PAD guidelines [19]. Since it relies on observation by the care provider, the patient may be in different states of alertness (Table 2.4).

BPS scale is a four-grade scale and includes three items (face expression, upper limb movement, compliance to mechanical ventilation); the objective signs (descriptors) define four different levels of pain and with text and illustrations. The final score represents the presence or absence of pain.

The total score ranges between 3 (no pain) and 12 (most pain). A further tool's evolution allows pain evaluation in non-intubated patients (BPS-NI) [20]. In this feature, the item "Vocalization" replaces the "Compliance with ventilation" one. The final four descriptors are equally scored in the two tools, thus allowing a comparison between ventilated and nonventilated patients.

**Table 2.4** BPS scale

| Item | Description | Score |
|------|-------------|-------|
| Facial expression | Relaxed | 1 |
| | Partially tightened (e.g., brow lowering) | 2 |
| | Fully tightened (e.g., eyelid closing) | 3 |
| | Grimacing | 4 |
| Upper limbs | No movement | 1 |
| | Partially bent | 2 |
| | Fully bent with finer flexion | 3 |
| | Permanently retracted | 4 |
| Compliance with ventilation | Tolerating movement | 1 |
| | Coughing but tolerating ventilation for most of the time | 2 |
| | Fighting ventilator | 3 |
| | Unable to control ventilation | 4 |

The CPOT includes evaluation of four different behaviors (facial expressions, body movements, muscle tension, and compliance with the ventilator for mechanically ventilated patients or vocalization for non-intubated patients) rated on a score between 0 and 2, the total score ranging between 0 and 8. The CPOT is feasible, easy to complete, and simple to understand (Table 2.5).

Assessing pain in patients with severe disorders of consciousness such as MCS and UWS is a great challenge, but it is possible with Nociception Coma Scale (NCS) (Table 2.6) which assesses similar components to the BPS and CPOT with good to excellent concurrent validity and interrater agreement [21]. Recent studies suggest that the visual subscale does not discriminate noxious stimuli, and its exclusion increased sensitivity from 46 to 73% with specificity of 97% and accuracy of 85% (NCS-R) [22]. A score of 4 on the NCS-R was identified as a threshold value to detect a response to noxious stimuli.

**Table 2.5** CPOT scale

| Indicator | Score | | Description |
|-----------|-------|---|-------------|
| Facial expressions | Relaxed, neutral | 0 | No muscle tension observed |
| | Tense | 1 | Presence of frowning, brow lowering, orbit tightening and levator contraction, or any other changes (e.g., opening eyes or tearing during nociceptive procedures) |
| | Grimacing | 2 | All previous facial movements plus eyelid tightly closed (the patient may present with mouth open or biting the endotracheal tube) |
| Body movements | Absence of movements or normal position | 0 | Does not move at all (doesn't necessarily mean absence of pain) or normal position (movements not aimed toward the pain site or not made for the purpose of protection) |
| | Protection | 1 | Slow, cautious movements, touching or rubbing the pain site, seeking attention through movements |
| | Restlessness/ agitation | 2 | Pulling tube, attempting to sit up, moving limbs/thrashing, not following commands, striking at staff, trying to climb out of bed |

**Table 2.5** (continued)

| Indicator | Score | | Description |
|---|---|---|---|
| Compliance with the ventilator (intubated patients) or Vocalization (extubated patients) | Tolerating ventilator or movement | 0 | Alarms not activated, easy ventilation |
| | Coughing but tolerating | 1 | Coughing, alarms may be activated but stop spontaneously |
| | Fighting ventilator | 2 | Asynchrony: blocking ventilation, alarms frequently activated |
| | Talking in normal tone or no sound | 0 | Talking in normal tone or no sound |
| | Sighing, moaning | 1 | Sighing, moaning |
| | Crying out, sobbing | 2 | Crying out, sobbing |
| Muscle tension Evaluation by passive flexion and extension of upper limbs when patient is at rest or evaluation when patient is being turned | Relaxed | 0 | No resistance to passive movements |
| | Tense rigid | 1 | Resistance to passive movements |
| | Very tense or rigid | 2 | Strong resistance to passive movements or incapacity to complete them |
| Total __/8 | | | |

**Table 2.6** Nociception Coma Scale

| | | |
|---|---|---|
| Motor response | Localization to noxious stimulation | 3 |
| | Flexion withdrawal | 2 |
| | Abnormal posturing | 1 |
| | None/flaccid | 0 |
| Verbal response | Verbalization (intelligible) | 3 |
| | Vocalization | 2 |
| | Groaning | 1 |
| | None | 0 |
| Visual response | Fixation | 3 |
| | Eyes movement | 2 |
| | Startle | 1 |
| | None | 0 |
| Facial expression | Cry | 3 |
| | Grimace | 2 |
| | Oral reflexive movement/startle response | 1 |
| | None | 0 |

The Behavioral Pain Scale (BPS) and the Critical-Care Pain Observation Tool (CPOT) are the most valid and reliable behavioral pain scales for monitoring pain in medical, postoperative, or trauma (except for brain injury) adult ICU patients who are unable to self-report and in whom motor function is intact and behaviors are observable [19].

## 2.4 Evaluation of Agitation and Sedation

Most patients in ICU receive sedative medication, often associated to painkillers to reduce anxiety and discomfort, improving the compliance to treatments. Anxiety and agitation are very common in ICU patients and associated to worsening clinical outcomes.

The concept of anxiety has been defined as comprising two components: trait anxiety and state anxiety. Trait anxiety corresponds to the individual personality trait of anxiety, namely, a relatively enduring disposition to feel stress, worry, and discomfort. State anxiety corresponds to the emotional (e.g., feelings of fear, worry, and apprehension) and physiological (e.g., tachycardia) manifestations of anxiety when faced with stressful stimuli. One could think of trait anxiety as chronic and state anxiety as acute anxiety [23].

Agitation is a state of extreme arousal, tension, irritability, and/or excessive psychomotor activity. It is described as excessive restlessness, characterized by nonpurposeful mental and physical activity due to internal tension and anxiety. However, no clear, concise, and universally accepted definition of agitation in ICU patients exists.

An optimal sedation level suitable for all critically ill patients doesn't exist. Daily assessment is required to define the exact need in every patient, evaluating clinical history, tolerance concerning forced posture and devices indwelled, compliance with ventilator and invasive procedure performed, presence of anxiety and agitation, and eventually possible side effects of sedative and analgesic treatments. There is a quite strong level of scientific evidence supporting a mild sedation, with the aim to improve the compliance to performed procedures and illness adjustment, keeping an early level of quiet wakefulness. Constant control in sedation level is associated to reduced mortality, length of stay in ICU, duration of mechanical ventilation, less hospital acquired infection, and decreasing in cost [24].

There are several scales available discussed in this chapter and compared in Table 2.7.

The Richmond Agitation-Sedation Scale (RASS) [25] consists of one value with response options ranging from +4 to −5. A score of 0 is considered alert and calm, while positive values correspond to increasing agitation and negative values correspond to progressively deep sedation. There are three steps to

**Table 2.7** Synopsis sedation/agitation scales in ICU (www.sedaicu.it)

| | Richmond Agitation-Sedation Scale (RASS) | Bloomsbury Sedation Score (Bloomsbury) | Ramsay Sedation Scale (RSS) | Motor Activity Assessment Scale (MAAS) | Riker Sedation-Agitation Scale (SAS) | Observer's Assessment of Alertness and Sedation (OAAS) | Nursing Instrument for the Communication of Sedation (NICS) |
|---|---|---|---|---|---|---|---|
| Combative | +4 | | | 6 | 7 | | +3 |
| Very agitation | +3 | | 1 | | 6 | | |
| Agitated | +2 | +3 | | 5 | | | +2 |
| Restless | +1 | +2 | | 4 | 5 | | +1 |
| Alert and calm | 0 | +1 | 2 | 3 | 4 | 5 | 0 |
| Drowsy | −1 | 0 | | | | 4 | −1 |
| Light sedation | −2 | | 3 | 2 | 3 | 3 | |
| Moderate sedation | −3 | −1 | 4 | | 2 | 2 | −2 |
| Deep sedation | −4 | −2 | 5 | 1 | | 1 | |
| Unarousable | −5 | −3 | 6 | 0 | 1 | 0 | −3 |

evaluate the patient: observation, verbal stimulation, and then physical stimulation. More aggressive stimulation results in a lower score. It has high reliability and validity in medical and surgical, ventilated and nonventilated, and sedated and nonsedated adult ICU patients; nurses described RASS as logical, easy to administer, and readily recalled. RASS application procedure is described in Table 2.8.

Bloomsbury Sedation Score (Bloomsbury) [26] contains a scale with a 7-point range between −3 (unarousable) and +3 (agitated and restless) and a categorization for natural sleep. A study aiming to develop a risk assessment tool for voluntary self-extubation in the ICU performed a post hoc analysis to determine the validity of the Bloomsbury compared with the Ramsay Scale [27]. Ramsay Sedation Scale (RSS) [28] has six different levels, according to patient arousability. It is an intuitively obvious scale and therefore lends itself to universal use,

**Table 2.8**  Procedure to perform RASS

| *Procedure* |
| --- |
| 1. Observe patient. Is patient alert and calm (score 0)? |
| Does patient have behavior that is consistent with restlessness or agitation (score +1 to +4)? |
| 2. If patient is not alert, in a loud speaking voice, state patient's name and direct patient to open eyes and look at speaker. Repeat once if necessary Can prompt patient to continue looking at speaker |
| Patient has eye opening and eye contact, which is sustained for more than 10 s (score −1) |
| Patient has eye opening and eye contact, but this is not sustained for 10 s (score −2) |
| Patient has any movement in response to voice, excluding eye contact (score −3) |
| 3. If patient does not respond to voice, physically stimulate patient by shaking shoulder and then rubbing sternum if there is no response to shaking shoulder |
| Patient has any movement to physical stimulation (score −4) |
| Patient has no response to voice or physical stimulation (score −5) |

not only in the ICU but wherever sedative drugs or narcotics are given. A disadvantage of the Ramsay Scale is that it does not provide any definition of the degree of agitation, while there are occasions when this may be important to record. The Richmond Agitation-Sedation Scale does take this into consideration.

Motor Activity Assessment Scale (MAAS) consists of a 7-point scale ranging between 0 (unresponsive to noxious stimuli) and 6 (dangerously agitated, uncooperative). MAAS is a valid and reliable sedation scale in mechanically ventilated patients in the surgical intensive care unit. This tool contains specific descriptors to differentiate between levels of sedation. It has demonstrated strong psychometric properties [29].

Riker Sedation-Agitation Scale (SAS) [30] is a common sedation assessment scale that has been validated in ventilated and nonventilated patients in medical and surgical ICUs. It consists of 7 items ranging between 1 (unarousable) and 7 (dangerous agitation).

The SAS scale must be applied following instructions in Table 2.9.

Observer's Assessment of Alertness and Sedation (OAAS) scale aims to assess the degree of suppression of consciousness and is widely used in anesthesia research literature to quantify the hypnotic effects of drugs. The OAAS is a 6-level score. Patients are considered responsive at an OAAS level of 5, 4, or 3 and are scored as unresponsive at an OAAS level 2, 1, or 0. Patients are considered to have loss of consciousness (LOC) at the transition between level 3 and level 2 [31].

Nursing Instrument for the Communication of Sedation (NICS) [32] is a 7-level scale ranging between −3 (unresponsive to deep stimulation) and +3 (dangerously agitated). NICS is a valid and reliable sedation scale in mixed population of intensive care unit patients. NICS ranked highest in nursing preference and ease of communication and may thus permit more effective and interactive management of sedation.

Recent extensive psychometric testing suggests that both Richmond Agitation-Sedation Scale (RASS) and Riker

Sedation-Agitation Scale (SAS) scored the highest for validity, reliability, feasibility, and relevance [19].

Ensuring patient comfort requires a multidisciplinary approach in addition to pharmacotherapy. This includes frequent communication and explanation to the patient by all staff directly involved in their care, both nurses and doctors, and relatives. Physiotherapy plays an important role as prolonged immobility may be painful, increases muscle catabolism, and increases the risk for sepsis and deep vein thrombosis. It has to be reduced by daily assessment and treatment. Basic needs, such as feeding and hydration, require addressing regularly to prevent the symptoms of hunger and thirst [33]. Educational initiatives are necessary to improve ICU practice, particularly for nurses unexperienced in ICUs [34].

## 2.5 Delirium Assessment in ICU

Delirium is a complex psychiatric syndrome characterized by disturbance of consciousness and cognitive functions, with perception deficits and altered sleep-wake cycle; it has a fluctuating course during time. In critically ill patients, it's very common and stressful; from 30% until 80% of ICU patients can show this syndrome [35]. The variations of the prevalence and incidence of ICU delirium depend on the criteria for its detection and on the cohorts of critically ill patients studied.

Delirium is a serious disorder associated with prolonged ICU and hospital length of stay, higher costs, and increased morbidity and mortality [36].

This syndrome has been studied for a long time in patients with heart diseases [37], and it has been considered as a priority in ICU patients from Kornfeld in 1967, with modern ICU [38], however being still difficult to diagnose and treat.

The current reference standard diagnostic criteria are the fifth edition of American Psychiatric Association's *Diagnostic and*

*Statistical Manual of Mental Disorders* (DSM-V) [39] and WHO's *International Classification of Diseases*, 10th Revision (ICD-10) [40]. According to DSM-V criteria, delirium is defined as the disturbance in attention and awareness and change in cognition that is not better accounted for by a pre-existing, established, or evolving dementia. The disturbance develops over a short period and tends to fluctuate during the course of the day, and there is evidence from the history, physical examination, or laboratory findings that the disturbance is caused by a direct physiologic consequence of a general medical condition, an intoxicating substance, medication use, or more than one cause. According to the WHO criteria, the diagnosis of delirium requires the following: clouding of consciousness with reduced ability to focus, sustain, or shift attention, disturbance of cognition, presence of psychomotor disturbances, disturbance of sleep or the sleep-wake cycle, rapid onset and fluctuations of the symptoms over the course of the day, and objective evidence from history, physical, and neurological examination

**Table 2.9** Procedure to perform SAS

| |
|---|
| 1. Agitated patients are scored by their most severe degree of agitation as described |
| 2. If patient is awake or awakens easily to voice ("awaken" means responds with voice or headshaking to a question or follows commands), that's a SAS 4 (same as calm and appropriate—might even be napping) |
| 3. If more stimuli such as shaking are required but patient eventually does awaken, that's SAS 3 |
| 4. If patient arouses to stronger physical stimuli (may be noxious) but never awakens to the point of responding yes/no or following commands, that's a SAS 2 |
| 5. Little or no response to noxious physical stimuli represents a SAS 1 |
| This helps separate sedated patients into those you can eventually wake up (SAS 3), those you can't awaken but can arouse (SAS 2), and those you can't arouse (SAS 1) |

or laboratory tests of an underlying cerebral or systemic disease (other than psychoactive substance-related) that can be presumed to be responsible for the clinical manifestations.

Three subtypes of delirium can be distinguished:

1. Hyperactive subtype: the patient is hyperalert or agitated.
2. Hypoactive subtype: the patient is hypoalert or lethargic.
3. Alternating or mixed subtype: characterized by alternating hyper- and hypoactive symptoms.

The hyperactive subtype, usually associated with delusions, hallucinations, agitation, and disorientation, occurs in approximately 1–2% of patients with delirium. The hypoactive subtype, characterized by lethargy, psychomotor slowing, and inappropriate speech or mood, occurs in approximately 35% of patients. In intensive care patients with delirium, the alternating or mixed subtype has the highest incidence rate and represents up to 60–70% of all cases of delirium. Especially, the hypoactive subtype is difficult to recognize, and the incidence/prevalence is therefore likely to be underreported. Because of the fluctuating course of delirium, it can be assumed that the alternating subtype is also underreported [41]. It's very important to distinguish between ICU delirium and dementia, which is characterized by a state of generalized cognitive deficits in which there is a deterioration of previously acquired intellectual abilities. Dementia usually develops over weeks, months, or even years with varying levels of cognitive impairment from mild to severe.

## 2.5.1 Risk Factors for the Development of ICU Delirium

Some illness and patients have an increased risk to develop delirium during ICU stay. Risk factors can be divided in predisposing and precipitating factors (Table 2.10). Predisposing factors are present before the admission in hospital and are correlated to

**Table 2.10** Risk factors

| Predisposing factors | Precipitating factors |
|---|---|
| Age > 70 | Restraint devices |
| History of depression and/or dementia and/or stroke | Inability to communicate if connected to a ventilator |
| Drug abuse | Visual or hearing impairment |
| Hypo-/hyperthermia | Invasive procedures |
| Hypo-/hypernatremia | Catheter indwelled (CVC, urinary catheter, NGT, orotracheal tube, etc.) |
| Hypo-/hyperthyroidism | Drug administration |
| Hepatic and/or renal failure | Pain |
| Septic and/or cardiogenic shock | Isolation |
| Emergency surgery | Sleep deprivation |
| Malnutrition | Stress |

patient clinical history. Precipitating factors are all the stimuli and any acute factor during the stay in ICU. After 24 h in ICU, it is possible to detect delirium in ICU using the PRE-DELIRIC model [42] or E-PRE-DELIRIC at the admission. The predictors that build this model are largely consistent with previously reported risk factors for delirium, including age, pre-existing dementia, history of alcoholism, and a high severity of illness at admission [43].

## 2.5.2  Detection

Early detection of ICU delirium is necessary to limit the destructive consequences of an untreated delirium: each subsequent day of this cerebral syndrome is correlated with a 10% increase in hospital mortality [41]. The early definition of ICU delirium referred to DSM-IV is based on which different evaluation scales have been developed, nowadays not anymore (Table 2.11).

**Table 2.11** Comparing DSM classification of delirium [44]

| DSM-V | DSM-IV |
|---|---|
| A. Disturbance in *attention* (i.e., reduced ability to direct, focus, sustain, and shift attention) and awareness (reduced *orientation to the environment*) | A. Disturbance of consciousness (i.e., reduced clarity of awareness of the environment) with reduced ability to focus, sustain, or shift attention |
| B. The disturbance develops over a short period of time (usually hours to a few days), *represents an acute change from baseline attention and awareness*, and tends to fluctuate in severity during the course of a day | B. A change in cognition or the development of a perceptual disturbance that is not better accounted for by a pre-existing, established, or evolving dementia |
| C. An additional disturbance in cognition (e.g., memory deficit, disorientation, language, visuospatial ability, or perception) | C. The disturbance develops over a short period of time (usually hours to days) and tends to fluctuate during the course of the day |
| D. *The disturbances in Criteria A and C are not better explained by a pre-existing, established, or evolving neurocognitive disorder and do not occur in the context of a severely reduced level of arousal such as coma* | D. There is evidence from the history, physical examination, or laboratory findings that the disturbance is caused by the direct physiological consequences of a general medical condition |
| E. There is evidence from the history, physical examination, or laboratory findings that the disturbance is *a direct* physiological consequence of another medical condition, *substance intoxication or withdrawal* (i.e., *due to a drug of abuse or to a medication), or exposure to a toxin or is due to multiple etiologies* | |

The Confusion Assessment Method for the ICU (CAM-ICU) and the Intensive Care Delirium Screening Checklist (ICDSC) are strongly recommended for delirium assessment by the 2013 PAD guidelines, although there are several scales available to assess this syndrome [19].

The CAM-ICU [45] is a part of the neurological evaluation which accounts different levels. First of all it is necessary to assess the level of consciousness by a validated scale (authors recommend the RASS). The second stage is the evaluation of content of consciousness. If the patient is sedated (RASS = −4 or −5), it is impossible to assess because of patient's unresponsiveness. These levels are defined as coma, and in these cases we don't use the CAM-ICU but we describe the patient as not evaluable.

If sedation is mild (RASS ≥ −3), patients show some responsiveness which enables to evaluate their thoughts and the presence of delirium.

The CAM-ICU analyzes four aspects:

1. Acute onset or fluctuating course
2. Inattention
3. Altered level of consciousness
4. Disorganized thinking

The ICDSC (Table 2.12) is a scale for delirium stratification, but it can also be used as a diagnostic scale, and the scale's application is easy and quick [46]. The ICDSC consists of eight observed variables that are compared with the assessment of the previous day, and increasing values on the ICDSC are compatible with severity stratification. In addition, the ICDSC is useful in the diagnosis of subsyndromal delirium [47].

If the score is 0, there is no delirium; from 1 to 3, there is "subsyndromal delirium;" and from 4 to 8, there is presence of delirium.

The ICDSC has been demonstrated to be a good scale to assess and monitor for delirium and may be preferred since it does not score changes in wakefulness and attention directly attributable to recent sedative medication as positive ICDSC points.

**Table 2.12** Intensive Care Delirium Screening Checklist (ICDSC)

| Category | Description | Points |
|---|---|---|
| *Altered level of consciousness* | (a) Drowsy and requires mild to moderate stimulation for response | +1 |
| | (b) Hypervigilant (no points are given for a sleeping state) | |
| *Inattention* | Patient displays a level of *inattention*, including distractibility by external stimuli, difficulty keeping up with conversations, or difficulty shifting focus | +1 |
| Disorientation | Evident mistake in time, person, or place | +1 |
| Hallucination, delusion, or psychosis | Any indication of hallucinations (grabbing for an unseen object), delusion, or gross impairment in reality testing | +1 |
| Psychomotor agitation or retardation | (a) Hyperactivity that requires use of sedative drugs or restraints to control potential danger to the patient | +1 |
| | (b) Hypoactivity or clinically noticeable psychomotor slowing | |
| Inappropriate speech or mood | Patient displays inappropriate speech or mood | +1 |
| Sleep/wake cycle disturbance | Patient sleeps <4 h during the night, has frequent awakenings (not related to medical staff-initiated awakenings), or sleeps throughout most of the day | +1 |
| Symptom fluctuation | Fluctuation of any of the manifestations of any item or symptom within a 24 h period (i.e., between shifts) | +1 |

Studies have demonstrated that the ICDSC has a high sensitivity (99%) but low specificity (64%) for the diagnosis of delirium when compared to formalized psychiatric assessment. The CAM-ICU has a lower sensitivity (93%), but higher specificity (96%) than ICDSC, and may correlate more strongly with patient outcome than ICDSC. The use of sedation and analgesia in the ICU can lead to diagnose a form of drug-induced, hypoactive delirium. Despite its better outcome, such deliric conditions deserves the same attention and promp treatment as other ICU delirium features.

ICU delirium assessment should be performed once per shift or whenever a mental status change occurs.

It's important to use validated tools when changes in sedative or analgesic medication occur, when anesthesia ends its effectiveness, when changes in state of conscience occur, or when patients show an acute change of their neurological state [48].

## 2.5.3   Prevention

Delirium management in ICU must be focused in underlying organic or metabolic cause. There's the need to restrict precipitating factors in patient with predisposing factors.

Prevention is carried out through nonpharmacological, environmental, and orientation strategies. It's important to optimize neuroactive therapy decreasing sedative administration.

Finally, after an optimal level in analgesia and sedations is reached, the suitable pharmacological antipsychotic treatment to prevent the cognitive and physical worsening should be considered.

Some acronyms have been created to guide nurses and doctors in case of ICU delirium.

What to THINK about when delirium is present:

- **T** Toxic situations, CHF, shock, dehydration, deliriogenic meds (tight titration), new organ failure(e.g., liver, kidney)
- **H** Hypoxemia
- **I** Infection/sepsis (nosocomial), immobilization
- **N** Nonpharmacological interventions (hearing aids, glasses, reorient, sleep protocols, music, noise control, ambulation)
- **K** K+ or electrolyte problems

In case of patient with delirium, attention is given to a series of condition under the acronym DrDRE:

- **D** Diseases (sepsis, COPD, CHF)
- **DR** Drug Removal (SATs and stopping benzodiazepines/narcotics)
- **E** Environment (immobilization, sleep and day/night, hearing aids, glasses)

To perform a differential diagnosis, the acronym I WATCH DEATH is used:

- **I**nfection (HIV, sepsis, pneumonia)
- **W**ithdrawal (alcohol, barbiturate, sedative-hypnotic)
- **A**cute metabolic (acidosis, alkalosis, electrolyte disturbance, hepatic failure, renal failure)
- **T**rauma (closed head injury, heatstroke, postoperative, severe burns)
- **C**NS pathology (abscess, hemorrhage, hydrocephalus, subdural hematoma, infection, seizures, stroke, tumors, metastases, vasculitis, encephalitis, meningitis, syphilis)
- **H**ypoxia (anemia, carbon monoxide poisoning, hypotension, pulmonary or cardiac failure)
- **D**eficiencies (vitamin B12, folate, niacin, thiamine)
- **E**ndocrinopathies (hyper-/hypoadrenocorticism, hyper-/hypoglycemia, myxedema, hyperparathyroidism)
- **A**cute vascular (hypertensive encephalopathy, stroke, arrhythmia, shock)
- **T**oxins or drugs (prescription drugs, illicit drugs, pesticides, solvents)
- **H**eavy metals (lead, manganese, mercury)

Every sedative can lead to delirium; especially benziodiazepines increase delirium recurrence more than propofol and dexmedetomidine. Another way to decrease delirium is to optimize treatment with painkillers: both the pain and excessive painkiller administration are associated to delirium onset.

Opioids are the first choice of medication to treat pain in ICU but have important side effects (hypercapnia, hypotension, depression in consciousness level).

Antipsychotics are the first choice to treat delirium after analyzing and solving every possible cause; they must be administered very carefully and stopped as soon as possible. Haloperidol can show different side effects (muscular tension, tremors, dyskinesia, drowsiness, thought disorder); other atypical antipsychotics (olanzapine, quetiapine, risperidone, etc.) show the same efficacy with less side effects.

Early mobilization (which may, in addition to its nonpharmacological intervention component, lighten sedation) appears to be the major beneficial strategy in preventing delirium in the ICU (Table 2.13) [49]. It has been demonstrated to reduce morbidity and mortality in ICU patients.

Moreover it's been demonstrated that the use of a protocol of nonpharmacological intervention in a medical intensive care unit (MICU) permits to decrease delirium incidence (15.7% vs. 9.4%, $P = 0.04$).

Finally, taking into consideration circadian rhythm is important to promote physiologic sleeping in its peculiar phases (REM and slow wave) which are usually reduced in case of critical illness. Literature give us the advice to keep the awake period during the daytime (i.e., using music or television and

**Table 2.13** Nonpharmacological interventions to prevent ICU delirium

- Early mobility
- Clock
- Reorientation
- Noise reduction
- Medication/procedure reschedule
- Open blinds
- Eye mask
- Dim hallways at night

discourage sleeping time during the day) and keep silence during the night, give the patient earplugs or eye masks, keep lights off if possible, reduce noise, and avoid unnecessary procedures.

A qualitative better sleeping is achieved decreasing sedative administration or giving the patient some melatonin in the evening.

A correct approach toward sleeping can decrease delirium prevalence and duration.

Take-Home Messages
- Neurological evaluation is an expertise of ICU nurses and doctors.
- Subjective pain evaluation is the gold standard; both nurses and doctors must know how to assess the pain depending on patient neurological condition and choose the right tool.
- Sedation should be tailored to the individual needs of the patient.
- Delirium is a common and serious disorder related to morbidity and mortality.

# References

1. Ludwig A. Altered states of consciousness. Arch Gen Psychiatry. 1966;15:225–34.
2. Sharshar T, Citerio G, Andrews PJ, Chieregato A, Latronico N, Menon DK, et al. Neurological examination of critically ill patients: a pragmatic approach. Report of an ESICM expert panel. Intensive Care Med. 2014;40:484–95. https://doi.org/10.1007/s00134-014-3214-y.
3. Stone JJ, Childs S, Smith LE, Battin M, Papadakos PJ, Huang JH. Hourly neurologic assessments for traumatic brain injury in the ICU. Neurol Res. 2014;36:164–9. https://doi.org/10.1179/1743132813Y.0000000285.
4. Samaniego EA, Mlynash M, Caulfield AF, Eyngorn I, Wijman CA. Sedation confounds outcome prediction in cardiac arrest survivors

treated with hypothermia. Neurocrit Care. 2011;15:113–9. https://doi.org/10.1007/s12028-010-9412-8.

5. Le Roux P, Menon DK, Citerio G, Vespa P, Bader MK, Brophy GM, et al. Consensus summary statement of the International Multidisciplinary Consensus Conference On Multimodality Monitoring In Neurocritical Care: a statement for healthcare professionals from the Neurocritical Care Society and the European Society of Intensive Care Medicine. Neurocrit Care. 2014;21(Suppl 2):S1–26. https://doi.org/10.1007/s12028-014-0041-5.

6. Haupt WF, Hansen HC, Janzen RW, Firsching R, Galldiks N. Coma and cerebral imaging. Spring. 2015;4:180. https://doi.org/10.1186/s40064-015-0869-y.

7. Bruno MA, Ledoux D, Lambermont B, Damas F, Schnakers C, Vanhaudenhuyse A, et al. Comparison of the Full Outline of Unresponsiveness and Glasgow Liege Scale/Glasgow Coma Scale in an intensive care unit population. Neurocrit Care. 2011;15:447–53. https://doi.org/10.1007/s12028-011-9547-2.

8. Laureys S, Celesia GG, Cohadon F, Lavrijsen J, León-Carrión J, Sannita WG, et al. European task force on disorders of consciousness. Unresponsive wakefulness syndrome: a new name for the vegetative state or apallic syndrome. BMC Med. 2010;8:68. https://doi.org/10.1186/1741-7015-8-68.

9. Chan MF, Matter I. Investigating nurses' knowledge, attitudes and self-confidence patterns to perform the conscious level assessment: a cluster analysis. Int J Nurs Pract. 2013;19:351–9. https://doi.org/10.1111/ijn.12077.

10. Teasdale G, Jennett B. Assessment of coma and impaired consciousness. A practical scale. Lancet. 1974;2:81–4.

11. Reith FC, Van den Brande R, Synnot A, Gruen R, Maas AI. The reliability of the Glasgow Coma Scale: a systematic review. Intensive Care Med. 2016;42:3–15. https://doi.org/10.1007/s00134-015-4124-3.

12. Riker RR, Fugate JE. Participants in the International Multi-Disciplinary Consensus Conference on Multimodality Monitoring. Clinical monitoring scales in acute brain injury: assessment of coma, pain, agitation, and delirium. Neurocrit Care. 2014;21(Suppl 2):S27–37. https://doi.org/10.1007/s12028-014-0025-5.

13. Wijdicks EF, Bamlet WR, Maramattom BV, Manno EM, McClelland RL. Validation of a new coma scale: the FOUR score. Ann Neurol. 2005;58:585–93. https://doi.org/10.1002/ana.20611.

14. Kramer AA, Wijdicks EF, Snavely VL, Dunivan JR, Naranjo LL, Bible S, Rohs T, Dickess SM. A multicenter prospective study of interobserver agreement using the Full Outline of Unresponsiveness score

coma scale in the intensive care unit. Crit Care Med. 2012;40:2671–6. https://doi.org/10.1097/CCM.0b013e318258fd88.

15. Gelinas C, Klein K, Naidech AM, Skrobik Y. Pain, sedation, and delirium management in the neurocritically ill: lessons learned from recent research. Semin Respir Crit Care Med. 2013;34:236–43. https://doi.org/10.1055/s-0033-1342986.

16. Breivik H, Borchgrevink PC, Allen SM, Rosseland LA, Romundstad L, Hals EK, Kvarstein G, Stubhaug A. Assessment of pain. Br J Anaesth. 2008;101:17–24. https://doi.org/10.1093/bja/aen103.

17. Payen JF, Bru O, Bosson JL, Lagrasta A, Novel E, Deschaux I, et al. Assessing pain in critically ill sedated patients by using a behavioral pain scale. Crit Care Med. 2001;29:2258–63.

18. Gelinas C, Fillion L, Puntillo KA, Viens C, Fortier M. Validation of the critical-care pain observation tool in adult patients. Am J Crit Care. 2006;15:420–7.

19. Barr J, Fraser GL, Puntillo K, Ely EW, Gelinas C, Dasta JF, et al. American College of Critical Care Medicine. Clinical practice guidelines for the management of pain, agitation, and delirium in adult patients in the intensive care unit. Crit Care Med. 2013;41:263–306. https://doi.org/10.1097/CCM.0b013e3182783b72.

20. Chanques G, Payen JF, Mercier G, de Lattre S, Viel E, Jung B, et al. Assessing pain in non-intubated critically ill patients unable to self report: an adaptation of the Behavioral Pain Scale. Intensive Care Med. 2009;35:2060–7. https://doi.org/10.1007/s00134-009-1590-5.

21. Schnakers C, Chatelle C, Vanhaudenhuyse A, Majerus S, Ledoux D, Boly M, et al. The Nociception Coma Scale: a new tool to assess nociception in disorders of consciousness. Pain. 2010;148:215–9. https://doi.org/10.1016/j.pain.2009.09.028.

22. Chatelle C, Majerus S, Whyte J, Laureys S, Schnakers C. A sensitive scale to assess nociceptive pain in patients with disorders of consciousness. J Neurol Neurosurg Psychiatry. 2012;83:1233–7. https://doi.org/10.1136/jnnp-2012-302987.

23. Castillo MI, Cooke ML, Macfarlane B, Aitken LM. In ICU state anxiety is not associated with posttraumatic stress symptoms over six months after ICU discharge: a prospective study. Aust Crit Care. 2015.; pii: S1036-7314(15)00106-X. doi: https://doi.org/10.1016/j.aucc.2015.09.003

24. Jackson DL, Proudfoot CW, Cann KF, Walsh T. A systematic review of the impact of sedation practice in the ICU on resource use, costs and patient safety. Crit Care. 2010;14:R59. https://doi.org/10.1186/cc8956.

25. Sessler CN, Gosnell MS, Grap MJ, Brophy GM, O'Neal PV, Keane KA, et al. The Richmond Agitation-Sedation Scale: validity and reli-

ability in adult intensive care unit patients. Am J Respir Crit Care Med. 2002;166:1338–44. https://doi.org/10.1164/rccm.2107138.

26. Moons P, Sels K, DeBecker W, DeGeest S, Ferdinande P. Development of a risk assessment tool for deliberate self-extubation in intensive care patients. Intensive Care Med. 2004;30:1348–55. https://doi.org/10.1007/s00134-004-2228-32.

27. Ramsay MA, Savege TM, Simpson BR, Goodwin R. Controlled sedation with alphaxalone-alphadolone. Br Med J. 1974;2:656–9.

28. Devlin JW, Boleski G, Mlynarek M, Nerenz DR, Peterson E, Jankowski M, et al. Motor Activity Assessment Scale: a valid and reliable sedation scale for use with mechanically ventilated patients in an adult surgical intensive care unit. Crit Care Med. 1999;27:1271–5.

29. Riker RR, Picard JT, Fraser GL. Prospective evaluation of the Sedation-Agitation Scale for adult critically ill patients. Crit Care Med. 1999;27:1325–9.

30. Chernik DA, Gillings D, Laine H, Hendler J, Silver JM, Davidson AB, et al. Validity and reliability of the observer's Assessment of Alertness/Sedation Scale: study with intravenous midazolam. J Clin Psychopharmacol. 1990;10:244–51.

31. Mirski MA, LeDroux SN, Lewin JJ 3rd, Thompson CB, Mirski KT, Griswold M. Validity and reliability of an intuitive conscious sedation scoring tool: the nursing instrument for the communication of sedation. Crit Care Med. 2010;38:1674–84. https://doi.org/10.1097/CCM.0b013e3181e7c73e.

32. Rowe K, Fletcher S. Sedation in intensive care unit. Contin Educ Anaesth Crit Care Pain. 2008;8:50–5. https://doi.org/10.1093/bjaceaccp/mkn005.

33. Ramoo V, Abdullah KL, Tan PS, Wong LP, Chua YP, Tang LY. Sedation scoring and managing abilities of intensive care nurses post educational intervention. Nurs Crit Care. 2015;22:141–9. https://doi.org/10.1111/nicc.12180.

34. Salluh JI, Soares M, Teles JM, Ceraso D, Raimondi N, Nava VS, et al. Delirium epidemiology in critical care (DECCA): an international study. Crit Care. 2010;14:R210. https://doi.org/10.1186/cc9333.

35. Jackson P, Khan A. Delirium in critically ill patients. Crit Care Clin. 2015;31:589–603. https://doi.org/10.1016/j.ccc.2015.03.011.

36. Curtin RG. The delirium noticed in cardiac disease. Trans Am Climatol Assoc. 1904;20:81–91.

37. Kornfeld DS. Psychiatric view of the intensive care unit. Br Med J. 1969;1:108–10.

38. American Psychiatric Association. Diagnostic and statistical manual of mental disorders. 5th ed. Washington DC: American Psychiatric Publishing; 2013.

39. WHO. The ICD-10 classification of mental and behavioral disorders: diagnostic criteria for research. Geneva: World Health Organization; 1993.
40. Peterson JF, Pun BT, Dittus RS, Thomason JW, Jackson JC, Shintani AK, et al. Delirium and its motoric subtypes: a study of 614 critically ill patients. J Am Geriatr Soc. 2006;54:479–84. https://doi.org/10.1111/j.1532-5415.2005.00621.x.
41. van den Boogaard M, Pickkers P, Slooter AJ, Kuiper MA, Spronk PE, van der Voort PH, et al. Development and validation of PRE-DELIRIC (PREdiction of DELIRium in ICu patients) delirium prediction model for intensive care patients: observational multicentre study. BMJ. 2012;344:e420. https://doi.org/10.1136/bmj.e420.
42. Wassenaar A, van den Boogaard M, van Achterberg T, Slooter AJ, Kuiper MA, Hoogendoorn ME, et al. Multinational development and validation of an early prediction model for delirium in ICU patients. Intensive Care Med. 2015;41:1048–56. https://doi.org/10.1007/s00134-015-3777-2.
43. European Delirium Association and American Delirium Society. The DSM-5 criteria, level of arousal and delirium diagnosis: inclusiveness is safer. BMC Med. 2014;12:141. https://doi.org/10.1186/s12916-014-0141-2.
44. Ely EW, Inouye SK, Bernard GR, Gordon S, Francis J, May L, et al. Delirium in mechanically ventilated patients: validity and reliability of the confusion assessment method for the intensive care unit (CAM-ICU). JAMA. 2001;286:2703–10.
45. Bergeron N, Dubois MJ, Dumont M, Dial S, Skrobik Y. Intensive Care Delirium Screening Checklist: evaluation of a new screening tool. Intensive Care Med. 2001;27:859–64.
46. Tomasi CD, Grandi C, Salluh J, Soares M, Giombelli VR, Cascaes S, et al. Comparison of CAM-ICU and ICDSC for the detection of delirium in critically ill patients focusing on relevant clinical outcomes. J Crit Care. 2012;27:212–7. https://doi.org/10.1016/j.jcrc.2011.05.015.
47. Mortensen AL, Mazer MA, McCarthy PJ, Rimawi RH. ICU delirium—attention to inattention. In: Ramzy H, editor. Bedside critical care guide. Foster City, CA: OMICS Group eBooks; 2014. p. 003–6.
48. Rivosecchi RM, Smithburger PL, Svec S, Campbell S, Kane-Gill SL. Nonpharmacological interventions to prevent delirium: an evidence-based systematic review. Crit Care Nurse. 2015;35:39–50. https://doi.org/10.4037/ccn2015423.
49. Rivosecchi RM, Kane-Gill SL, Svec S, Campbell S, Smithburger PL. The implementation of a nonpharmacologic protocol to prevent intensive care delirium. J Crit Care. 2016;31:206–11. https://doi.org/10.1016/j.jcrc.2015.09.031.

# Chapter 3
# Respiratory and Ventilatory Assessment

**Alberto Lucchini, Christian De Felippis, and Stefano Bambi**

## 3.1 Introduction

The basic treatment of acute and chronic respiratory failure grounds on the mechanical ventilatory support. However, this kind of treatment could arouse ventilator-induced lung injury (VILI) [1]. Some recommended evidence-based ventilatory strategies are available to avoid potential adverse effect, especially in patient developing adult respiratory distress syndrome (ARDS) [2, 3]:

- Low tidal volume (TV) (≤6 mL/kg of ideal body weight); plateau pressure (P-plat) <30 cmH$_2$O—to prevent volutrauma, barotrauma, and biotrauma
- Recruitment maneuvers—to open the lungs
- Positive end-expiration pressure (PEEP)—to keep lungs open
- Prone positioning—to improve gas exchanges through improvement of ventilation in the lung dorsal areas
- Early-assisted mechanical ventilation (MV)—to prevent the disuse and the weakness of diaphragm

© Springer International Publishing AG, part of Springer Nature 2018    59
I. Comisso et al., *Nursing in Critical Care Setting*,
https://doi.org/10.1007/978-3-319-50559-6_3

- Sedation and paralysis (in the earliest phases of severe ARDS)—to ease the patient's adaptation to MV
- Noninvasive ventilation (NIV)—to avoid intubation

Putting these key points into practice during the treatment of ARDS requires a continuous monitoring of patient-pulmonary ventilator interaction, in order to avoid potential adverse effects and iatrogenic damage. In the next sections, all the basic leading principles about MV settings and monitoring will be discussed.

## 3.2 Basic Monitoring Tools

### 3.2.1 Pulse Oximetry

Pulse oximetry is a technique to perform a continuous monitoring of peripheral oxygen saturation and heart rate. The reading obtained through a probe uses a sensor containing two different light sources (red and infrared) plus a photodetector able to read the light wave length, ranging from 650 to 940 nm. Light's absorption doesn't rule out between oxygenated and deoxygenated blood and tissue pigmentation. Then, only the pulsatile wave form will be calculated. Any fluctuations regarding the light's absorption are related to vascular bed's status. The pulsation modifies the amount of arterial blood during short periods of time. Because the arterial blood is the only light-absorbing component, it can be isolated and calculated.

Oxygen saturation can be defined as a ratio between oxygenated hemoglobin ($HbO_2$) and the total amount of hemoglobin ($HbO_2$ + Hb + carboxyhemoglobin + methemoglobin + sulfhemoglobin). Red and infrared lights emitted by diodes pass through tissues, and are subsequently read by a photodetector, and then converted into electrical signal. Signal is amplified, processed, and finally showed on a display as a numeric value of $SpO_2$ plus heart rate.

Several anatomical sites fit for a proper reading by the probe. Main limitations refer to correct positioning of probe's sides itself, to the pulsatile arteriolar bed, and the thickness of tissues crossed by the lights. Common anatomical sites are the finger, nose, earlobe, and great toe. Different types of probes are available as wrap style sensor or clip style sensor. It's fundamental to apply the right probe for the right site.

Several factors can affect the correct reading of pulse oximetry. Movements of the patient disturb reading, and then a potential desaturation should be ruled out, discriminating between reading artifacts and a real desaturation event. In these cases, the comparison between the heart rate values displayed from the electrocardiogram trace and from the pulse oximetry could be helpful. Nail polish could lead to reading artifacts due to its capability to adsorb different light waves: it should be removed prior to commence any monitoring actions [4, 5]. Incorrect positioning of the probe could lead to venous stasis and a lower saturation levels reading due to an increase in the pulsatile venous bed.

Nevertheless, the reading cannot rule out between hemoglobin and carboxyhemoglobin resulting in an overrated estimation of the values. Patient suspected for carbon monoxide poisoning or jaundice should be monitored via arterial blood gas (ABG) sample tested by laboratory.

Prolonged monitoring time requires a probe's site swap on a regular basis (every 4 h or less, according to patient's skin conditions), to avoid skin and tissue (pressure ulcers, burns) damages.

## 3.2.2 End-Tidal Carbon Dioxide (EtCO₂) Monitoring

EtCO$_2$ is defined as the concentration or partial pressure of carbon dioxide (PaCO$_2$) measured in "mmHg" (millimeter of mercury), or CO$_2$ percentage inside respiratory gases. Usually, PaCO$_2$ ranges from 35 to 45 mmHg. EtCO$_2$ reflects cardiac output (CO) and pulmonary blood flow. As soon as CO$_2$ moves from alveolar capillary network into airways, the capnograph detects its concentration or partial pressure in the respiratory gases. During cardiopulmonary resuscitation, the amount of CO$_2$ reflects the pulmonary bloodstream. Capnography is referred to a visualization of a graphic waveform of CO$_2$ concentration (Fig. 3.1).

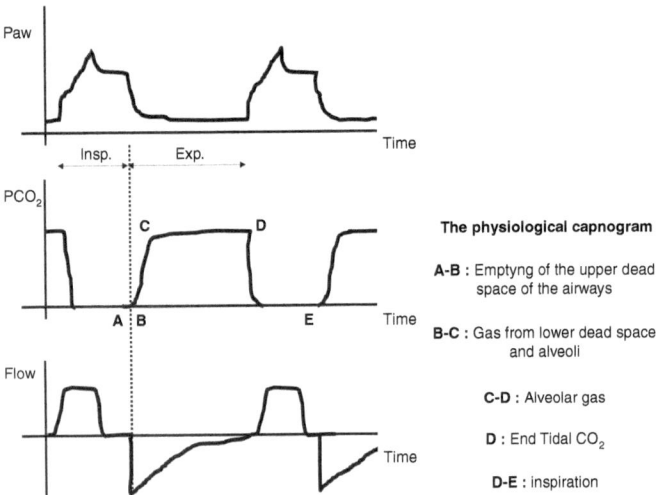

**Fig. 3.1** Relationship between capnography, airway pressure, and gas flow

Usually the normal gap between $PaCO_2$ and $EtCO_2$ is 4–5 mmHg, as expression of ventilatory wasted space known as "dead space."

The capnography measurement can be implemented through two kinds of technologies: "mainstream" and "sidestream" (Fig. 3.2).

The mainstream technology is available for intubated patients only. A sample cell ("cuvette") and an adaptor are located in line on ventilator circuit between the endotracheal tube and "Y-shaped" connector, so the respiratory gases are nearly real-time detected and measured. The disadvantages are additional weight on the airway lines, additional dead space, and reading failure due to bronchial secretions or excessive condensation.

The sidestream technology is based on a continuous sampling of gases from the breathing circuit. A tiny gauge-sized plastic tube positioned via a connector delivers the gas sample into a sampling cell within the monitor. Lightweight is probably its best advantage, although it can be easily obstructed by bronchial secretions, mouth secretions, or condensation.

Microstream technology is the ultimate evolution of capnography's monitoring. It is suitable for intubated patients. Advantages are smaller sampling volume needed and accuracy in detecting $CO_2$ levels from low expiratory flows.

Figure 3.2 shows a waveform capnography.

The main indications for $EtCO_2$ monitoring are:

- Continuous monitoring about quality of mechanical ventilation.
- Verification of artificial airway device placement.
- Monitoring of circulation during cardiopulmonary resuscitation. In fact, the sudden and steady increment of $PetCO_2$ is an indicator of ROSC.

Capnography wave changes are induced by some clinical problems, as illustrated in Fig. 3.3 [6–8].

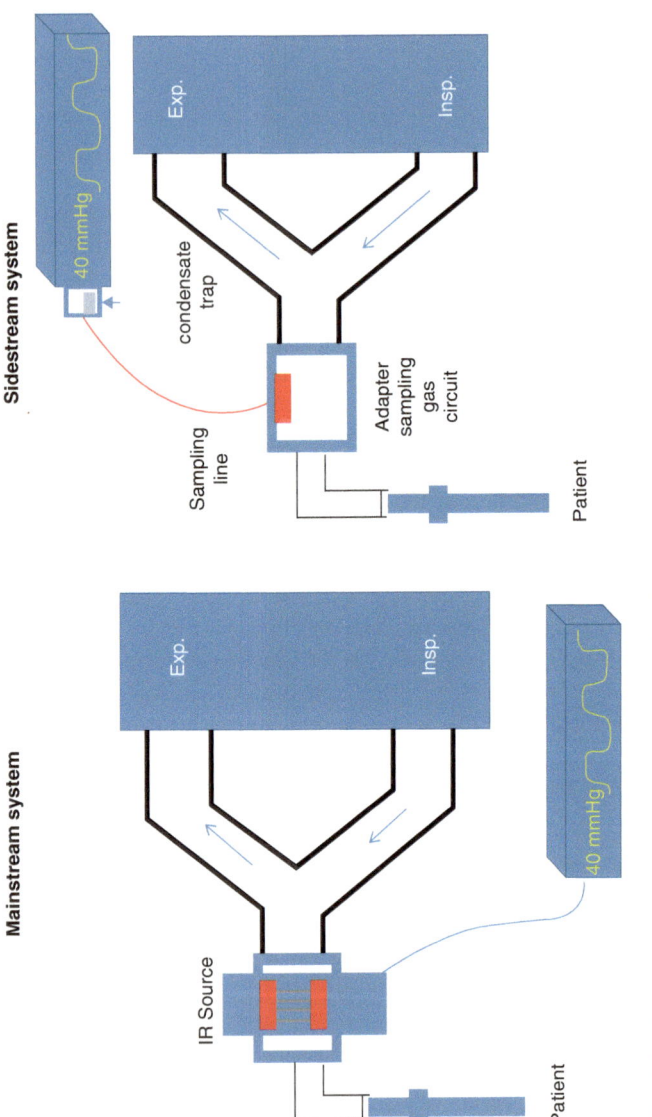

**Fig. 3.2** Mainstream and sidestream technology for EtCO$_2$ measurement

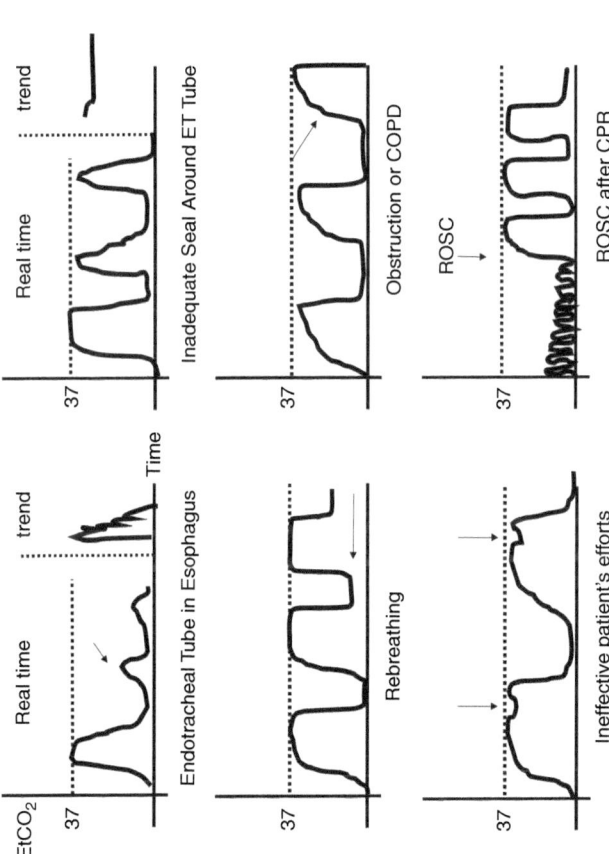

**Fig. 3.3** Capnography waves in different clinical situations

## 3.3    Basic Monitoring During MV

### *3.3.1    Basic Principles*

Modern pulmonary ventilators can be divided into two main units:

- Control unit, consisting of the display section with the control section
- Patient unit, consisting of the pneumatic section and the power section

The basic features of a modern ventilator are showed in Fig. 3.4. The various components are numbered from 1 to 10 (from 1 to 5, inspiratory line; from 6 to 12, expiratory line).

### *3.3.2    Ventilator Waveform Monitoring*

Monitoring of respiratory mechanics via scalar waves (scalar plot airway pressure, volume, or flow against time) provides important information and/or red flags to the bedside nurse in ICU. Several studies have shown that a better understanding and interpretation of ventilatory graphic waveforms by ICU nurses can result in a shorter time of weaning from MV support [9].

Waveform analysis is performed through three different ventilatory aspects: airway pressure, airway flow, and airway volume versus time. Graphically, time measure is the X-axis, while the other abovementioned factors are plotted in the Y-axis [10].

#### 3.3.2.1    Pressure-Time Waveform

On volume-controlled mode two different pressures can be distinguished: peak pressure (Pmax) and plateau pressure. Pmax is

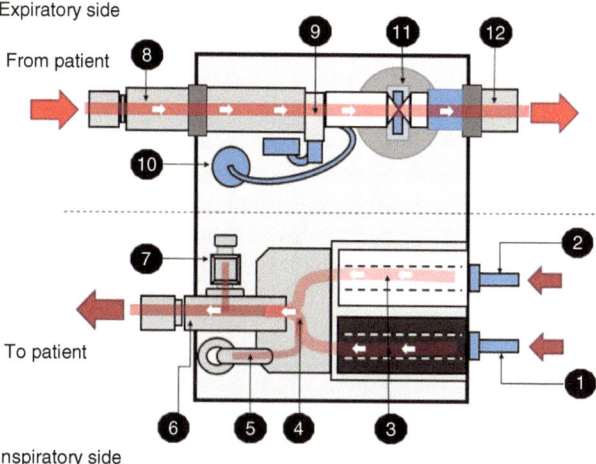

**Fig. 3.4** Ventilator components. (1) Gas inlet for medical air. The connected air must have a pressure between 2 and 6.5 bar. (2) Gas inlet for oxygen. The connected oxygen must have a pressure between 2 and 6.5 bar. (3) The gas flow delivered to the patient system is regulated by the inspiratory valves. Generally, there is one inspiratory valve unit for each kind of gas. The inspiratory valves are regulated by a feedback control system. (4) The gases are mixed in the inspiratory mixing chamber. (5) The pressure of the mixed gas delivered to the patient (inspiratory pressure—Pmax, Pplat) is measured by the inspiratory pressure transducer. The transducer is generally protected by an antibacterial filter. (6) The inspiratory pipe leads the mixed gas from ventilator mixing chamber to the patient system. The inspiratory pipe also contains the safety valve, a holder for the $O_2$ cell, and the inspiratory outlet. The spring-loaded safety valve will open in case of a power failure and/or if the inspiratory pressure exceeds 100 cmH$_2$O. (7) The oxygen concentration inside the inspiratory pipe is measured by the $O_2$ cell. (8) The patient system's expiratory gas tube is connected at the expiratory inlet. The expiratory inlet can contain a moisture trap or can be protected by a warming system. (9) The gas flow through the expiratory limb is measured by the expiratory flow transducer. Patient trigger efforts, indicated by a decreasing in the continuous flow, are sensed by this expiratory flow transducer. (10) The expiratory pressure is measured by the expiratory pressure transducer. The transducer is protected by a bacteria filter. Patient trigger efforts, indicated by a pressure drop, are sensed by this expiratory pressure transducer. (11) The pressure of the gas (PEEP) in the patient system is regulated by expiratory valve. The expiratory valve is regulated by a feedback control system. (12) The gas from the patient system leaves the ventilator via this expiratory outlet. The outlet contains a non-return valve, which is a part of the patient triggering system

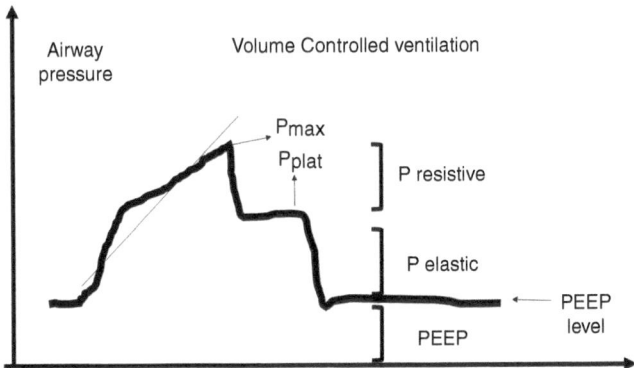

**Fig. 3.5** Pressure-time waveform. The difference between peak pressure (Pmax) and plateau pressure (Pplat) defines resistive pressure, whereas the difference between plateau pressure and PEEP defines the elastic pressure. Analysis of the airway pressure shape during phase of constant flow inflation (VC mode) can be used to calculate stress index

determined by both pulmonary resistance and compliance, while the plateau pressure is related only to the static compliance (elastic pressure) of the lung. Stress index factor (indicating the overstretching of lungs during MV) can be obtained by analyzing the ascending wave's shape during a constant flow phase.

On pressure control ventilation mode, the shape of graphic wave will be different: the ventilator will provide the inspiratory peak pressure, keeping it constant throughout the settled inspiratory timing (Fig. 3.5).

If the aim of a controlled ventilation mode is a complete management of patient's respiratory rate, every spontaneous breath triggered by the patient should be avoided. Therefore, strictly monitoring of ventilator graphics becomes crucial to recognize potential trigger asynchronies. In both controlled ventilation modes (pressure/volume), these unplanned spontaneous breaths lead to a modification of the inspiratory/

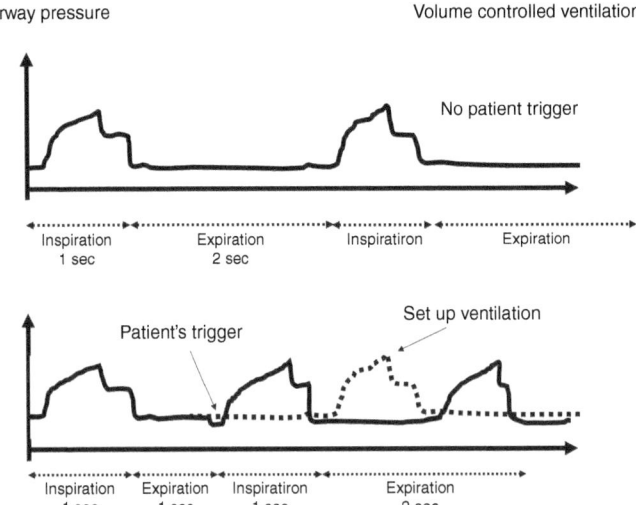

**Fig. 3.6** Comparison between a machine-based and a patient's trigger-based delivery of TV [11]

expiratory ratio, affecting its timing and resulting in a potential "'air-trapping" effect (Fig. 3.6).

### 3.3.2.2 Flow-Time Waveform

The flow-rate scalar wave is made by two distinct parts, the positive side originated by the ventilator itself (managed by the machine) and the negative side, or expiratory flow (ruled by patient's conditions). From a graphical point of view, time is shown (seconds) on the horizontal axis (X), while the airway flow (Lt/min) provided by the machine is showed on the vertical axis (Y).

On volume-controlled mode, the inspiratory tracing is shaped by the ventilatory settings. As before mentioned, the patient's related variable on volume-controlled mode is the airway pressures (Ppeak and PPlat). The amount of airway flow is dependent from ventilator settings. The flow is the resultant of the ventilation settings (e.g., controlled volume, TV 500 mL, with RR = 20 e $Ti$ = 1'—Flow = 500 mL in 1'). As result, the trend of waveforms will be square-shaped, keeping it during the entire inspiratory timing with a quick no-flow step at the end of it. Then the expiratory timing is split into two parts; the high initial expiratory peak flow is followed by its gradual releasing.

On pressure-controlled mode the expiratory wave still remains the same (lead by patient), while the inspiratory will be affected by alterations. In order to reach the settled pressure value as quick as possible, the flow waveform results in a regular decreasing shape (after the flow peak) due to a progressive lacking of space available into the lungs. Monitoring of the TV and minute volume is performed by the visualization of graphic time-volume waveform.

From a nursing perspective, two factors seem to be crucial in the monitoring of waveforms.

The presence of bronchial secretions, in absence of collection condense trap, will result in a "sawtooth" pattern on scalar trace. According to latest guidelines, the detection of this ventilatory patient's status is a lead indicator to perform a bronchial suctioning [12, 13].

It is possible to recognize this situation also from a different graphic monitoring, as known as "loop" waveform, a real-time analysis between flow and volume able to provide the right timing to commence the suctioning maneuver.

Loops plot pressure and flow against volume (P/V, F/V) and allow the practitioner to analyze the inspiratory and expiratory phases of each breath using either flow-volume or pressure-volume tracings. In flow-volume loop, volume is plotted on the X-axis and flow on the Y-axis. Positive flow from a positive-pressure breath often appears above the horizontal axis, with expiratory flow below the axis, but this pattern may be reversed, depending on the ventilator being used (Fig. 3.7).

If the expiratory portion doesn't return to baseline before the start of the next breath, "air trapping" or PEEP$_i$ could be present (Fig. 3.8) [14].

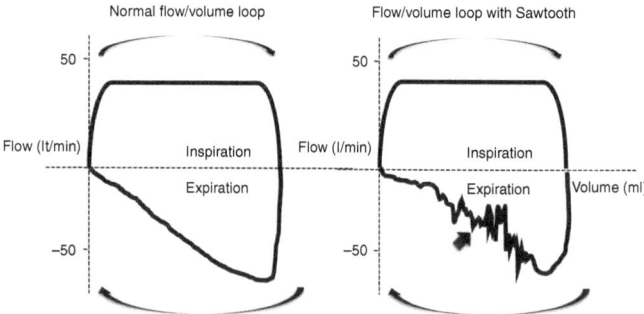

**Fig. 3.7** Normal flow-volume loop (left) and flow/volume loop with sawtooth (right)

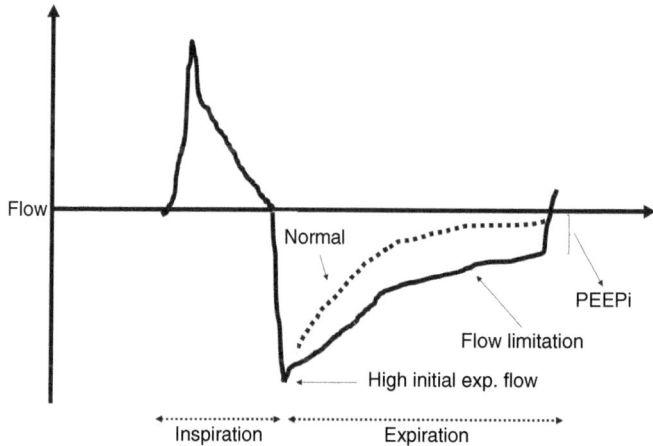

**Fig. 3.8** Flow-volume waveform in patient with iPEEP

### 3.3.2.3 Time-Volume Waveform

Time-volume graphic trace shows on the Y-axis the amount of gas volume provided. Two relevant aspects are related with this topic: basically, it allows to monitor the volume as a real-time checking during volume-controlled ventilatory setting, but at the same time it provides an evaluation and monitoring of the real amount of volume on pressure-controlled settings. If at the end of the inspiratory phase the volume's amount fails to be zeroed, a leakage from the tubing should be considered.

### 3.3.2.4 Other Advanced Respiratory Monitoring Parameters

There are some other important parameters that can be used by ICU nurses in their advanced respiratory assessment of critically ill patients. These parameters require special competencies and skill to be employed in the clinical practice (Table 3.1).

## 3.4 Monitoring During Invasive Spontaneous Ventilation

### 3.4.1 The Weaning Process

Because of the potential risks related to MV, weaning process should begin as soon as possible. Nevertheless, an excessive early planned extubation is not recommended, resulting in weaning failure and consequent reintubation associated with poor outcome and increased mortality rates.

In order to prevent delayed weaning and extubation failure, scientific literature suggests [21]:

**Table 3.1** Advanced ventilatory assessment parameters

| Parameter | Description |
| --- | --- |
| Compliance respiratory system (Cpl,rs or respiratory system compliance) | Compliance is defined as the ratio between volume and pressure. Regarding the pulmonary system, TV represents the volume variable, while delta pressure (plateau pressure minus PEEP) is the real pressure generated from machine to deliver that gas volume |
| | Cpl,rs stand for the ventilated lung parenchyma and stiffness of chest wall, and the normal physiologic values are 1.2–1.5 mL/cmH$_2$O/kg |
| Auto-positive end-expiratory pressure (PEEPi) | Presence of PEEPi is due to an incomplete emptying of the lungs. PEEPi formula is total PEEP (pressure at the end of expiration—measured by performing an expiratory pause of 3 s with patient on controlled ventilation) minus set PEEP |
| | PEEPi can be related to clinical findings (COPD, asthma, etc.) or direct consequence of inaccurate respiratory setting by clinicians [15] |
| | In case of flow limitation (COPD patients), PEEPi can get reduced by low levels of external PEEP. In case of flow obstruction PEEPi, (bronchial secretions, ET tube diameter size, I/E ratio reversed), the external PEEP cannot affect the PEEPi. PEEPi is strictly related to the patient's respiratory pattern |
| Esophageal pressure (Pes) | A tight correlation appears to exist between pressures inside pleural space and esophageal pressure. The most common way to perform a bedside measurement is throughout an esophageal balloon filled with air, with the balloon-tipped catheter connected to a pressure transducer kit as a part of a multiparameter monitoring system (Fig. 3.9—left) |
| | From a nursing point of view, Pes monitoring can detect patient-ventilator asynchrony in invasive or noninvasive ventilatory support [16] |

(continued)

**Table 3.1** (continued)

| Parameter | Description |
| --- | --- |
| Diaphragmatic function | Trigger pneumatic signal is based on airway pressure, flow, and volume. It represents a communicative link between machine and patient's demand, able to drive, control, and synchronize both inspiratory and expiratory cycling. Inspiratory trigger commences the inspiratory phase of ventilation, while the expiratory trigger rules the expiratory one. Lately, a new way of trigger detection appeared called (by its acronyms) NAVA (neurally adjusted ventilatory assist) [17–19]. Basically, NAVA's triggering principle is based on the electric diaphragm activity (Edi): it's the best electrical signal to get analyzed in order to estimate respiratory drive and trigger off and cycle off the delivery of mechanical ventilation; Edi is definitely more accurate, reliable, and faster compared to conventional signal before mentioned. Detection of signal is possible via a dedicated NG tube equipped with electrodes on its distal end. This dedicated NG tube able to detect the diaphragmatic activity and then provide the ventilatory NAVA supports can be used itself as a valid monitoring tool for asynchronies when it's matched with a graphic monitoring of ventilation: flow and pressure (Fig. 3.9—right) Moreover, it could be very helpful to early detect a multifactor syndrome defined as VIDD (ventilator-induced diaphragmatic dysfunction) [20] mainly characterized by loss of contractile force and muscular mass. Diaphragmatic dysfunction is common in patients mechanically ventilated, and it's one of the main reasons for weaning failure |

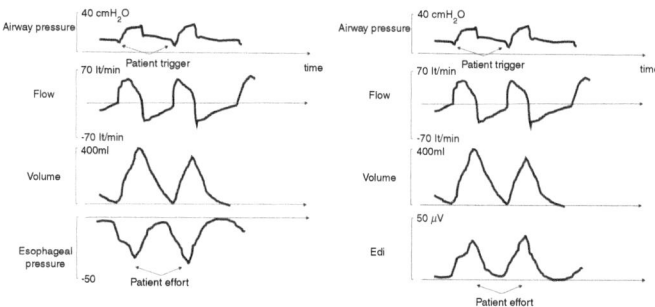

**Fig. 3.9** Graphic waveforms with esophageal pressure (*left*) and with Edi monitoring (*right*)

1. Predictive measurement tools for weaning

2. Trial of unassisted breathing (CPAP with tube resistance compensation or T-tube trial)

3. Trial of extubation

During pressure support ventilation (PSV), the clinical goal is to best balance the use and abuse of patient's respiratory muscles, avoiding functional muscular failure due to excessive WOB.

The respiratory over-assistance should be prevented [22] because the only patient-machine's interaction is related to the trigger activation, without any other muscular effort. It's working like a pressure-controlled ventilation mode set on patient trigger. On the contrary, inadequate PS with a full muscular involvement could lead to fatigue and finally muscular respiratory failure.

Therefore, different monitoring tools should be considered in order to help bedside nurse in titrating the most suitable PSV, avoiding over- and underestimated PSV, index of muscular fatigue, and detection of maximum inspiratory pressure. Analyzing all those elements the ICU nurse can manage an advanced patient's respiratory assessment to get the best respiratory weaning pathway, from the very beginning (VC ventilation off) until the full patient recovery (successful extubation) (Table 3.2).

**Table 3.2** Weaning process advanced assessment parameters

| Parameter | Description |
|---|---|
| $P_{0.1}$ | The airway occlusion pressure ($P_{0.1}$) is a reliable index of patient's breath neuromuscular driving correlated with WOB (work of breathing) as well. $P_{0.1}$ is defined as the negative airway pressure generated during the first 100 ms of an occluded inspiration |
|  | $P_{0.1}$ is an estimate of the neuromuscular drive but as index could be easily affected from external stimuli, especially from patient's level of sedation: detection and measurement should be performed in a very quiet and relaxed environment. Common range of values is 1–1.5 cmH$_2$O. Using $P_{0.1}$ as lead indicator and avoiding over-assistance or under-assistance, the pressure support range of values will be settled according to a $P_{0.1}$ between 2 and 4 cmH$_2$O. On a PS ventilation $P_{0.1}$ index less than 1.5 reflects patient's respiratory muscles completely unloaded. $P_{0.1}$ index, according to literature, appears to be not reliable on patients with major neurological impairment or severe muscular force deficit (MIP <10 cmH$_2$O) |
| Maximum inspiratory pressure (MIP) or negative inspiratory pressure (NIF) | MIP index is a marker about the strength of inspiratory muscles, mainly the diaphragm, as reflection of negative pressure generated against an occluded airway |
|  | A bedside calculation example should consider the baseline PEEP plus any possible PEEPi |
|  | The clinical procedure for determining this marker is very dependent on patient's efforts and his/her previous education: a maximal inspiratory effort is required from the participant, while the operator is performing a manual expiratory hold for 30 s at least. For not collaborative patients, it appears helpful to extend the apnea time in order to the maximal effort. Normal range of values is 80/100 cmH$_2$O, but most of the pulmonary ventilators available cannot read those negative pressure, usually no more than −45 cmH$_2$O |

**Table 3.2** (continued)

| Parameter | Description |
|---|---|
| Pressure muscle index (PMI) | Pressure muscle index (PMI) represents the pressure elastic recoil of lungs detected at the end of an inspiratory occlusion [23]. PMI value is obtained following this equation: |
| | PMI = PPlat − (PEEP + PS) |
| | In order to perform an end-inspiratory occlusion maneuver, the operator should switch the ventilator mode on pressure support mode alone (avoiding any controlled mode ventilation or synchronized intermittent mandatory breaths because pressing the inspiratory hold button results into a delivery of mandatory breath). This marker allows the practitioner to assess the inspiratory muscle activity related to PS setting |
| | Excess of PS should be recognized and avoided because it leads the patient to a loss of respiratory muscle mass and contractile force, especially the diaphragm. If there's no contraindication, PS level can be settled in order to obtain a PMI value between 2 and 6 cmH$_2$O |
| | Good practice suggests to prevent PMI equal or less than zero, as manifestation of over-support, to repeat the maneuver three times in a short timing of minutes to get a reliable value |
| | From a graphic point of view in Fig. 3.10, as a result of an inspiratory occlusion, the pressure scalar should increase when the PMI is positive |

## 3.5 Pressure and Flow Monitoring to Assess Asynchrony

MV support aims to realize a harmonious patient-ventilator interaction. Patient-ventilator asynchronies (PVA) can be defined as a mismatch between patient's respiratory efforts and the machine interaction or cycling (Table 3.3—Fig. 3.13a-f). PVA are frequent during assisted MV, but often physicians and nurses fail to detect them, especially the less evident ones. PVA events in ICU can affect patients' out-

**Table 3.3** Patient-ventilator asynchronies

| Kind of asynchrony | Description |
| --- | --- |
| Ineffective inspiratory efforts (IIE) | Basically, ineffective inspiratory efforts are defined by a muscular activation drive by patient not followed by a trigger activation |
| | Figure 3.11a shows IIE from a graphic point of view |
| | Graphically speaking, asynchrony is detectable on flow and pressure scalar: monitoring the expiratory flow can show the drop to baseline for a short time, without a switch to inspiration phase but simple returning to expiration, plus a temporary PEEP rising on pressure scalar. This phenomenon is common when an overrated pressure support produces a decrease of natural respiratory drive |
| Double triggering | Double triggering [26] is defined as two ventilator insufflations delivered within one inspiratory effort of the patient. Graphically it's displayed as two inspiratory efforts split by a minimal, almost none, expiration. This type of asynchrony is common when inspiratory cycling timing is stretched (weaning from ARDS, poor Cpl,rs). When the machine cycles into exhalation, the continuing muscular contraction results in a second effort sense and a breath delivery, during a prolonged inspiratory time. Double triggering is shown in Fig. 3.11b |
| | The basic intervention to fix the double triggering asynchrony is prolonging the time of pressure support inspiratory ramp (Fig. 3.11c) |
| Early cycling-off | Premature cycling is the reason behind the double triggering asynchrony but without switching into a secondary inspiratory cycle [26] |
| | Visually monitoring the exhalation flow waveform will show a sudden decreasing line before returning into expiratory phase |
| | On pressure scalar, the detection of pressure drop ("stacking of breath") at the end of inspiratory time will occur behind the PEEP level settled (Fig. 3.11d) |

**Table 3.3** (continued)

| Kind of asynchrony | Description |
| --- | --- |
| Autotriggering | Autotriggering on PSV is defined as a delivery of breath by the machine without a trigger stimuli performed by the patient [26]. However, this phenomenon may occur on controlled ventilation as well: despite the I/E ratio settled, the ventilator delivers an extra TV |
| | Pressure scalar is the graphic to monitoring for its detection. On PS, even with high-sensitive trigger, the patient's neural demand is a negative deflection just before the waveform. The absence of patient's triggering results in a square pattern of PS waveform (Fig. 3.11e) |
| | Events which may mimic a false trigger are air leakage (fistula, chest tube on suction), poor Cpl,rs, water condensation in tubing hoses, heartbeat transmission due to very poor lung compliance |
| Late cycling-off | A ventilator failure in the cycling inspiration to expiration detection keeps the inspiratory cycle while the patient needs to exhale [26]. This kind of issue is due to the mechanism itself of triggering during PS ventilation. On normal respiratory mechanics, the cycle setting is 25% of peak inspiratory flow; vice versa, in case of obstructive mechanics (COPD), modifications in the inspiratory flow curve lead to the 25% level being reached later. Visually this kind of asynchrony appears to be different according to invasive versus noninvasive ventilation |
| | In intubated patients, graphics will show a pressure increase above the set pressure support level, resulting into a pressure-cycle response to the patient's active exhalation and efforts (Fig. 3.11f) |
| | On the other hand, air leakage issues produce a never-ending inspiratory flow, preventing the expiratory trigger activation |

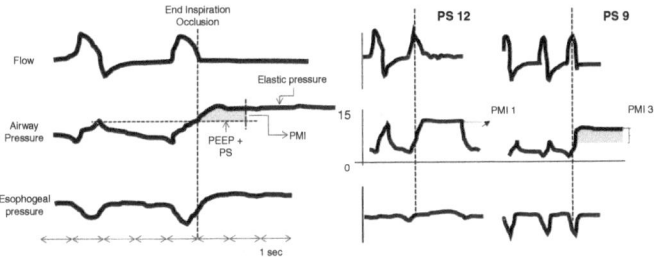

**Fig. 3.10** PMI detection during pressure support ventilation

come, prolong MV and hospital LOS, and increase mortality [24]. Moreover, several studies have shown a relationship between asynchronies and poor quality of sleep in ICU patients [25]. Recognizing PVA is an advanced competence for nurses.

## 3.6 Noninvasive Ventilation Monitoring and Management

Respiratory assessment in ICU patients undergoing NIV requires to take in account not only the patients' conditions but also the interfaces, the management of gas flow, humidification, noise adverse effects, interface-related pressure ulcers, and the patient-breathing circuit interactions.

### 3.6.1 Helmet CPAP

CPAP (continuous positive airway pressure) ventilation principle is based on a constant positive airway pressure delivered throughout the whole respiratory cycle. It can be delivered via

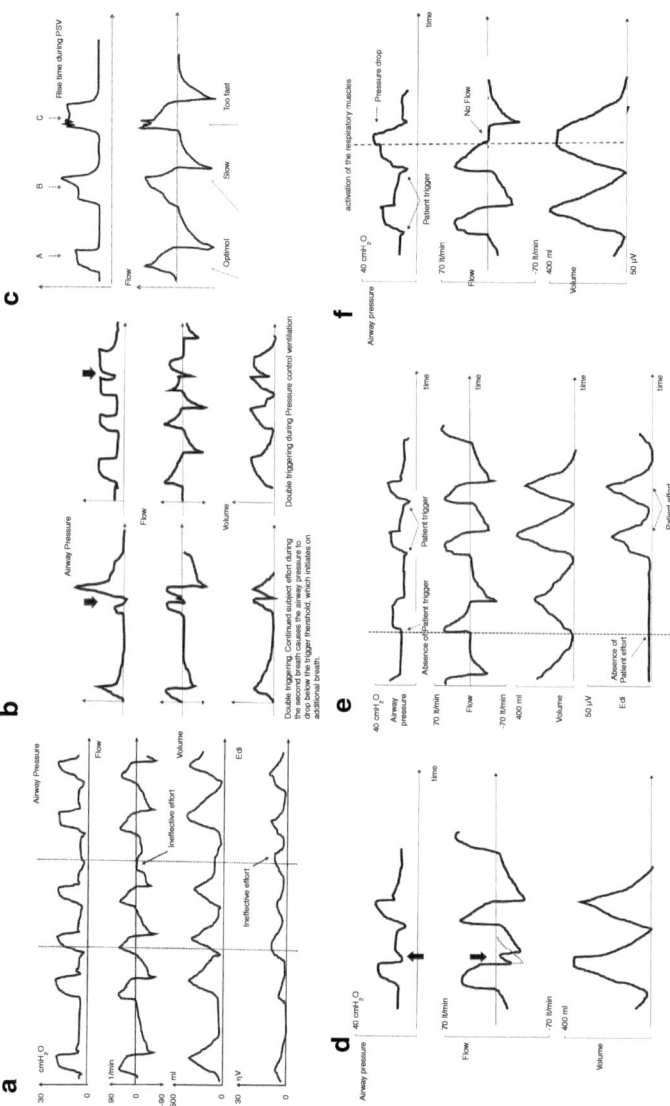

**Fig. 3.11** Patient-ventilator asynchronies

endotracheal intubation (invasive airway) or via facial mask/ helmet (noninvasive interface).

Literature promotes noninvasive CPAP in case of acute cardiogenic pulmonary edema, ARDS (adult respiratory distress syndrome), posttraumatic acute respiratory failure, and postoperative hypoxemia. Moreover, it appears to be a useful respiratory support as a bridge to complete weaning after extubation. Nowadays in immunocompromised patients, it represents the first-line choice in case of hypoxemic respiratory failure [27, 28].

During the 1980s, noninvasive CPAP therapy was only delivered via facial mask. The limits were its timing: a short length of stay in situ (no more than 2 h), due to the high pressures generated onto facial skin, tissues, and bones structures, resulting in an intermittent application of this support [29]. In order to deal with these limitations, during the early 1990s, a new NIV delivery interface was developed in Italy: the CPAP helmet. It's a reusable, single patient interface, made of a clear plastic hood on a hard-plastic ring with a multi-sized silicon-polyvinyl chloride soft collar, to fit a wide range of necks' dimensions. Its capability to provide a permanent pneumatic seal keeps a continuous positive pressure throughout the whole respiratory cycle. Inlet for fresh gases and outlet for PEEP valve (mechanical or water) should be available. A correct management of the helmet is helpful to minimize claustrophobia, preserving full visual contact and communication with healthcare providers and patient's significant others [30, 31].

Basic principles of helmet monitoring are related to gas flow regulation, circuit handling, patient surveillance, noise reduction, helmet anchorage, and gas humidification [32, 33].

### 3.6.1.1   Gas-Flow Management

Despite the helmet's size, the total amount of inlet gas flow shouldn't be lower than 30 L/min. Literature has clearly proved that under the aforementioned gas flow cutoff limit, carbon dioxide rebreathing occurs inside the helmet [29].

As far as the unplanned disconnection takes place, from the helmet inlet, after 240 s the $CO_2$ level detected is ranging from 50 to 60 mmHg, depending on the size of CPAP helmet in use. Due to these safety issues, several of CPAP helmets available on markets are equipped with anti-suffocation or safety valves. These safety valves remain closed due to the pressure generated inside the helmet by the PEEP. When any accidental disconnection occurs, the loss of pressure opens the valve, allowing the patient to breath ambient air. The PEEP cutoff limit for opening these valves is 3 $cmH_2O$. These safety valves cannot prevent the hazardous of unplanned disconnections, but they contribute to reduce risks as demonstrated 240 s after disconnection: carbon dioxide value is around 20 mmHg [33].

The use of an ICU pulmonary ventilator to deliver CPAP through helmets is not recommended. Limitations are, even in case of high performance pneumatic pressure ventilators, related to the inability to deliver continuous flows over 30 L/min, fatally leading to $CO_2$ rebreathing [33].

### 3.6.1.2   Basic Monitoring on CPAP: Patient and Circuit

The basic monitoring of patient on a CPAP helmet should consider as follows [31]:

• Oxygen saturation $SpO_2$
• Heart rate
• Blood pressure

Checking the gastric residual volume represents a key point as well during CPAP. Airway pressurization can lead to gastric distention due to bloating of stomach. Even if potential inhalation hazard is far from happening due to free space available in the helmet, a nasogastric tube placement should be considered, especially when CPAP therapy discontinuation is not allowed. Nasogastric tube placement is mandatory only if the CPAP therapy via helmet is continued without time breaks allowed. Otherwise, if discontinuity of therapy (also to orally feed the patient) is permitted, nasogastric tube positioning should be avoided.

In healthy subjects, the esophageal valve occlusion is able to oppose against external pressure until 25–30 cmH$_2$O [33], avoiding abdominal bloating and gastric distention, but those pressure levels are not within the CPAP range of pressure delivering. Instead, nasogastric tube represents the real determinant factor for the lower esophageal sphincter failure.

### 3.6.1.3  Noise Reduction

The gas airflow moving through the restricted area of flexible CPAP tubing hose generates turbulence and, subsequently, noise levels. This phenomenon is more evident for Venturi-based devices. For those reasons the use of precautions is essential to reduce noise levels inside CPAP helmets, especially for long-term therapy [32, 34].

Several options are available:

- Hose tubing with inner smooth surface. The choice of smooth interior wall hoses rather than corrugated type allows to avoid flow turbulence and the consequent reduction of the gas flow noise.
- HME filter: its usual purpose as a gas humidifier is intentionally avoided (absence of reverse flow direction). Basically, the inner membrane works like an engine exhaust muffler, resulting in a real noise reduction.
- Earplugs: blocking the noise wave transmission. It's necessary to educate the patient about experiencing a sort of ear

pressurization feeling, similar to scuba diving, because it is not unusual and is related to the pressure generated inside the helmet.

### 3.6.1.4  Helmet Anchorage

From a physical point of view, the pressure inside the helmet results in a vertical thrust of itself. To manage this issue, several solutions are available [31]:

- Armpit strap
- Band fastened on bedsides
- Counterbalance system

Armpit straps represent the basics of all possible options. Extremities of both straps are secured onto the rigid part of the helmet, while the midportion passes under the patient's armpit. Indications for this kind of system are 2 h at least CPAP delivering and PEEP levels less than 10 $cmH_2O$ in order to avoid pressure ulcers, venous stasis, and clotting phenomena in the axillary region. PEEP levels between 5 and 10 $cmH_2O$ generate a traction force more than 2 kg against each armpit's tissue, leading into an axillary discomfort experience.

Bed rails and bedsides can be used as anchorage structure for band fixing lines (usually with a cross-shaped layout). Despite its reliability, this choice results in a major limitation for patient's freedom of movement. This leads to distress/frustration and then less collaborative behavior.

The counterweight system requires the armpit straps abovementioned but in a modified way of use. In this setting, the midportion of the strap passes over patient's shoulders. For each strap, a 2 kg weight is attached as a counterbalance (e.g., skeletal traction counterweight). This kind of anchorage does not constrain the patient's freedom of movements (Fig. 3.12).

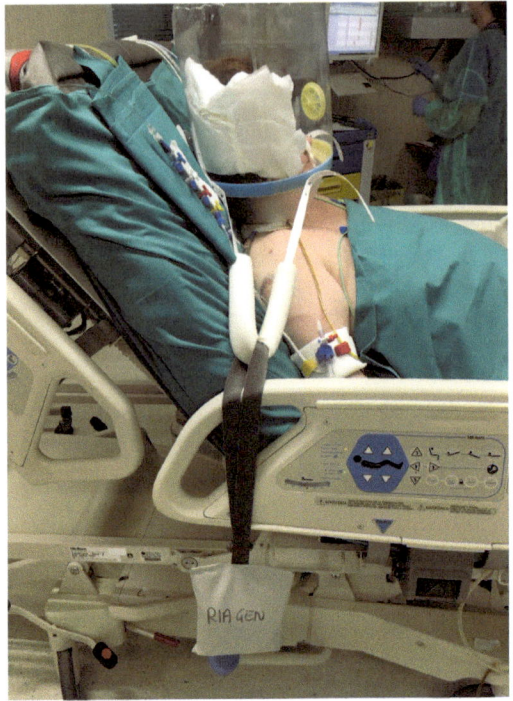

**Fig. 3.12** Patient with helmet CPAP and counterweight system

### 3.6.1.5 Airway Humidification

Invasive ventilation (tube or tracheostomy) completely bypasses the natural process of air filtering and humidification; in the noninvasive one, those physiological processes are fully active.

However, gases for medical purpose are not equivalent to natural fresh air: temperature and moisture of natural air are basically influenced by environment's climate, while the medical gases usually have a temperature range of 10–20 °C and a humidity level lower than 3% [35].

According to the International Consensus Conferences in Intensive Care Medicine's statement about noninvasive positive-pressure ventilation in acute respiratory failure [36], the minimal water content in 1 L of air, to prevent alterations of physiological humidification's process, is 10 mg.

Early detection of patients at risk during NIV via helmet is necessary. Lately, it has been showed that helmet CPAP performed by high flow rate of gas delivery (>40 L/min) needs the use of an active humidifier, especially for a long-term CPAP therapy.

Technical issues are related to the employment of active humidifiers with high flow delivery: the conventional setup for invasive ventilation doesn't fit for this option.

An optimal active humidification setup for a ventilated patient via ET tube requires a temperature of heater equal to 35 °C plus a relative humidity of 100% and 37 °C for gases on inspiratory inlet. Those parameters will result in a temperature of 37° and a relative humidity of 80%.

The air temperature inside the helmet space fueled by raw medical gas with no moisture and no temperature treatment is around 29–30 °C [37]. Gas delivery at 37 °C will lead to condensation on the inner side of helmet, increasing patient's discomfort. Due to this technical reason, the clinical goal about humidification setting for CPAP helmet is to keep a gas relative humidity of 100%, according to a comfortable temperature of helmet environment before mentioned (29–30 °C) [32].

Humidifier outlet chamber temperature setting could be titrated (if NIV option is available) to 28 °C with 100% of relative humidity, while the distal inlet at the helmet is settled on 30 °C. Those settings provide a proportional amount of water fitted for the helmet inner temperature, due to a rising of temperature inside the hosing line and reducing the moisture buildup before the helmet inlet.

If HME filter as noise reduction system is in place, it will be connected between the medical gas source and the heater chamber inlet. Otherwise the filter itself would be a real block to moisture due to its technical nature.

## 3.6.2   Monitoring During Mask-PSV

NIV can be delivered via different interfaces. The most common and widespread type remains the full-face mask, a first-line choice for patients who require urgent rescue respiratory support, no matter the primary cause (acute or chronic respiratory failure) [38, 39]. Graphic monitoring and delivery of this kind of ventilatory support differ from the nasal NIV mask, usually a typical interface for at-home chronic therapy support (e.g., sleep apnea) [40].

The NIV failure rate is equal to 25%, especially in COPD exacerbation: however, the abovementioned rate can be deeply affected by timing of commence and quick response to treatment.

The facial mask represents the most used device in the literature about studies on NIV, due to its minimal dead space volume when compared with the inner volume of a CPAP helmet interface.

Despite being the most available interface, the NIV-PSV main issues are related to air leakage due to incomplete seal. Nowadays this problem is not completely solved, even if the technological achievements are improving the interface device, especially pneumatic sealing and comfort, thanks to a fully adjustable facial mask [41–43]. Air leakage itself deeply affects the expiratory trigger and could lead into a complete loss of synchrony between patient and ventilator. It's useful to remind how triggering influences PSV (Fig. 3.13):

- Inspiratory: provides synchronization between patient and machine
- Expiratory: provides the switch of inspiratory/expiratory cycling

A continuous and real-time monitoring of patient-machine synchrony is required to set a reliable inspiratory trigger and a performant expiratory trigger. The software standard configura-

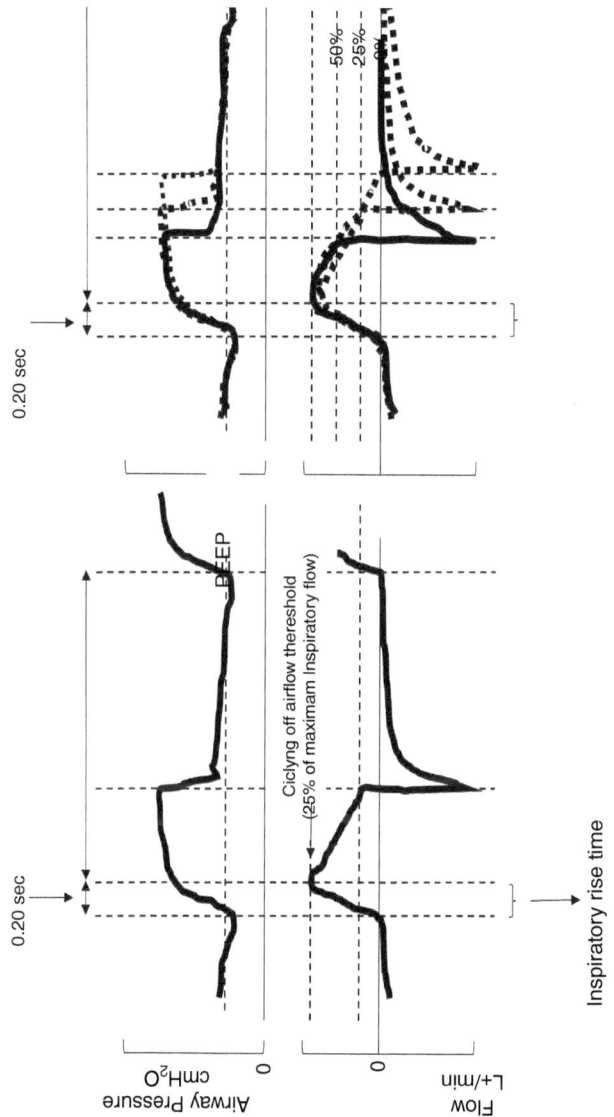

**Fig. 3.13** Expiratory trigger settings

tion is common for both invasive ventilation and NIV, and it demands an expiratory cycling at 25–30% of inspiratory peak flow. So, put into practice, for a peak flow of 50 L/min, the cycling for expiration will run at 12.5 L/min of scalar flow. But on NIV support, the possible large amount of air leakage (compared to invasive) mimics a fistula that doesn't allow to reach that threshold. This condition keeps the inspiratory cycling constantly switched on. This mismatch leads to a full asynchrony where the natural expiratory reflex of the patient is totally denied by a closed expiratory valve and a never-ending inspiratory flow ("inspiratory hang-up" phenomenon). Without interventions, a paradox situation will occur: the patient's efforts to exhale against the flow will result into an increased WOB, neutralizing all the benefits and purpose of PS ventilation.

All the before mentioned asynchronies, previously analyzed in Sect. 3.5, are equivalent also for NIV support, mainly as result of not perfect air leakage management (Fig. 3.14).

Table 3.4 shows most common NIV asynchronies and how to reduce or eliminate air leakage.

Table 3.5 shows the interventions to prevent the interface-related complications during NIV [42–44].

The setting of the ventilator during NIV for COPD patients is often intricate, since the altered respiratory mechanics, together with the presence of air leaks, can deeply interfere with the synchrony between the patient and the machine. During NIV, patient-ventilator mismatching can determine a bad tolerance to NIV and, consequently, its failure.

The close observation of the ventilator graphics (i.e., flow and pressure waveforms) can be used to detect a gross patient-ventilator mismatching. It has been suggested, but never directly assessed, that the systematic use of ventilator signals on the screen may be useful in depicting asynchronies and at the same time in driving the operator in setting modifications [45].

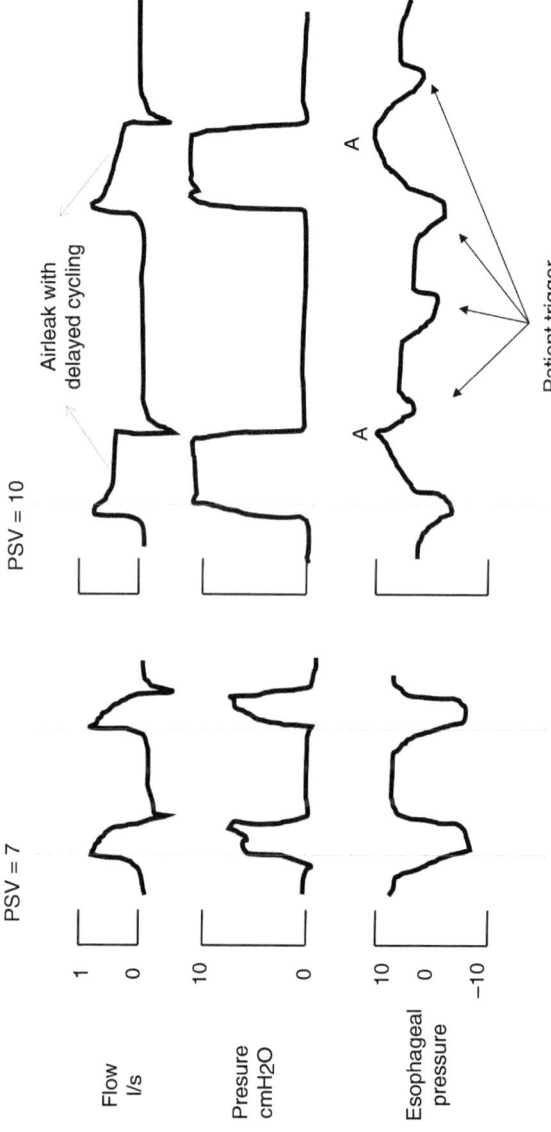

**Fig. 3.14** Hang-up problems during noninvasive PSV ventilation

**Table 3.4** Patient-ventilator asynchronies during NIV with PSV and mask

| Asynchrony/problem | Signs | Actions |
|---|---|---|
| Autotriggering | Detection of autotriggering | Reduction of air leaks and/or reduction of inspiratory trigger sensitivity:<br>1. Reduce inspiratory trigger sensitivity<br>2. Switch to pressure trigger<br>3. Improve mask sealing |
| Ineffective efforts | Individuation of ineffective efforts | Titration of pressure support, inspiratory and expiratory triggers, and PEEP ext :<br>1. Reducing PSV<br>2. Check setting of expiratory trigger<br>3. Assess PEEP settled vs. PEEPi |
| Late cycling-off | Pressure increase at the end of inspiratory cycle or flow and pressure prolonged plateau | Reduction of air leaks and/or titration of expiratory trigger or setting of maximal inspiratory time:<br>1. Rising of expiratory trigger cycling (>25%)<br>2. Treat air leakage (NG tube in place)<br>3. Tighten mask sealing |
| Early cycling-off | Convex pattern of expiratory flow waveform and concavity of pressure waveform | Titration of expiratory trigger:<br>Lower the threshold expiratory trigger (<25%) |

**Table 3.4** (continued)

| Asynchrony/problem | Signs | Actions |
|---|---|---|
| Not balanced PEEPi | Expiratory flow that does not reach zero prior to inspiration or ineffective efforts | Titration of PEEPext: As a general rule, changes in PS were carried out by steps of 2 cmH$_2$O and changes in inspiratory and expiratory triggers by steps of 5–10% |

**Table 3.5** Interface-related complications in mask-PSV NIV

| Target | Action | Monitoring |
|---|---|---|
| Preventing pressure ulcers | • Ultrathin hydrocolloid layer as protective film between skin and interface<br>• Turnover of different mask interface layout<br>• Fill the inflatable cushion with water instead of air | • Skin inspection<br>• Evaluation of nasal bridge and orbital region |
| Improving skin tissue-mask layout sealing | • Wide set of size availability<br>• Wide spectrum of mask shape layout<br>• Denture should be worn | • Detect air leakage<br>• Tvi/Tve comparison<br>• Flow reading<br>• Volume reading |
| Improve patient's comfort | • Progressive PS buildup: CPAP only first<br>• Assessment of synchronization<br>• Increment PSV step by step of 2 cmH$_2$O | • Patient's feedback<br>• Pain assessment |
| Improve patient-machine synchrony | • Gradual commence of PSV<br>• Expiratory cycling titration<br>• Inspiratory cycling titration<br>• Improved mask sealing<br>• Check delivery time of PSV (Fig. 3.15) | • Look for asynchronies<br>• Check Tvi/Tve ratio<br>• Pes availability may be helpful |

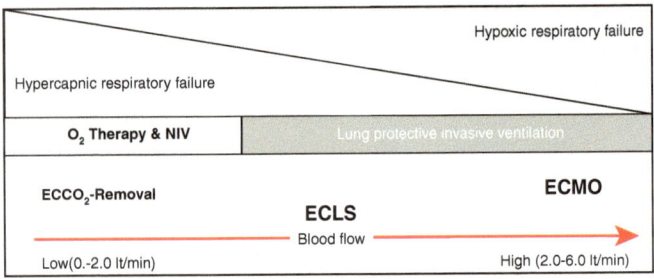

**Fig. 3.15** Indications for extracorporeal life support in respiratory failure

## 3.7 Monitoring During Extracorporeal Membrane Oxygenation (ECMO) Support

### 3.7.1 The Need for ECMO Support

ARDS and ALI are both distinguished by rapid onset and mismatch in gas exchange, as result of a widespread injury to vascular-alveolar membrane. Even if recent data showed a reduction of its incidence, mortality rate seems to be constant, with a value of 40% [46].

MV is a mandatory therapy supporting and providing adequate alveolar ventilation throughout the entire respiratory distress process. A lot of studies have shown the potential side effects of MV (e.g., VILI) requiring different strategies like the protective ventilation: low airway pressure and low TV are associated with a better surviving rate [3]. Nevertheless, some patients with a badly rapid onset developing widespread lung injury not manageable with MV only are far from getting adequate $CO_2$ removal and oxygenation to survive [3]. To improve their survival, several rescue life-saving therapies are performed as ventilatory recruiting maneuver, prone positioning, nitric oxide inhalation, high-frequency oscillation ventilation, and extracorporeal oxygenation techniques.

Putting all the abovementioned therapies in place basically requires access to high-level technology and adequate knowledge and know-how, plus a background experience promoted by strong skills and organizations, usually available in selected referral ECMO centers. The most effective and challenging supportive technique is the extracorporeal membrane oxygenation (ECMO) [47].

ECMO support allows to achieve the best protective ventilation available (TV and respiratory rate can be extremely decreased), due to its capability to balance $O_2$ and $CO_2$ blood levels. A recent trial (CESAR, UK) has shown a greater survival rating for those patients admitted to a referral ECMO center [48]. Early commence and timing are crucial for the effective implementation of other rescue therapies and may positively affect patients' outcome [49].

Nowadays, in addition to respiratory failure treatment, the ECMO support appears to be useful in obstructive and restrictive pathologies and, as advanced treatment, in case of cardiac arrest or cardiogenic shock [50]. Basic principle of ECMO circuit is founded on a forced drainage of blood flow via a centrifugal pump, pushed throughout an artificial gas exchanger (membrane lung), and then returned oxygenated to patient's bloodstream.

The veno-venous approach indicated for respiratory failure management usually drains blood from a great vessel from venous side and returns it in proximity of the right atrium. Because only the venous side is affected by extracorporeal circulation, there's no significant impact to hemodynamics.

VV cannula configuration, according to the type of drainage cannula (multistage or cannula with conventional design) and to VV configuration (femoro-femoral or femoro-jugular), is shown in Fig. 3.16. The returning cannulas normally have holes only in a short portion near to their tip. There are no issues in choosing multistage cannulas both for drainage and reinfusion if a femoro-jugular approach is applied. If a femoro-femoral approach is chosen, a different kind of venous cannula must be used, because the side holes will generate a consistent recirculation of oxygenated blood from the returning cannula to the drainage one [51].

Recirculation in the femoro-femoral approach can be minimized maintaining the drainage cannula below the diaphragm and above the renal veins and the returning cannula in the atrium (or just below it).

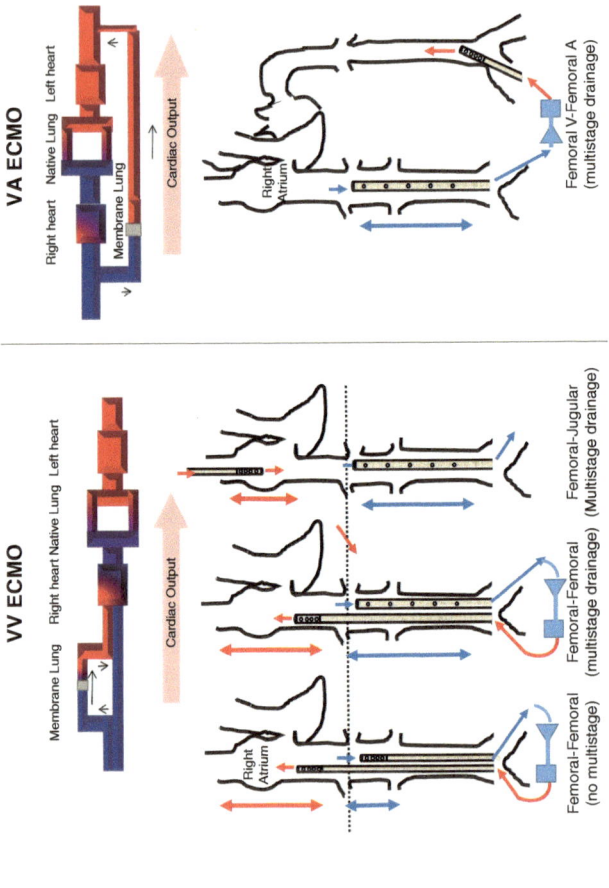

**Fig. 3.16** Different ECMO approaches: VV versus VA

**Table 3.6** VV ECMO versus VA ECMO: Advantages and disadvantages

| | VA ECMO | VV ECMO High flow (>3 L/min) | VV ECMO Low flow (1–2 L/min) |
|---|---|---|---|
| Pump | + | + | + |
| Circulatory support | + | − | − |
| $O_2$ delivery | + | + | − |
| $CO_2$ removal | + | + | + |
| Right ventricular loading | − | No effect | No effect |
| Left ventricular loading | + | No effect | No effect |
| Arterial thrombosis risk | + | − | − |

In the venoarterial approach (VA ECMO), the drainage areas remain the same as for the VV one, while the returning cannula site is femoral artery. This configuration can lead to a lacking perfusion that can determine ischemia of the limb. To avoid this problem, a distal perfusion cannula as a comprehensive part of the circuit can be inserted to revert the ischemic phenomena [52].

Table 3.6 summarizes the main difference between VV ECMO and VA ECMO approaches.

## 3.7.2 Circuit Monitoring During ECMO

The latest ECMO circuit is equipped with low resistance and high-efficiency gas exchange membrane lung. From a theoretical point of view, the ECMO circuit (no matter what approach) should be a very linear system, reducing any connection use at minimum (Fig. 3.17).

In the act of monitoring ECMO, three issues appear to be essential:

• ECMO flow or blood flow (BF): oxygenation directly derives from BF rate. Good practice suggests to keep it at the minimal value able to provide adequate patient's oxygenation.

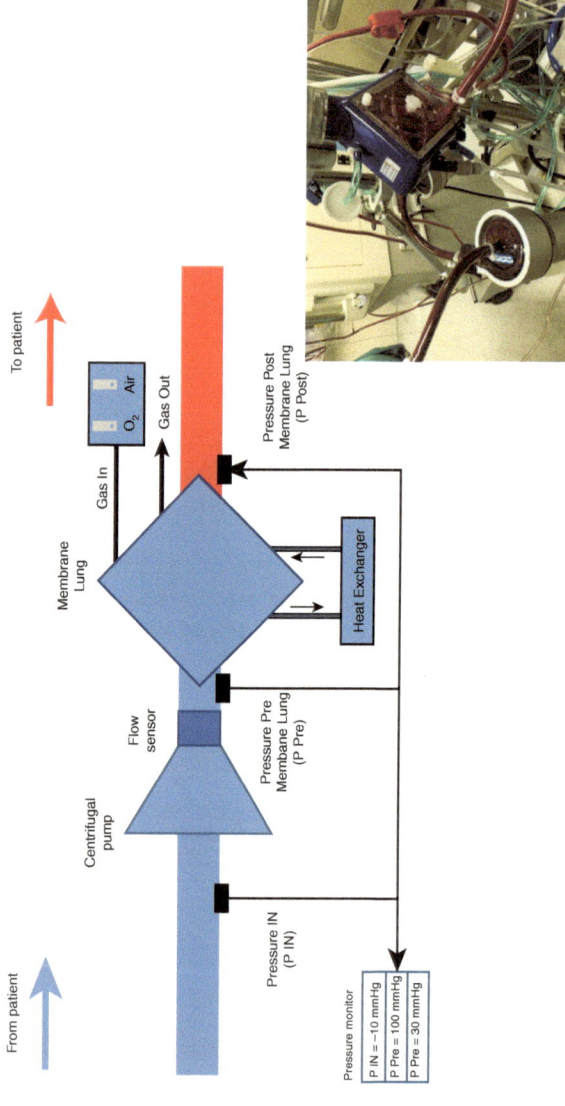

**Fig. 3.17** Standard ECMO circuit scheme with pressure monitoring sites and sampling point for blood checks

- Gas flow (GF): $CO_2$ removal depends on sweep gas flow rate and on ventilatory setting.
- Fraction of inspired oxygen ($FiO_2$) of GF: initial $FiO_2$ setting is equal to 1 of, then gradually reduced according to patient's oxygenation improvements.

Daily assessment of ECMO circuit by a perfusionist plus a continuous monitoring by the ICU bed nurse is strongly recommended [53–55]. Before any nursing care routine, a visual inspection is suggested and all the actions described in Table 3.7 at column "Monitoring" as well as Table 3.8.

**Table 3.7** Key point for monitoring ECMO performance

| Key point | Gold standard | Monitoring |
|---|---|---|
| How is the membrane lung performing? | $FiO_2$ equal to 1 should provide a range value of $PaO_2$ postoxygenator greater than 300/400 mmHg | At least once daily sampling as monitoring comparison pre- and postoxygenator arterial blood gas analysis should be performed |
| What BF is achieved? | Monitoring venous inlet pressure (P in): it should not exceed negative values of 100 mmHg. Any withdrawal impairment should be managed via a boost in the RPM causing augmentation of negative pressure | Pump's pressure in and RPM related. Extreme negative pressure leads into a BF reduction: a typical swinging movement of the drainage cannula occurs. Check fluid balance status and patient's position |
| Any clot presence in the circuit? | An ECMO circuit should be clot-free on a visual assessment. A comparison between pre- and postoxygenator pressure should not record any sudden spike in gap values. Keep those reference ranges ACT = 180–220 s PTT INR 1.5 e 2 AT III > 70% | Visual inspection of circuit with a source of light every shift. All the circuit pressures monitored (P in, P Pre, e P Post). Sampling for ACT, aPTT, and platelets every 8 h at least. Daily check of ATIII |

P In: pressure before centrifugal pump
P in Membrane Lung: pressure before centrifugal pump
P out: pressure after membrane lung

**Table 3.8** Signs for suspicion about the presence of clots in the ECMO circuit

| Issue | Signs | Action to take |
|-------|-------|----------------|
| Clots inside the pump | Changes of pump's noise<br>Recognizable clots visually<br>Augmentation of plasmatic Hb value | Change of centrifugal pump's housing or the whole ECMO circuit<br>Heparin dosage augmentation |
| Clots inside the membrane lung | Spikes of pressure values inside membrane oxygenator<br>Postoxygenator $PaO_2$ reduction and $PaCO_2$ increment<br>Visual detection of clots in the oxygenator | Change of membrane lung or the whole ECMO circuit<br>Heparin dosage augmentation |

Take-Home Messages

- Respiratory assessment of critically ill patients should be performed through clinical and instrumental tools, with a multimodal approach. $SpO_2$ and $EtCO_2$ are both standard in the basic respiratory assessment.
- Potential MV complications and methods to reduce ventilator-induced lung injury should be considered in all patients undergoing invasive MV support.
- Asynchronies are prevalent in ICU patients and negatively related to outcome, ranging from prolonged MV, prolonged ICU and hospital stays, and increased mortality.
- Detection of asynchronies mostly relies on a mismatch between surrogates of the patient inspiratory effort and the ventilator cycling.
- Nursing surveillance is required to provide a safe and effective level of care for the patient receiving mechanical ventilation.
- Patients undergoing ECMO should be monitored to prevent artificial lung-related complications.

# References

1. Nieman GF, Satalin J, Andrews P, Habashi NM, Gatto LA. Lung stress, strain, and energy load: engineering concepts to understand the mechanism of ventilator-induced lung injury (VILI). Intensive Care Med Exp. 2016;4:16. https://doi.org/10.1186/s40635-016-0090-5. Epub 2016 Jun 18

2. ARDS Definition Task Force, Ranieri VM, Rubenfeld GD, Thompson BT, Ferguson ND, Caldwell E, Fan E, et al. Acute respiratory distress syndrome: the Berlin definition. JAMA. 2012;307:2526–33. https://doi.org/10.1001/jama.2012.5669.

3. Bein T, Grasso S, Moerer O, Quintel M, Guerin C, Deja M, et al. The standard of care of patients with ARDS: ventilatory settings and rescue therapies for refractory hypoxemia. Intensive Care Med. 2016;42:699–711. https://doi.org/10.1007/s00134-016-4325-4.

4. Jubran A. Pulse oximetry. Crit Care. 2015;19:27. https://doi.org/10.1186/s13054-015-0984-8.

5. Nitzan M, Romem A, Koppel R. Pulse oximetry: fundamentals and technology update. Med Devices (Auckl). 2014;7:231–9. https://doi.org/10.2147/MDER.S47319.

6. Walsh BK, Crotwell DN, Restrepo RD. Capnography/capnometry during mechanical ventilation: 2011. Respir Care. 2011;56:503–9. https://doi.org/10.4187/respcare.01175.

7. Thompson JE, Jaffe MB. Capnographic waveforms in the mechanically ventilated patient. Respir Care. 2005;50:100–8.

8. Kodali BS, Urman RD. Capnography during cardiopulmonary resuscitation: current evidence and future directions. J Emerg Trauma Shock. 2014;7:332–40.

9. Jordan J, Rose L, Dainty KN, Noyes J, Blackwood B. Factors that impact on the use of mechanical ventilation weaning protocols in critically ill adults and children: a qualitative evidence-synthesis. Cochrane Database Syst Rev. 2016;10:CD011812. https://doi.org/10.1002/14651858.CD011812.pub2.

10. Brochard L, Martin GS, Blanch L, Pelosi P, Belda FJ, Jubran A, et al. Clinical review: respiratory monitoring in the ICU—a consensus of 16. Crit Care. 2012;16:219. https://doi.org/10.1186/cc11146.

11. Mehta S, Cook DJ, Skrobik Y, Muscedere J, Martin CM, Stewart TE, et al. A ventilator strategy combining low tidal volume ventilation, recruitment maneuvers, and high positive end-expiratory pressure does not increase sedative, opioid, or neuromuscular blocker use in adults with acute respiratory distress syndrome and may improve patient comfort. Ann Intensive Care. 2014;4:33–7. https://doi.org/10.1186/s13613-014-0033-9.

12. Sole ML, Bennett M, Ashworth S. Clinical indicators for endotracheal suctioning in adult patients receiving mechanical ventilation. Am J Crit Care. 2015;24:318–24. https://doi.org/10.4037/ajcc2015794.

13. AARC Clinical Practice Guidelines. Endotracheal suctioning of mechanically ventilated patients with artificial airways 2010. American Association for Respiratory Care. Respir Care. 2010;55:758–6.

14. Hough CL, Kallet RH, Ranieri VM, Rubenfeld GD, Luce JM, Hudson LD. Intrinsic positive end-expiratory pressure in Acute Respiratory Distress Syndrome (ARDS) Network subjects. Crit Care Med. 2005;33(3):527.

15. Vitacca M, Lanini B, Nava S, Barbano L, Portal R, Clini E, et al. Inspiratory muscle workload due to dynamic intrinsic PEEP in stable COPD patients: effects of two different settings of non-invasive pressure-support ventilation. Monaldi Arch Chest Dis. 2004;6:81–5. https://doi.org/10.4081/monaldi.2004.704.

16. Mauri T, Yoshida T, Bellani G, Goligher EC, Carteaux G, Rittayamai N, et al. Esophageal and transpulmonary pressure in the clinical setting: meaning, usefulness and perspectives. Intensive Care Med. 2016;42:1360–73. https://doi.org/10.1007/s00134-016-4400-x.

17. Moerer O, Barwing J, Quintel M. Neurally adjusted ventilatory assist (NAVA). A new mode of assisted mechanical ventilation. Anaesthesist. 2008;57:998–1005. https://doi.org/10.1007/s00101-008-1412-0.

18. Navalesi P, Colombo D, Della Corte F. NAVA ventilation. Minerva Anestesiol. 2010;76:346–52.

19. Piquilloud L, Vignaux L, Bialais E, Roeseler J, Sottiaux T, Laterre PF, et al. Neurally adjusted ventilatory assist improves patient-ventilator interaction. Intensive Care Med. 2011;37:263–71. https://doi.org/10.1007/s00134-010-2052-9.

20. Petrof BJ, Hussain SN. Ventilator-induced diaphragmatic dysfunction: what have we learned? Curr Opin Crit Care. 2016;22:67–72. https://doi.org/10.1097/MCC.0000000000000272.

21. Rose L, Schultz MJ, Cardwell CR, Jouvet P, McAuley DF, Blackwood B. Automated versus non-automated weaning for reducing the duration of mechanical ventilation for critically ill adults and children: a Cochrane systematic review and meta-analysis. Crit Care. 2015;19:4. https://doi.org/10.1186/s13054-015-0755-6.

22. Vagheggini G, Mazzoleni S, Vlad Panait E, Navalesi P, Ambrosino N. Physiologic response to various levels of pressure support and NAVA in prolonged weaning. Respir Med. 2013;107:1748–54. https://doi.org/10.1016/j.rmed.2013.08.013.

23. Bellani G, Patroniti N, Weismann D, Galbiati L, Curto F, et al. Measurement of pressure-time product during spontaneous assisted breathing by rapid interrupter technique. Anesthesiology. 2007;106:484–90.

24. Blanch L, Villagra A, Sales B, Montanya J, Lucangelo U, Luján M, et al. Asynchronies during mechanical ventilation are associated with mortality. Intensive Care Med. 2015;41:633–41. https://doi.org/10.1007/s00134-015-3692-6.
25. Delisle S, Ouellet P, Bellemare P, Tétrault JP, Arsenault P. Sleep quality in mechanically ventilated patients: comparison between NAVA and PSV modes. Ann Intensive Care. 2011;1:42–6.
26. Murias G, Lucangelo U, Blanch L. Patient-ventilator asynchrony. Curr Opin Crit Care. 2016;22:53–9. https://doi.org/10.1097/MCC.0000000000000270.
27. Cavaliere F, Conti G, Costa R, Spinazzola G, Proietti R, Sciuto A, et al. Exposure to noise during continuous positive airway pressure: influence of interfaces and delivery systems. Acta Anaesthesiol Scand. 2008;52:52–6. https://doi.org/10.1111/j.1399-6576.2007.01474.x.
28. Patel BK, Wolfe KS, Pohlman AS, Hall JB, Kress JP. Effect of noninvasive ventilation delivered by helmet vs face mask on the rate of endotracheal intubation in patients with acute respiratory distress syndrome: a randomized clinical trial. JAMA. 2016;315:2435–4. https://doi.org/10.1001/jama.2016.6338.
29. Bellani G, Patroniti N, Greco M, Foti G, Pesenti A. The use of helmets to deliver non-invasive continuous positive airway pressure in hypoxemic acute respiratory failure. Minerva Anestesiol. 2008;74:651–6.
30. Patroniti N, Foti G, Manfio A, Coppo A, Bellani G, Pesenti A. Head helmet versus face mask for non-invasive continuous positive airway pressure: a physiological study. Intensive Care Med. 2003;29:1680–7. https://doi.org/10.1007/s00134-003-1931-8.
31. Ferrario D, Lucchini A. Helmet delivered CPAP for in-patients. Minerva Anestesiol. 2002;68:481–4.
32. Lucchini A, Valsecchi D, Elli S, Doni V, Corsaro P, Tundo P, et al. The comfort of patients ventilated with the helmet bundle. Assist Inferm Ric. 2010;29(4):174–83.
33. Milan M, Zanella A, Isgrò S, Deab SA, Magni F, Pesenti A, et al. Performance of different continuous positive airway pressure helmets equipped with safety valves during failure of fresh gas supply. Intensive Care Med. 2011;37:1031–5. https://doi.org/10.1007/s00134-011-2207-3.
34. Trevisanuto D, Camiletti L, Udilano A, Doglioni N, Zanardo V. Noise levels during neonatal helmet CPAP. Arch Dis Child Fetal Neonatal Ed. 2008;93:F396–7. https://doi.org/10.1136/adc.2008.140715.
35. American Association for Respiratory Care, Restrepo RD, Walsh BK. Humidification during invasive and noninvasive mechanical ventilation: 2012. Respir Care. 2012;57:782–8. https://doi.org/10.4187/respcare.01766.

36. American National Standards Institute; American Society of Anesthesiologists. Standard for humidifiers and nebulizers for medical use. ANSI. 1979;Z79:9.
37. Chiumello D, Chierichetti M, Tallarini F, Cozzi P, Cressoni M, Polli F, et al. Effect of a heated humidifier during continuous positive airway pressure delivered by a helmet. Crit Care. 2008;12:R55. https://doi.org/10.1186/cc6875.
38. Nava S, Ceriana P. Patient-ventilator interaction during noninvasive positive pressure ventilation. Respir Care Clin N Am. 2005;11:281–9. https://doi.org/10.1016/j.rcc.2005.02.003.
39. Moerer O, Beck J, Brander L, Costa R, Quintel M, Slutsky AS, et al. Subject-ventilator synchrony during neural versus pneumatically triggered non-invasive helmet ventilation. Intensive Care Med. 2008;34:1615–23. https://doi.org/10.1007/s00134-008-1163-z.
40. Lemyze M, Mallat J, Nigeon O, Barrailler S, Pepy F, Gasan G, et al. Rescue therapy by switching to total face mask after failure of face mask-delivered noninvasive ventilation in do-not-intubate patients in acute respiratory failure. Crit Care Med. 2013;41:481–8. https://doi.org/10.1097/CCM.0b013e31826ab4af.
41. Bambi S. Noninvasive positive pressure ventilation: an ABC approach for advanced nursing in emergency departments and acute care settings. Dimens Crit Care Nurs. 2009;28:253–63. https://doi.org/10.1097/DCC.0b013e3181b3ffdc.
42. Bambi S, Peris A, Esquinas AM. Pressure ulcers caused by masks during noninvasive ventilation. Am J Crit Care. 2016;25:6. https://doi.org/10.4037/ajcc2016906.
43. Nava S, Navalesi P, Gregoretti C. Interfaces and humidification for noninvasive mechanical ventilation. Respir Care. 2009;54:71–84.
44. Pisani L, Carlucci A, Nava S. Interfaces for noninvasive mechanical ventilation: technical aspects and efficiency. Minerva Anestesiol. 2012;78:1154–61.
45. Di Marco F, Centanni S, Bellone A, Messinesi G, Pesci A, Scala R, et al. Optimization of ventilator setting by flow and pressure waveforms analysis during noninvasive ventilation for acute exacerbations of COPD: a multicentric randomized controlled trial. Crit Care. 2011;15:R283. https://doi.org/10.1186/cc10567.
46. Bellani G, Laffey JG, Pham T, Fan E, Brochard L, Esteban A, et al. Epidemiology, patterns of care, and mortality for patients with acute respiratory distress syndrome in intensive care units in 50 countries. JAMA. 2016;315:788–800. https://doi.org/10.1001/jama.2016.0291.

47. Luciani GB, Hoxha S, Torre S, Rungatscher A, Menon T, Barozzi L, et al. Improved outcome of cardiac extracorporeal membrane oxygenation in infants and children using magnetic levitation centrifugal pumps. Artif Organs. 2016;40:27–33. https://doi.org/10.1111/aor.12647.

48. Peek GJ, Mugford M, Tiruvoipati R, Wilson A, Allen E, Thalanany MM, et al. Efficacy and economic assessment of conventional ventilatory support versus extracorporeal membrane oxygenation for severe adult respiratory failure (CESAR): a multicentre randomised controlled trial. Lancet. 2009;374:1351–63. https://doi.org/10.1016/S0140-6736(09)61069-2.

49. Patroniti N, Zangrillo A, Pappalardo F, Peris A, Cianchi G, Braschi A, et al. The Italian ECMO network experience during the 2009 influenza A(H1N1) pandemic: preparation for severe respiratory emergency outbreaks. Intensive Care Med. 2011;37:1447–5. https://doi.org/10.1007/s00134-011-2301-6.

50. Gattinoni L, Carlesso E, Langer T. Clinical review: extracorporeal membrane oxygenation. Crit Care. 2011;15:243. https://doi.org/10.1186/cc10490.

51. Pesenti A, Zanella A, Patroniti N. Extracorporeal gas exchange. Curr Opin Crit Care. 2009;15:52–8. https://doi.org/10.1097/MCC.0b013e3283220e1f.

52. Avalli L, Sangalli F, Migliari M, Maggioni E, Gallieri S, Segramora V, et al. Early vascular complications after percutaneous cannulation for extracorporeal membrane oxygenation for cardiac assist. Minerva Anestesiol. 2016;82:36–4.

53. Chauhan S, Subin S. Extracorporeal membrane oxygenation—an anaesthesiologist's perspective—part II: clinical and technical consideration. Ann Card Anaesth. 2012;15:69–82. https://doi.org/10.4103/0971-9784.91485.

54. Posluszny J, Rycus PT, Bartlett RH, Engoren M, Haft JW, Lynch WR, et al. Outcome of adult respiratory failure patients receiving prolonged ($\geq$14 days) ECMO. Ann Surg. 2016;263:573–8. https://doi.org/10.1097/SLA.0000000000001176.

55. Lubnow M, Philipp A, Foltan M, Bull Enger T, Lunz D, Bein T, et al. Technical complications during veno-venous extracorporeal membrane oxygenation and their relevance predicting a system-exchange—retrospective analysis of 265 cases. PLoS One. 2014;9:e112316. https://doi.org/10.1371/journal.pone.0112316.

# Chapter 4
# Cardiovascular Assessment

Irene Comisso and Alberto Lucchini

## 4.1 Introduction

In healthy people, cardiovascular system allows blood to reach the organ and tissues, providing oxygen and nutrients, and blood flow from peripheral tissues removes toxins and carbon dioxide ($CO_2$).

In intensive care unit (ICU) patients, cardiovascular function often results strongly compromised, thus determining the need for advanced monitoring and support. Instrumental monitoring is one of the most important components of cardiovascular function assessment, together with scores (such as the APACHE II or SOFA) and clinical observation. Since clinical scores and direct observation are not reliable enough to assess adequately the changes of patients' status during time, instrumental monitoring systems have found a rapid development in clinical practice whose main application, in the beginning, has been in anesthesia practices, where basic monitoring has been assumed as standard by several societies [1]. During the last three decades, more and more sophisticated devices to assess cardiovascular parameters have been tuned fine, allowing clinicians to

© Springer International Publishing AG, part of Springer Nature 2018     107
I. Comisso et al., *Nursing in Critical Care Setting*,
https://doi.org/10.1007/978-3-319-50559-6_4

obtain (even with relatively easy training) complementary information, that all together outline the general situation of the patient. Nonetheless, it has to be considered that cardiovascular monitoring (CM) is often invasive and expensive and requires sufficient expertise in device insertion and data interpretation. Similarly, not all monitoring devices are appropriated in different clinical situations. On these bases, a progressive implementation model [2] for CM monitoring in ICU has been proposed, defining three levels of complexity for CM, that should be adopted on a continuum according to the patient condition.

## 4.2 General Considerations

From a general point of view, you can consider the characteristics of a CM according to its continuity and invasiveness. According to the system used, the same parameter can be evaluated continuously or intermittently (central venous pressure obtained via a pressure transducer or a water manometer). Invasiveness refers to the extent of a barrier violation. Electrocardiogram is a noninvasive monitoring, while blood pressure obtained through a transducer is considered invasive (or minimally invasive), and pulmonary artery catheter represents the maximal invasivity. Precision and accuracy are also important variables to be considered. Precision indicates how a measurement produces the same result each time it is repeated under the same conditions [3]. Accuracy reflects how close is the actual measurement to the real value [3].

Basic monitoring includes those parameters recorded in all critically ill patients, while advanced monitoring comprises those who are introduced in specific critical conditions (Table 4.1). As it can be easily understood, cardiovascular parameters should always be evaluated with the respiratory ones, since there is a strict interaction between the two systems

**Table 4.1** Characteristics of main parameters monitorized in ICU patients

|  | Basic | Advanced |
| --- | --- | --- |
| ECG | 3–5 leads continuous ECG | 12-lead ECG |
| Pump function | Invasive or noninvasive blood pressure | Intermittent or continuous cardiac output |
| Oxygen | $SpO_2$, $ScvO_2$ | $SvO_2$ |
| Volemia/filling pressures | PVC | PAOP (wedge pressure) Stroke volume, intrathoracic blood volume/global end-diastolic volume |

that is enhanced in critically ill patients undergoing to mechanical ventilation (MV).

Assessment of cardiovascular function in ICU patients consists of four evaluation points:

- Electrical activity
- Pump function effectiveness
- Oxygen transportation and consumption
- Volemia

## 4.3 Electrical Activity

Continuous ECG monitoring allows nurses and clinicians to quickly identify arrhythmia and promptly respond to such events.

The development of electrocardiographic (ECG) monitoring began during the first three decades of the twentieth century, with 3-lead ECG recording [4]. Further developments allowed the diagnosis of bundle branch block and cardiac ischemia, and in 1954 the standardization of 12-lead electrode positioning was released [4]. Current standard for cardiac monitoring within coronary care units include heart rate and rhythm, ST-segment analysis, and QT-interval measurement [4].

ECG leads are classified as unipolar, with one registering and one indifferent electrode (aVR, aVF, aVL, and the six precordial leads V1–V6), and bipolar, with a positive and a negative electrode (the original Einthoven leads, I, II, III) [5].

Heart contraction is made possible by polarization and depolarization of muscle fibers. Evaluation of electrical activity through a 3- or 5-lead electrocardiogram (ECG) provides easy and immediate information about stimulus conduction through the heart, although a more accurate evaluation is only possible by 12-lead ECG. Cardiac cycle begins with spontaneous depolarization of sinus node cells, whose depolarization wave diffuses through the whole myocardial muscle, followed by atrial contraction (P wave). Atrial contraction allows ventricular filling. Electrical impulse reaches then the atrioventricular node (P-R interval) and is then diffused to ventricular cells, who undergo a depolarization process (QRS interval), with subsequent ventricular contraction. Finally, atrial and ventricular depolarization occur (the first is masked by the second because of its highest electrical potential) (T wave) (Fig. 4.1) [5].

Normally, ECG analysis is based on six points (Table 4.2):

- Presence/absence of electrical activity. This point may reflect a simple artifact (due, e.g., to electrodes disconnection), or highlight the presence of asistolia, or other condi-

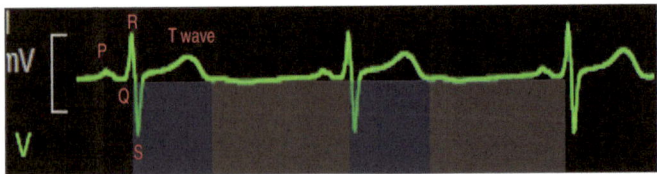

**Fig. 4.1** Normal ECG visualization

**Table 4.2** Steps for ECG interpretation and features

| | Normal ECG findings | Arrhythmic features |
|---|---|---|
| Electrical activity and heart rate | Normal ECG features (see Fig. 4.1) Normal HR ranges between 60 and 100 beats per minute (BPM) | Asystole: no electrical activity is visible, and ECG lead reconnection has been excluded Pulseless electrical activity: when electrical activity is not followed by mechanical contraction Bradycardia describes a HR < 60 BPM Tachycardia describes a HR > 60 BPM |
| R-R interval | Regular interval, its duration depending from HR | In atrial fibrillation (AF), the most frequent arrhythmia, electrical atrial activity is disorganized, and only a few electrical impulses reach the ventricles |
| P wave | P wave present, sinus rhythm | In AF and in ventricular tachycardia, P waves are not identifiable |
| Relationship between P wave and QRS complex | Normally, the interval between P wave and QRS complex is <0.2 s; a P wave is always followed by a QRS complex | The relationship between P wave and QRS complex is inconstant in second third degree atrioventricular block |
| ST-segment elevation | ST segment aligned with the isoelectric line | ST segment alterations may be related to ischemic conditions |
| P-R interval | 0.12–0.2 s | P-R interval is prolonged in first and second grade atrioventricular block and is absent in third grade atrioventricular block |

tions in which electrical activity is absent (such as pulseless electrical activity, i.e., an electrical activity not followed by cardiac muscle contraction). Electrical activity results in heart rate (HR), expressed as number of QRS complexes in a minute

- Cardiac rhythm, highlighted by the R-R interval
- Presence of P wave, defining the presence or absence of atrial activity
- Relationship between P wave and QRS complex
- QRS width
- ST-segment elevation [6].

Avoidance of artifacts during ECG monitoring includes checking the correct positioning of the leads, since reversal between left and right arms or arms and legs can occur, thus leading to polarity inversion [7]. Artifacts can also be induced by patient's tremors [7].

## 4.4 Pump Function Effectiveness

Heart works as a pump in the circulatory system, being responsible, together with aortic compliance (what is called "Windkessel effect"—see arterial pressure monitoring paragraph) of continuous blood flow through vessels.

### 4.4.1 Cardiac Output

Cardiac output defines the amount of blood flowing through heart's chambers during 1 min and is expressed by the equation:

$$CO = HR \times SV$$

In healthy individuals, cardiac output ranges around 5 L/min. To easiest compare cardiac output in differently sized people, values are indexed over body surface area, thus determining the cardiac index (CI). CO is one of the most important hemodynamic parameters using in ICU patients, since blood flow through arteries is one of the determinants of oxygen delivery toward cells. It is possible to determine CO through Fick's principle or by dye dilution.

Fick's principle states that blood flow through an organ (or the whole body) can be measured from three variables:

- Amount of marker substance taken up by the organ per unit time
- Concentration of marker substance in arterial blood supplying the organ
- Concentration of marker substance in venous blood leaving the organ

Therefore, determining oxygen consumption ($VO_2$) per unit time, and dividing it by arteriovenous oxygen content difference, provides cardiac output measurements, as expressed in the formula:

$$VO_2 = (CO \times C_a) - (CO \times C_v)$$

Dye dilution has a wider bedside applicability, if compared with Fick's principle, and it is based on the concept that an indicator injected through a vessel at known volume and concentration can be detected downstream. Its concentration at detection site depends on blood flow per unit time. Further application of this principle consists in using cold normal saline solution and recording blood temperature variations using a thermistor. This is one of the applications of Swan-Ganz catheter (also called pulmonary artery catheter—PAC), originally conceived to determine pulmonary artery and wedge pressure. PAC was introduced in clinical practice in 1970 [8] and, up to the mid-1980s, remained the most advanced cardiovascular monitoring system in ICU. It is a 110 cm catheter, provided with different lumens (Fig. 4.2):

- Distal lumen opens out in pulmonary artery and provides continuous pulmonary artery pressure (PAP) reading.
- Proximal lumen opens out in right atrium and provides continuous central venous pressure (CVP) reading.
- Thermistor lumen provides continuous blood temperature reading.
- Balloon lumen inflates a balloon close to the distal lumen; its occlusion stops blood flow through the pulmonary artery and provides a balloon downstream pressure reading (from the PAP lumen). This pressure reflects on left atrium pressure and is called wedge pressure (WP).

Cardiac output is determined with the thermodilution technique, according to the Stewart-Hamilton equation:

$$Q = \frac{V\left(T_b - T_1\right) K_1 K_2}{T_b\left(t\right)^{dt}}$$

where

- $V_1$ = injected volume.
- $T_b$ = blood temperature (at pulmonary artery).
- $T_1$ = injected dye temperature.
- $K_1$ = density factor.
- $K_2$ = computation constant.

To obtain a reliable curve, some issues have to be considered: the indicator mixing has to be rapid (bolus injection) and complete; blood flow and baseline temperature have to be constant; bolus volume should produce an adequate temperature variation [9].

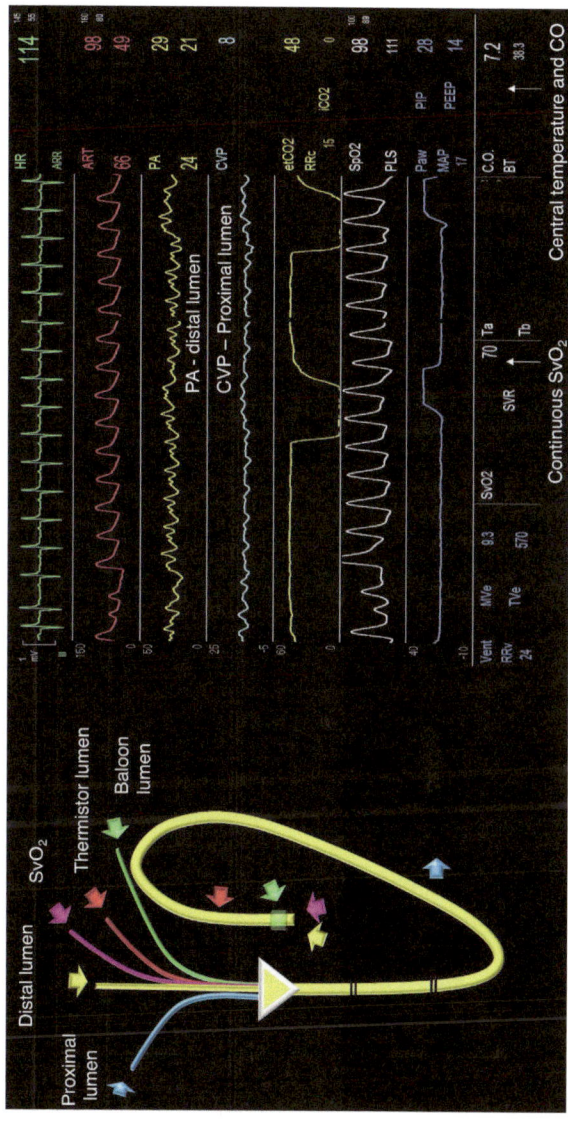

**Fig. 4.2** Swan-Ganz catheter and wave visualization

Valvular insufficiency (tricuspid and pulmonary) may lead to CO underestimation, as backward flow might result in dye recirculation. Furthermore, flow variations are physiologically observed during different respiratory cycle phases (both in spontaneous breathing and mechanical ventilation), thus requiring 3–5 bolus injections.

As other invasive devices, PAC requires maximum sterile barrier precautions during its insertion. Its use in ICU patients is limited to situations in which CO monitoring is necessary together with PAP. Several studies [10–13] evaluated the relationship between PAC application and patients' survival, demonstrating no substantial benefit, but a high risk of complications (arrhythmia, endocarditis, valve damage, pulmonary artery embolus) related with PAC positioning. PAC positioning also seemed to be related to higher mortality in ICU patients, probably depending on strict indications to its positioning that refer to more severe clinical conditions.

Technologies' developments allowed introduction of new devices dedicated to cardiac output monitoring. A modified PAC was introduced in the early 1990s. This device is provided with a thermal filament which is warmed at 8 min intervals. Filament's warming increases blood temperature, whose variation is detected downstream by catheter's thermistor: practically, the catheter works with an inverse thermodilution curve. This device has the same invasiveness of a traditional PAC but with some advantages: particularly, inverse thermodilution is a semicontinuous measurement and allows clinicians to an easier and more prompt identification of clinical conditions changes [14].

Other technologies developed during recent years to determine cardiac output found wider application in ICU and high-risk surgical patients. These methods are classified as less invasive (requiring a femoral or radial artery catheter and a central venous catheter) [15] or minimally invasive (requiring a radial artery catheter) and are based on pulse contour analysis algorithms. Some of them require calibration, while others do not. The most important advantage of these methods lays in continuous cardiac output measurement (which is determined beat by beat), immediately reflecting changes in hemodynamic condition. Furthermore, these technologies provide adjunctive parameters (related to volemia and fluid responsiveness). Likewise, some limitations for their applications have to be considered, since minimally invasive methods' reliability seems to be affected by hyperdynamic conditions and atrial fibrillation [16].

Indeed, wider importance and application has been reached during recent years by noninvasive measurements, including transthoracic echocardiography [17, 18].

Cardiac output measurements' methods have been validated toward PAC (which is considered the gold standard).

Currently, CO measurement is mainly indicated in high-risk surgical patients (such as cardiac surgery or liver transplant), in patients with septic shock and acute respiratory distress syndrome [16].

## 4.4.2 Arterial Pressure Monitoring

Arterial blood pressure (ABP) represents the force exerted from blood on arterial walls and derives from interaction between three factors: hydrostatic pressure (which, in turn, is related to the height of blood column and its density), hemodynamic pressure (coming from the strength of heart contraction), and kinetic energy (related to blood progression within cardiovascular system) [19]. In ICU patients, arterial blood pressure is usually measured using invasive catheters, which are generally inserted in large vessels (such as radial or femoral artery). The catheter is connected to an electronic pressure transducer using a tubing system filled with normal saline solution. The electronic transducer allows conversion of mechanical pressure wave into an electric one. Intra-arterial catheters provide more reliable data, compared with oscillometric systems. Furthermore, values obtained using these devices are continuous, providing clinicians immediate information concerning clinical stability variations and responses to treatments. Arterial catheters also allow collection of arterial blood without the need for peripheral puncture. Finally, analysis of the arterial waveform might highlight adjunctive information regarding patient's volemia and predict fluid responsiveness.

When measuring arterial blood pressure, three values are considered and displayed on the monitor: systolic (SBP), diastolic (DBP), and mean (MBP) pressure. SBP is the peak pressure reached during the cardiac cycle, resulting from interaction of several factors (EDV, SV, heart contractility force, blood density, arterial walls compliance); DBP is the trough during cardiac cycle and is mainly determined by arterial walls compliance [19, 20]. MAP is defined as mean pressure (usually equated as MAP = (SBP + 2DBP)/3) during cardiac cycle, and it is considered a hemodynamic target during resuscitation maneuvers [20]. The difference between SBP and DBP is called pulse pressure (PP), and it determines the peripheral palpability of arterial pressure wave (e.g., at radial, pedidial, or femoral site) [20].

When visualizing an arterial pressure waveform, several components can be identified [19] (Fig. 4.3):

- Anacrotic limb, corresponding to pressure increase due to left ventricle contraction; it ends with the top rounded, also called anacrotic shoulder.
- Dicrotic limb, corresponding to a decrease in pressure; it ends with the dicrotic notch, which reflects the closure of aortic valve.
- After closure of aortic valve, ABP still decreases until it reaches diastolic value; time and slope of this curve portion depend on heart rate and arterial compliance.

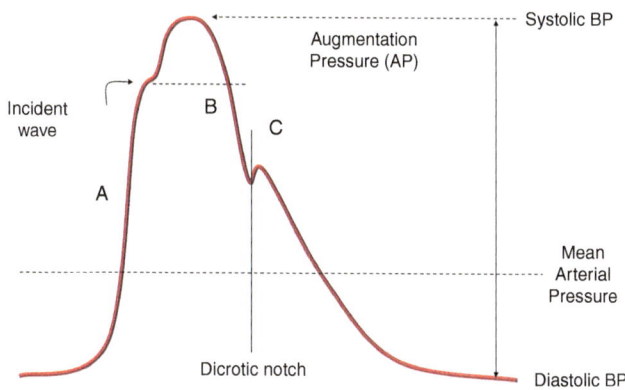

**Fig. 4.3** Arterial waveform. $A$ = anacrotic limb; $B$ = dicrotic limb; $C$ = dicrotic notch

It is important to consider that ABP results not only from ventricular ejection force but also from the reflection waves directed toward the heart. Moreover, arterial wall's structure works as a reservoir, which is filled during systole, and releases blood during diastole, thus allowing continuous blood flow over the whole cardiac cycle (Windkessel effect). Arterial waveforms significantly differ according to the measurement site, since the reflection wave effect becomes more evident as more distant from aortic root the measurement is performed. Furthermore, reduction in aortic elasticity can result in increased and earlier reflection wave. Patient's position during measurement can also affect measured values, due to the effects of the hydrostatic column (therefore, in a standing position, arterial pressure measured at foot level will be higher than the one at neck level).

Analysis of arterial waveform found important implications during the 1990s, when algorithms considering pulse contour analysis allowed continuous measurement of cardiac output. Adjunctive considerations were conducted on pressure and stroke volume variation during respiratory cycle. The underlying consideration is that nearly 50% of patients (defined as preload nonresponders) don't show a positive response to fluid challenge during shock resuscitation [21]. Considering that fluid overload may lead to pulmonary and cerebral edema, it's easy to understand the need to develop criteria and parameters to guide fluid bolus administration and early identify patients potentially nonresponding to these treatments [22].

After preparing the required supplies (pressure bag, normal saline bag, monitoring kit), setting an arterial transducer is detailed in Table 4.3.

During preparation of an arterial line, some important principles have to be considered:

- Tube length should not exceed 120 cm; tubes should be stiffer than the ones used to administer fluids, in order to reduce pressure wave dispersion through the tube walls.
- Avoid air bubbles within tubing system: small ones can lead to reduced signal resonance (with falsely high SBP readings), while large ones will reduce signal amplification (with falsely

**Table 4.3** Steps to set the pressure transducer

| Action | Rationale |
| --- | --- |
| Insert aseptically the spike into the bag, and fill almost half of the drip chamber | Avoid fluid contamination and air bubbles into the tube |
| Turn the stopcock off to the patient, and pull the fast-flush device | Priming the tube portion to the transducer system |
| Turn the stopcock off to the transducer and pull the fast-flush device | Priming the tube portion to the patient |
| Remote any remaining air bubble keeping the fast-flush device open | Avoid air in the system |
| Place normal saline bag inside a pressure bag, and inflate it to 250–300 mmHg | Keep a small continuous flush and avoid blood reflux |

low DBP) [19, 21]. Similarly, clots should be prevented by continuous tube-flushing (obtained through a 300 mmHg pressurized normal saline bag), and catheter kinking avoided through adequate dressing.

Accuracy of the measurement requires to apply some principles summarized in Table 4.4 [19, 23].

A simple evaluation of dynamic response can be obtained by performing a square wave test (Table 4.5) and by observing the resultant oscillations (Fig. 4.4). In order to perform this assess-

**Table 4.4** Principles to obtain accurate invasive pressure values

| | |
|---|---|
| Zeroing | Refers to attributing a "zero point" to the measurement, above which an invasive pressure is measured; the "zero point" normally refers to atmospheric pressure; after zeroing the transducer system, it will be possible to associate numeric values to the pressure wave |
| Leveling | Refers to positioning of the transducer system: when measuring cardiovascular pressures, the transducer level should be at fifth intercostal space on the midaxillary line or the sternal angle (where the sternum and second rib attach); in first case, the patient is required to be supine, and in the second, measurements can be obtained even at 60° elevation |
| | When pulmonary artery pressure is measured, the phlebostatic axis is defined by the midpoint between the anterior and posterior surfaces of the chest at the fourth intercostal space when the patient is supine |
| | When the transducer is under the phlebostatic axis, the measured value will be higher than the real pressure; conversely, when it is over the phlebostatic axis, the measured value will be lower than the real pressure |
| Damping | Refers to the dynamic response of the system to a sudden, high pressure (obtained releasing the transducer's fast-flush valve). Underdamped systems overestimate systolic pressure and underestimate diastolic pressures. Conversely, overdamped systems will underestimate systolic pressures and overestimate diastolic pressures (Fig. 4.4) |

**Table 4.5** Square wave testing

| Step | Action |
| --- | --- |
| 1 | Activate snap or pull tab on flush device |
| 2 | Observe square wave generated on bedside monitor |
| 3 | Count oscillations after square wave |
| 4 | Observe distance between the oscillations |

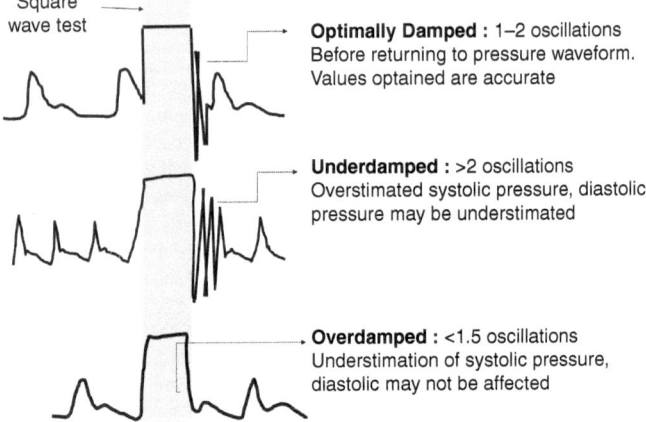

Square wave test

**Optimally Damped** : 1–2 oscillations
Before returning to pressure waveform.
Values optained are accurate

**Underdamped** : >2 oscillations
Overstimated systolic pressure, diastolic
pressure may be understimated

**Overdamped** : <1.5 oscillations
Understimation of systolic pressure,
diastolic may not be affected

**Fig. 4.4** Square wave test with optimally damped signal, underdamped and overdamped signal, during arterial invasive monitoring

ment accurately, a flush device that can be activated rapidly and then released is required. A flush device that does not close rapidly after activation (squeeze or press type) may not close the restrictor quickly and may produce erroneous results.

The same consideration can be applied for other blood pressure measured using a transducer (pulmonary artery pressure and central venous pressure).

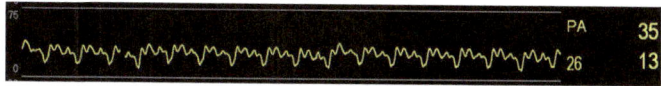

**Fig. 4.5** Pulmonary artery pressure waveform

### *4.4.3 Pulmonary Artery Pressure*

PAP values are detected through the distal lumen of a PAC. PAP wave is in some way similar to the systemic arterial pressure one, but values are lower, ranging between 20 and 30 mmHg for systolic pulmonary pressure and 5 and 10 mmHg for diastolic. PAP monitoring aims to identify and manage pulmonary hypertension (PH), a threatening condition that may lead to increased cardiac workload [23, 24] (Fig. 4.5).

Usually, PH is defined as a mean arterial pressure ≥25 mmHg at rest, measured by right heart catheterization [25]. Precapillary pulmonary artery hypertension (PAH) requires the measurement of wedge pressure and can be induced from lung diseases. The diagnostic criteria pointed out during the fourth World Symposium on Pulmonary Hypertension keep the pulmonary artery wedge pressure cutoff for the definition of precapillary PAH at ≤15 mmHg [25]. Several conditions (both congenital and disease related) have been associated with PAH [26].

PAH pathogenesis derives from an imbalance between vasodilators and vasoconstrictors molecules and can be enhanced by the reaction with some drugs.

## 4.5 Oxygen Transportation and Consumption

Oxygen is used by cells during metabolic processes, being transported by blood hemoglobin to peripheral tissues. Blood oxygen content is expressed by the equation:

$$CaO_2 = (1.34 \times Hb \times SaO_2) + (0.003 \times PaO_2)$$

It is therefore easy to understand how alteration of a single or multiple factor may affect oxygen availability. Anemia correction, oxygen fraction increasing, and cardiac function improvement are all interventions aiming to increase the amount of available blood oxygen. Oxygen extraction from cells depends on several factors, such as cells perfusion and metabolic activity. In ICU patients, some factors (fever, burns, shivering, and infectious and inflammatory reactions) may increase oxygen extraction, while other conditions (neuromuscular blockade, deep sedation, microvascular thrombosis, shunt) might decrease it.

Venous oxygen saturation is defined as the percentage of venous hemoglobin saturated by oxygen; venous oxygen saturation values normally range between 60 and 80% and vary according to measurements' districts. It can be measured collecting a blood sample from distal lumen of a central venous catheter (which is called central venous oxygen saturation—$ScvO_2$) in jugular or subclavian vein or Swan-Ganz catheter (which is called mixed venous oxygen saturation—$SvO_2$) [27]. Accurate $ScvO_2$ measurement might depend from distant positioning of catheter's tip from right atrium.

$SvO_2$ is considered as most accurate, since it reflects oxygen consumption at whole organs, including coronary and pulmonary circulation, while $ScvO_2$ provides an index of oxygen consumption at higher portions of the body. Studies have shown a good correlation between $ScvO_2$ and $SvO_2$, the first generally overestimating the second by 3–8% [28], but in patients with septic shock, the bias between the two measurements might be significantly higher, leading to misinterpretation of falsely high oxygen availability [29, 30] and suggesting that trends are more helpful than single values in estimating patients response to treatments. Venous oxygen saturation has been evaluated as consistent endpoint in studies [31] evaluating fluid challenge resuscitation in severe sepsis and septic shock, showing a consistent mortality reduction, particularly when treatment was initiated prior that severe organ damages emerge.

Decreased venous oxygen saturation (<60.8% [32]) may depend from insufficient oxygen delivery or increased oxygen extraction at cellular level [33]. Increased venous oxygen saturation (>77.4% [32]) usually reflects a decreased consumption (e.g., during general anesthesia or in severe hypothermic conditions) or a delivery exceeding cells requirements [33].

## 4.6   Volemia

Determination of patient's volemia might be crucial to manage a cardiovascular dysfunction condition and may help in differentiating the most appropriate therapeutic choice, particularly targeting the administration of fluids and inotropes.

### 4.6.1   Filling Pressures: Central Venous Pressure and Pulmonary Artery Occlusion Pressure

Central venous pressure (CVP) is defined as the pressure measured through a venous catheter whose tip is positioned close to the right atrium. CVP can be defined as the pressure resulting from the interaction between venous return and cardiac function. CVP has been widely used as a surrogate indicator of the volemic status of patients, according to the principle that a larger volume reflects on a higher pressure inside atrium. This principle is normally true in healthy subjects, nonetheless, it cannot be always considered true in ICU patients, in which many factors interact, determining alterations in CVP measurements. For example, several conditions common for ICU patients (such as pneumothorax, pericardial tamponade, heart failure) can result in high CVP readings, who often do not really reflect a normovolemic status.

CVP can both be measured using a transducer or a water manometer (in this case the observed value won't be continuous). As for any invasive pressure, leveling and zeroing procedures are required (Table 4.4). The transducer should be positioned at right atrium level (with patient supine on a flat position, or with head of bed elevated by 30°, 45°, or 60°, since the right atrium is anterior and round, and its midpoint remains at the same vertical distance below the sternal angle). The atrium position on the chest is normally identified by intersection of midaxillary line and fourth intercostal space (more easier, 5 cm below the sternal angle) [20].

CVP waveform (Figs. 4.6 and 4.7) is composed of three prominent positive waves (a, c, and v) and two prominent negative waves (x and y descents). The "a" wave is generated by atrial contraction; the "c" wave is due to backward closure of the tricuspid valve (onset of systole), and "v" wave reflects atrial

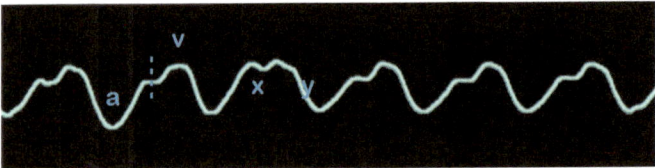

**Fig. 4.6** Central venous pressure waveform. Dotted line shows the ideal site for measurement

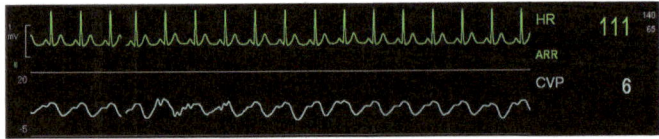

**Fig. 4.7** Central venous pressure waveform pooled together with the ECG waveform. Observe waves a (right after the P wave and before the QRS complex on the ECG, expression of atrial contraction) and v (corresponding to the descent T on the ECG, expression of atrial filling)

filling during diastole; the "x" descent comes from the fall in atrial pressure during atrial relaxation, while the "y" descent comes from a fall in atrial pressure (onset of diastole, emptying of atrium in the ventricle) [34]. To obtain a more reliable measurement, CVP should be obtained at the end of expiration, in order to reduce the effects of transmural pressure. The preferred site for measurement is the leading edge of the "c" wave (generally approximated by the base of the "a" wave) [35].

Pulmonary artery occlusion pressure (PAOP), also known as pulmonary artery wedge pressure (PAWP), is obtained performing right heart catheterization using a Swan-Ganz catheter. During its positioning, the Swan-Ganz catheter balloon is inflated in the right atrium until it reaches the wedging position that means the occlusion of a pulmonary artery branch. Balloon's inflation should follow some simple principles, to avoid severe complications: the air volume used should range between 1 and 1.5 mL. Recent summarized recommendations report that repeated inflations and deflations of the balloon should be avoided, since they have been associated to pulmonary artery's rupture [25]. PAWP values normally range between 5 and 12 mmHg, with a slight increase (up to 15 mmHg) related with age. Its measurement should always be standardized to an ideal position, with patient lying supine and the transducer at mid-thoracic line, halfway between the anterior sternum and the bed surface (left atrium) [25].

PAWP has been considered for a long time a surrogate marker of left ventricular preload, according to the principle that under normal (and static) conditions it is equivalent to left atrial pressure, which, in turn, equates to left ventricular end-diastolic pressure (LVEDP) [36]. This assumption remains actually true only in the absence of particular conditions, such as mitral valve and left ventricular wall pathologies, and when the effect of intrathoracic pressures is minimized (that means at end of expiration). Such criteria strongly limit the effective applicability of this measurement as preload index; therefore the association with other measurements is required [36].

### 4.6.2    Volumetric Indicators

The need for assessing volemia in critically ill patients gave course to development of the so-called "volumetric indicators" that usefully guide clinicians in fluid replacement. Volemia is defined as the total blood flowing through the circulatory system. Hypovolemic conditions can be both absolute and relative. The first is characterized by an important circulating volume loss (hemorrhage or dehydration due, e.g., to fever, burns, renal failure, vomiting, or diarrhea). The second is attributable to redistribution of volume in third space (such as in capillary leak syndrome) or in body cavities (such as in pulmonary edema, ascites, pleural effusion). In relative hypovolemia, an imbalance of fluid homeostasis between capillary and interstitial space (which is normally controlled by electrolytes and protein concentration) is observed.

Recent developments in hemodynamic monitoring devices offer relatively easy-to-use solutions to assess blood volumes at the bedside. The principle on which these measurements are based refers to dilution of a thermal indicator (in the past, it was a colorimetric one) injected at a known temperature through a central vein and detected though a thermistor placed in arterial catheter. This technique is known as transpulmonary thermodilution. The analysis of the thermodilution curve provides the so-called "mean transit time" (MTt) that defines mean time needed for passage of every indicator's molecule. After injection, thermal indicator distributes to intrathoracic thermal volume (ITTV), clinically represented by global end-diastolic volume (GEDV), extravascular lung water (EVLW), and pulmonary blood volume (PBV) (Table 4.6).

In healthy subjects, intrathoracic blood volume (ITBV) (resulting from summation of GEDV and PBV) represents approximately 26% of global blood volume. ITBV can be mathematically derived from GEDV [37] (Table 4.6).

**Table 4.6** Volumetric measurements

| Intrathoracic thermal volume (ITTV) | ITTV = MTt × CO | Total amount of blood and water inside chest |
|---|---|---|
| Total pulmonary volume (TPV) | | Total amount of blood and water inside lungs |
| Global end-diastolic volume (GEDV) | ITTV-TPV | Sum of the volume of the four cardiac chambers |
| Intrathoracic blood volume (ITBV) | 1.25 × GEDV [37] | Sum of the volume in cardiac chambers and pulmonary vascular bed |
| Extravascular lung water (EVLW) | ITTV-ITBV | Amount of water within the lung interstitial space |

GEDV, whose normal values range between 600 and 800 mL/m$^2$, includes the volume of the four cardiac chambers and the blood volume between the injection site (via a CVC at the superior vena cava) and the thermistor (femoral artery) [38]. As for CO measurement, uneven dye mixing (aortic aneurism, intracardiac shunt, vascular pulmonary bed reduction) may lead to incorrect volumetric esteem.

ITBV and GEDV (indexed on body surface area, ITBVI, and GEDVI) are used as preload indexes in several ICU and anesthesia conditions (sepsis, solid organ transplant) and have shown a better performance in guiding fluid and inotropic therapy, compared to previously used CVP and PAWP.

During lung transplantation, ITBVI showed a good correlation with stroke volume index (SVI), while only poor correlation was found between ITBVI and PAOP [39]. Similar results were obtained in hyperdynamic patients undergoing liver transplantation [40]. ITBVI was also found to be a better preload indicator than cardiac filling pressures (CVP and PAOP) in patients with sepsis or septic shock [41]. Extravascular lung water (EVLW) is a bedside measurement of the amount of lung water outside the vascular compartment. Practically, it is a measurement of the amount of pulmonary edema (defined as the difference between PTV and ITBV), previously assessed by radiologic imaging (such as chest X-ray, computerized tomography, and magnetic resonance imaging) [42].

The gold standard for EVLW measurement is the ex vivo gravimetry, obtained weighting lungs before and after their dry out [42]. Obviously, this method is inapplicable in alive patients. Dye dilution methods allowed bedside measurement of EVLW from the 1980s, and further thermal dilution had a wide diffusion [43]. Recently, estimation of EVLW has also been conducted by using the chest ultrasound, showing good performances in terms of sensitivity (81%) and specificity (90.9%) [44], although pulmonary edema detection may be limited from the lung region where it is performed [45].

The initially fixed cutoff value indexed on body surface area of 7 mL/kg body weight [46] has been recently increased to 10 mL/kg [47]. Recently, indexation of EVLW (EVLWI) to predicted body weight (rather than actual body weight) has been proposed, to avoid underestimation of EVLW in obese patients, and in those who develop positive fluid balance, it has been introduced, showing a better correlation with lung injury scores and oxygenation. Also, EVLW indexed on predicted body weight had a better correlation with patients' outcome [48]. Other authors also suggested EVLW indexation to patient's height, as it is considered the main determinant of lung volume [49]. EVLWI measurement using transpulmonary thermodilution might be overestimated by lung resection and underestimated by pulmonary embolism [45].

Currently, EVLW is not included in ARDS as defined by Berlin criterion, although diagnosis might be improved by using it [45].

EVLW guides clinicians when acting fluid, diuretic, and inotropic therapy, in addition to organ support treatments, such as mechanical ventilation and continuous renal replacement therapy. EVLW demonstrated prognostic power, because its mean value is higher in non-survivor critically ill patients [50]. Fluid therapy oriented on EVLW values seems to reduce ICU length of stay and mechanical ventilation duration [51]. Recently, EVLW has been investigated in patients with acute postoperative hypoxemic respiratory failure treated with noninvasive ventilation (NIV). Before starting NIV, EVLW was found to be significantly lower in patients who did not later require intubation ($8.6 \pm 1.08$ vs. $11.8 \pm 0.99$, $P < .01$) [52]. Similarly, after 1 h from beginning NIV treatment, EVLW significantly decreased in patients who did not require intubation ($8.6 \pm 1.08$ vs. $6.2 \pm 0.96$, $P < .01$) [52].

Take-Home Messages
1. Cardiovascular monitoring provides data to adequately frame hemodynamic condition, but it cannot itself change patient's outcome.
2. Proper treatment decisions need reliable data. Therefore, appropriate technique (particularly concerning transducer's leveling, zeroing, and signal's damping) has to be applied.
3. No single data should be used to implement clinical decisions: every measurement should be considered together with other available ones and with global patient's condition (including other vital functions' assessment). Similarly, trend values should be considered to assess patient's responses to treatments.
4. Monitoring devices should be chosen according to patient's condition and staff confidence with their use and interpretation.

# References

1. Thompson JP, Mahajan RP. Monitoring the monitors—beyond risk management. Br J Anaesth. 2006;97:1–3. https://doi.org/10.1093/bja/ael139.
2. Hofer CK, Cecconi M, Marx G, della Rocca G. Minimally invasive haemodynamic monitoring. Eur J Anaesthesiol. 2009;26:996–1002.
3. JCGM 200:2008. International vocabulary of metrology—basic and general concepts and associated terms (VIM). http://www.bipm.org/utils/common/documents/jcgm/JCGM_200_2008.pdf. Accessed 30 Jul 2017.
4. Hannibal GB. It started with Einthoven: the history of the ECG and cardiac monitoring. AACN Adv Crit Care. 2011;22:93–6. https://doi.org/10.1097/10.1097/NCI.0b013e3181fffe4c.
5. Petty BG. Basic electrocardiography. New York: Springer; 2015. https://doi.org/10.1007/978-1-4939-2413-4.
6. Drew BJ, Califf RM, Funk M, et al. Practice standards for electrocardiographic monitoring in hospital settings: an American Heart Association scientific statement from the Councils on Cardiovascular Nursing, Clinical Cardiology, and Cardiovascular Disease in the Young: endorsed by the International Society of Computerized Electrocardiology and the American Association of Critical-Care Nurses. Circulation. 2004;110:2721–46. https://doi.org/10.1161/01.CIR.0000145144.56673.59.
7. Baranchuk A, Shaw C, Alanazi H, Campbell D, Bally K, Redfearn DP, et al. Electrocardiography pitfalls and artifacts: the 10 commandments. Crit Care Nurse. 2009;29:67–73. https://doi.org/10.4037/ccn2009607.
8. Swan HJ, Ganz W, Forrester J, Marcus H, Diamond G, Chonette D. Catheterization of the heart in man with use of a flow-directed balloon-tipped catheter. N Engl J Med. 1970;283:447–51. https://doi.org/10.1056/NEJM197008272830902.
9. Moise SF, Sinclair CJ, Scott DH. Pulmonary artery blood temperature and the measurement of cardiac output by thermodilution. Anaesthesia. 2002;57(6):562.
10. Richard C, Warszawskj J, ANguel N, Deye N, Combes A, Barnoud D, et al. Early use of the pulmonary artery catheter and outcomes in patients with shock and acute respiratory distress syndrome: a randomized controlled trial. JAMA. 2003;290:2713–20. https://doi.org/10.1001/jama.290.20.2713.
11. Harvey S, Harrison DA, Singer M, Ashcroft J, Jones CM, Melbourne D, et al. Assessment of the clinical effectiveness of pulmonary artery

catheters in management of patients in intensive care (PAC-Man): a randomized controlled trial. Lancet. 2005;366:472–7. https://doi.org/10.1016/S0140-6736(05)67061-4.

12. Sandham JD, Hull RD, Brant RF, Knox L, Pineo GF, Doig CJ, et al. A randomized, controlled trial of the use of pulmonary-artery catheter in high risk surgical patients. N Engl J Med. 2003;348:5–14. https://doi.org/10.1056/NEJMoa021108.

13. Wheeler AP, Bernard GR, Thompson BT, Shoenfeld D, Wiedmann HP, deBoisblanc B, et al. Pulmonary artery versus central venous catheter to guide treatment of acute lung injury. National Heart, Lung and Blood Institute Acute Respiratory Distress Syndrome (ARDS). N Engl J Med. 2006;354:2213–24. https://doi.org/10.1056/NEJMoa061895.

14. McGee WT, Headley JM, Frazier JA. Quick guide to cardiopulmonary care. 2014. http://ht.edwards.com/scin/edwards/eu/sitecollectionimages/products/pressuremonitoring/ar11206-quickguide3rded.pdf. Accessed 7 Nov 2016.

15. Cottis R, Magee N, Higgins DJ. Haemodynamic monitoring with pulse-induced contour cardiac output (PiCCO) in critical care. Intensive Crit Care Nurs. 2003;19:301–7.

16. de Waal EE, Wappler F, Buhre WF. Cardiac output monitoring. Curr Opin Anaesthesiol. 2009;22:71–7. https://doi.org/10.1097/ACO.0b013e32831f44d0.

17. Mayer J, Suttner S. Cardiac output derived from arterial pressure waveform. Curr Opin Anaesthesiol. 2009;22:804–8. https://doi.org/10.1097/ACO.0b013e328332a473.

18. Sakka SG. Hemodynamic monitoring in the critically ill patient—current status and perspective. Front Med. 2015;2:44. https://doi.org/10.3389/fmed.2015.00044.

19. McGhee BH, Bridges EJ. Monitoring arterial blood pressure: what you may not know. Crit Care Nurse. 2002;22:60–4, 66–70. 73 passim

20. Pittman JA, Ping JS, Mark JB. Arterial and central venous pressure monitoring. Int Anesthesiol Clin. 2004;42:13–30.

21. Augusto JF, Teboul JL, Radermacher P, Asfar P. Interpretation of blood pressure signal: physiological bases, clinical relevance, and objectives during shock states. Intensive Care Med. 2011;37:411–9. https://doi.org/10.1007/s00134-010-2092-1.

22. Michard F, Teboul JL. Predicting fluid responsiveness in ICU patients: a critical analysis of the evidence. Chest. 2002;121:2000–8.

23. Keckeisen M. Monitoring pulmonary artery pressure. Crit Care Nurse. 2004;24:67–70.

24. Bridges EJ. Pulmonary artery pressure monitoring: when, how and what else to use. AACN Adv Crit Care. 2006;17:286–305.

25. Hoeper MM, Bogaard HJ, Condliffe R, Frantz R, Khanna D, Kurzyna M, et al. Definitions and diagnosis of pulmonary hypertension. J Am Coll Cardiol. 2013;62:D42–50. https://doi.org/10.1016/j. jacc.2013.10.032.

26. Simonneau G, Gatzoulis MA, Adatia I, Celermajer D, Denton C, Ghofrani A, et al. Updated clinical classification of pulmonary hypertension. J Am Coll Cardiol. 2013;62:D34–41. https://doi.org/10.1016/j. jacc.2013.10.029.

27. Goodrich C. Continuous central venous oximetry monitoring. Crit Care Nurs Clin North Am. 2006;18:203–209., x. https://doi.org/10.1016/j. ccell.2006.01.005.

28. Walley KR. Use of central venous oxygen saturation to guide therapy. Am J Respir Crit Care Med. 2011;184:514–20. https://doi.org/10.1164/ rccm.201010-1584CI.

29. Kopterides P, Bonovas S, Mavrou I, Kostadima E, Zakynthinos E, Armaganidis A. Venous oxygen saturation and lactate gradient from superior vena cava to pulmonary artery in patients with septic shock. Shock. 2009;31:561–7. https://doi.org/10.1097/ SHK.0b013e31818bb8d8.

30. Varpula M, Karlsson S, Ruokonen E, Pettilä V. Mixed venous oxygen saturation cannot be estimated by central venous oxygen saturation in septic shock. Intensive Care Med. 2006;32:1336–43. https://doi. org/10.1007/s00134-006-0270-y.

31. Rivers E, Nguyen B, Havstad S, Ressler J, Muzzin A, Knoblich B, et al. Early goal-directed therapy collaborative group. Early goal-directed therapy in the treatment of severe sepsis and septic shock. N Engl J Med. 2001;345:1368–77. https://doi.org/10.1056/NEJMoa010307.

32. Reid M. Central venous oxygen saturation: analysis, clinical use and effects on mortality. Nurs Crit Care. 2013;18:245–50. https://doi. org/10.1111/nicc.12028.

33. Perz S, Uhlig T, Kohl M, Bredle DL, Reinhart K, Bauer M, Kortgen A. Low and supranormal central venous oxygen saturation and markers of tissue hypoxia in cardiac surgery patients: a prospective observational study. Intensive Care Med. 2011;37:52–9. https://doi.org/10.1007/ s00134-010-1980-8.

34. Magder S. How to use central venous pressure measurements. Curr Opin Crit Care. 2005;11:264–70.

35. Magder S. Central venous pressure monitoring. Curr Opin Crit Care. 2006;12:219–27. https://doi.org/10.1097/01.ccx.0000224866.01453.43.

36. Robin E, Costecalde M, Lebuffe G, Vallet B. Clinical relevance of data from the pulmonary artery catheter. Crit Care. 2006;10(Suppl 3):S3. https://doi.org/10.1186/cc4830.

37. Sakka SG, Rühl CC, Pfeiffer UJ, Beale R, McLuckie A, Reinhart K, et al. Assessment of cardiac preload and extravascular lung water by single transpulmonary thermodilution. Intensive Care Med. 2000;26:180–7.

38. Kapoor PM, Bhardwaj V, Sharma A, Kiran U. Global end-diastolic volume an emerging preload marker vis-a-vis other markers—have we reached our goal? Ann Card Anaesth. 2016;19:699–704. https://doi.org/10.4103/0971-9784.191554.

39. Della Rocca G, Costa GM, Coccia C, Pompei L, Di Marco P, Pietropaoli P. Preload index: pulmonary artery occlusion pressure versus intrathoracic blood volume monitoring during lung transplantation. Anesth Analg. 2002;95:835–43.

40. Della Rocca G, Costa MG, Coccia C, Pompei L, Pietropaoli P. Preolad and haemodynamic assessment during liver transplantation: a comparison between the pulmonary artery catheter and transpulmonary indicator dilution technique. Eur J Anaesthesiol. 2002;19:868–75.

41. Sakka SG, Bredle DL, Reinhart K, Meier-Hellmann A. Comparison between intrathoracic blood volume and cardiac filling pressures in the early phase of hemodynamic instability of patients with sepsis or septic shock. J Crit Care. 1999;14:78–83.

42. Lange NR, Schuster DP. The measurement of lung water. Crit Care. 1999;3:R19–24. https://doi.org/10.1186/cc342. DOI:10.1186/cc342.

43. Shyamsundar M, Attwood B, Keating L, Walden AP. Clinical review: the role of ultrasound in estimating extra-vascular lung water. Crit Care. 2013;17:237. https://doi.org/10.1186/cc12710.

44. Volpicelli G, Skurzak S, Boero E, Carpinteri G, Tengattini M, Stefanone V, et al. Lung ultrasound predicts well extravascular lung water but is of limited usefulness in the prediction of wedge pressure. Anesthesiology. 2014;121:320–7. https://doi.org/10.1097/ALN.0000000000000300.

45. Jozwiak M, Teboul JL, Monnet X. Extravascular lung water in critical care: recent advances and clinical applications. Ann Intensive Care. 2015;5:38. https://doi.org/10.1186/s13613-015-0081-9.

46. Tagami T, Kushimoto S, Yamamoto Y, Atsumi T, Tosa R, Matsuda K, et al. Validation of extravascular lung water measurement by single transpulmonary thermodilution: human autopsy study. Crit Care. 2010;14:R162. https://doi.org/10.1186/cc9250.

47. Tagami T, Sawabe M, Kushimoto S, Marik PE, Mieno MN, Kawaguchi T, et al. Quantitative diagnosis of diffuse alveolar damage using extravascular lung water. Crit Care Med. 2013;41(9):2144–50. https://doi.org/10.1097/CCM.0b013e31828a4643.

48. Craig TR, Duffy MJ, Shyamsundar M, McDowell C, McLaughlin B, Elborn JS, et al. Extravascular lung water indexed to predicted body

weight is a novel predictor of intensive care unit mortality in patients with acute lung injury. Crit Care Med. 2010;38:114–20. https://doi.org/10.1097/CCM.0b013e3181b43050.

49. Huber W, Mair S, Götz SQ, Tschirdewahn J, Siegel J, Schmid RM, et al. Extravascular lung water and its association with weight, height, age, and gender: a study in intensive care unit patients. Intensive Care Med. 2013;39:146–50. https://doi.org/10.1007/s00134-012-2745-3.

50. Sakka SG, Klein M, Reinhart K, et al. Prognostic value of extravascular lung water in critically ill patients. Chest. 2002;122:2080–6.

51. Mitchell JP, Schuller D, Calandrino FS, Schuster DP. Improved outcome based on fluid management in critically ill patients requiring pulmonary artery catheterization. Am Rev Respir Dis. 1992;145:990–8. https://doi.org/10.1164/ajrccm/145.5.990.

52. Redondo Calvo FJ, Bejarano Ramirez N, Uña Orejon R, Villazala Garcia R, Yuste Peña AS, et al. Elevated extravascular lung water index (ELWI) as a predictor of failure of continuous positive airway pressure via helmet (helmet-CPAP) in patients with acute respiratory failure after major surgery. Arch Bronconeumol. 2015;51:558–63. https://doi.org/10.1016/j.arbres.2015.01.012.

# Chapter 5
# Early Mobility, Skin, and Pressure Ulcer Risk Assessment

Gian Domenico Giusti, Angela Peghetti, Irene Comisso, and Stefano Bambi

## 5.1 Introduction

Bed rest is one of the main therapeutic prescriptions in many diseases. Nonetheless, in ICU, prolonged bed rest and immobility are associated with many complications, including muscular atrophy, pressure ulcers (PUs), atelectasis, and bone demineralization [1]. Moreover, a meta-analysis about the effects of bed rest in 15 different conditions and medical procedures showed that bed rest is not always effective and may be associated with different damages, especially toward rehabilitative purposes [2].

In recent years, the increase of critically ill patients' survival rates highlighted the need to focus on the quality of life and the sequelae related to ICU stay and in hospital stay. Moreover, there is the necessity to implement all the preventive and rehabilitative interventions aimed to avoid physical, social, and psychological limitations [3]. For this reason, it's fundamental to prevent the events that may worsen the outcomes of ICU patients.

In this chapter, we will consider some of the complications that may occur during the prolonged bed rest, analyze the

© Springer International Publishing AG, part of Springer Nature 2018    137
I. Comisso et al., *Nursing in Critical Care Setting*,
https://doi.org/10.1007/978-3-319-50559-6_5

benefits of early mobilization interventions, and discuss the main pressure ulcer issues in ICU (definition, assessment, treatment).

Hospital-acquired pressure ulcers (HAPU), also known as "pressure ulcers," "pressure sores," "pressure injuries," or "bedsores," are one of the top five adverse events (AE) currently being reported among patients during their hospital stay [4]. The *weakness* in ICU patients can persist for many years after discharge from hospital [5], and although the etiology of *weakness* is multifactorial, early mobilization in ICU can help to reduce the muscular atrophy, the weakness itself, and the deconditioning associated with prolonged bed rest.

## 5.2    Intensive Care Unit-Acquired Weakness (ICU-AW)

In the past few years, critical illnesses in ICU (from myocardial infarction to surgical complications) required a mandatory complete immobility. ICU staff believed that bed rest could reduce the oxygen consumption, improve the tissue oxygenation, maintain the correct alignment of spine and bones, and decrease to a minimum the effects of trauma. However, the adverse effects of prolonged immobility are now well known and concern all the body systems (Fig. 5.1). Early mobilization may help to reduce some of these adverse effects [6].

ICU-AW is defined as a "syndrome of generalized limb weakness that develops while the patient is critically ill and for which there is no alternative explanation other than the critical illness itself" [7]. The etiology of ICU-AW is multifactorial, with several studies establishing independent risk factors for its development [1].

The reported incidence of ICU-AW varies according to the different definitions given to this syndrome, the diagnostic

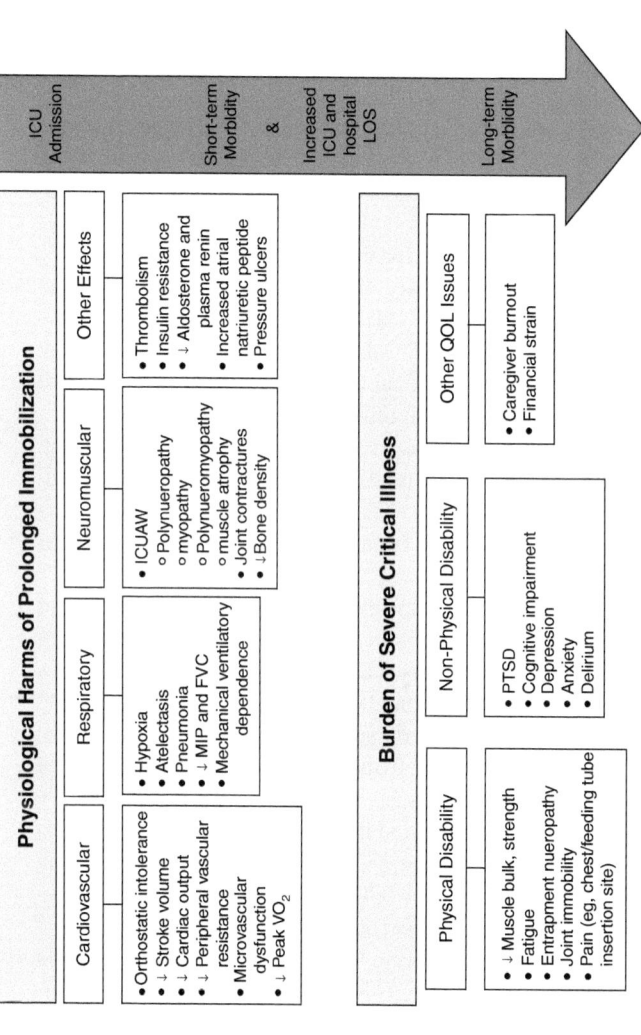

**Fig. 5.1** Physiological sequelae of immobilization and the burden of severe critical illness. FVC, forced vital capacity; ICU-AW, ICU-acquired weakness; MIP, maximum inspiratory pressure; PTSD, post-traumatic stress disorder; VO$_2$, oxygen consumption [7]

modalities used, and the specific population studied. A key issue in determining the incidence of ICU-AW is the struggle in ascertaining the development of neuromuscular weakness during the ICU stay, as opposed to weakness due to a preexisting condition (e.g., myasthenia gravis) and/or a specific etiology (e.g., new cerebrovascular accident). ICU-AW may be unrecognized in general critically ill populations, but it is prevalent in the chronic critically illnesses and in patients requiring prolonged MV [8].

Among the risk factors for the development of the ICU-AW, there are the disease severity, the presence of *systemic inflammatory response syndrome* (SIRS), and an organ failure associated with neuromuscular disorders. Also, MV duration, ICU-LOS, blood biochemical alterations (such as hypo- and hyperglycemia), and the administration of total parenteral nutrition (TPN) increase the risk of ICU-AW development. Furthermore, using of potentially myotoxic or neurotoxic medications, such as corticosteroids and non-depolarizing neuromuscular blocking agents, has been associated with neuromuscular abnormalities [1].

Mechanisms leading to the ICU-AW are complex and involve many physiopathological processes. On healthy subjects, for example, bed rest leads to a reduction in quadriceps force of around 1–1.5% a day [9], and this percentage increases significantly in sick or elderly subjects. In addition to the immobility, critical care patients often show signs of malnutrition during their ICU stay, because of malabsorption due to primary pathology, hypercatabolic and hypermetabolic stress, leading to protein loss [10]. Malnutrition is considered as a contributing factor to the occurrence of ICU-AW. Therefore, nutritive support in ICU is essential to correct nutritional deficits.

Patients with ICU-AW have an increased duration of MV and LOS. After 7 days of MV, 25–33% of patients experience clinically evident neuromuscular weakness [1].

## 5.2.1  Prevention and Treatment of Immobility

There are few treatment options to prevent or treat the ICU-AW. A proper glycaemia control seems to be the only intervention related to the decrease in the onset of this syndrome [11]. Minimizing patient's exposure to corticosteroids and/or neuromuscular blocking agents may be prudent until future studies will clarify the role of these medications in the development of ICU-AW [12].

A potential therapeutic option to reduce ICU-AW is the avoidance of bed rest via early mobilization in the ICU setting. Mobility is a basic nursing care, which is essential in maintaining patients' safety and prevention of bed rest induced complications. Mobility can improve gas exchanges, decrease incidence of ventilator-associated pneumonia and the occurrence of MV support, and decrease ICU and hospital LOS [12].

Physiotherapy carried out in ICU varies from hospital to hospital and among different typologies of ICUs. Furthermore, there is a wide range of interventions that can be carried out ranging from passive physiotherapy to kinetic therapy, or transferring the patient from bed to chair. In some case, patients are helped to brief walk within the ICU [8]. Usually more challenging physiotherapy (e.g., walking) is rarely performed in ICU because of the huge nurses' workload and the reduced number of physiotherapists dedicated to this activity [8].

Physiotherapy is also affected by the level of sedation: critical care patients are often deeply sedated especially if mechanically ventilated. Deep sedation is related to the increasing number of MV days that prevents their participation to the activities [13]. Periodic interruptions of sedation and the implementation of awakening tests can improve an early mobilization (see Chap. 17). Also, a multidisciplinary focus to perform an early mobilization program after the *physiologic stabilization* (Fig. 5.2) from cardiological, respiratory, and neurological impairments is desirable [14].

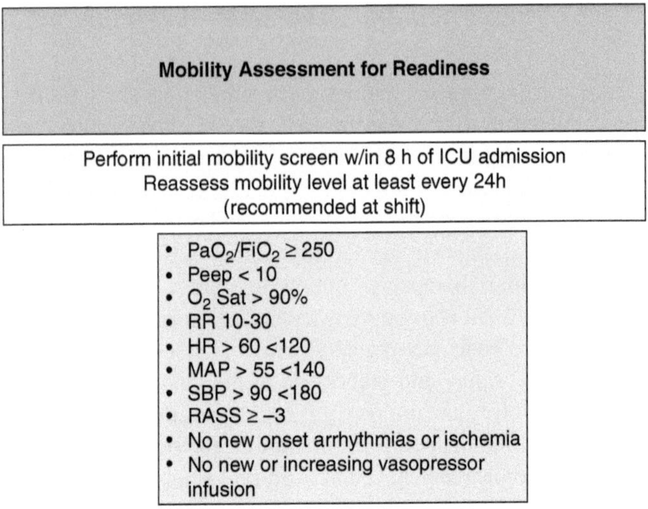

**Mobility Assessment for Readiness**

Perform initial mobility screen w/in 8 h of ICU admission
Reassess mobility level at least every 24h
(recommended at shift)

- $PaO_2/FiO_2 \geq 250$
- Peep < 10
- $O_2$ Sat > 90%
- RR 10-30
- HR > 60 <120
- MAP > 55 <140
- SBP > 90 <180
- RASS $\geq -3$
- No new onset arrhythmias or ischemia
- No new or increasing vasopressor infusion

**Fig. 5.2** Assessment of patients' readiness for mobility. Modified from Asfour [6]

## 5.3 Skin and Pressure Ulcer Risk Assessment

### 5.3.1 Definition

ICU patients are exposed to an increased risk for PUs' development due to circulatory impairment, hemodynamic instability, vasopressors, diminished sensory perception, and organ failure [15]. PUs are "ulcers caused by a prolonged pressure exerted on the epidermis, the dermis and the underlying tissues, up to engage in more serious cases the muscles and bones when the same position is maintained for a long period of time, such as, for example, in case of the bedridden patient" [16]. Body areas corresponding to bone protrusions are most frequently affected and become ischemic when pressure is maintained constant for a period that varies from person to person. Moreover, PUs' development depends on age and underlying diseases, as well as on a series of intrinsic and extrinsic factors discussed later.

The term *pressure injury* (PI) replaces *pressure ulcer* in the National Pressure Ulcer Advisory Panel Pressure Injury Staging System, according to the NPUAP (Table 5.1).

**Table 5.1** New definition and classification of PIs [17]

---

*Pressure injury*

A pressure injury is a localized damage to the skin and/or underlying soft tissue, usually over a bony prominence or related to a medical or other devices. The injury can be present as intact skin or an open ulcer and may be painful. The injury occurs as a result of intense and/or prolonged pressure, or pressure in combination with shear. The tolerance of soft tissue for pressure and shear may also be affected by microclimate, nutrition, perfusion, comorbidities, and conditions of the soft tissue

*Stage 1. Pressure injury: non-blanchable erythema of intact skin*

Intact skin with a localized area of non-blanchable erythema, which may appear differently in darkly pigmented skin. Presence of blanchable erythema or changes in sensation, temperature, or firmness may precede visual changes. Color changes do not include purple or maroon discoloration; these may indicate deep tissue pressure injury

*Stage 2. Pressure injury: partial-thickness skin loss with exposed dermis*

Partial-thickness loss of skin with exposed dermis. The wound bed is viable, pink or red, moist, and may also present as an intact or ruptured serum-filled blister. Adipose tissue (fat) is not visible and deeper tissues are not visible. Granulation tissue, slough, and eschar are not present. These injuries commonly result from adverse microclimate and shear in the skin over the pelvis and shear in the heel. This stage should not be used to describe moisture-associated skin damage (MASD) including incontinence-associated dermatitis (IAD), intertriginous dermatitis (ITD), medical adhesive-related skin injury (MARSI), or traumatic wounds (skin tears, burns, abrasions)

*Stage 3. Pressure injury: full-thickness skin loss*

Full-thickness loss of skin, in which adipose (fat) is visible in the ulcer and granulation tissue and epibole (rolled wound edges) are often present. Slough and/or eschar may be visible. The depth of tissue damage varies by anatomical location; areas of significant adiposity can develop deep wounds. Undermining and tunneling may occur. Fascia, muscle, tendon, ligament, cartilage and/or bone are not exposed. If slough or eschar obscures the extent of tissue loss, this is an unstageable pressure injury

---

(continued)

**Table 5.1** (continued)

*Stage 4. Pressure injury: full-thickness skin and tissue loss*

Full-thickness skin and tissue loss with exposed or directly palpable
  fascia, muscle, tendon, ligament, cartilage or bone in the ulcer.
  Slough and/or eschar may be visible. Epibole (rolled edges),
  undermining, and/or tunneling often occur. Depth varies by
  anatomical location. If slough or eschar obscures the extent of tissue
  loss this is an unstageable pressure injury

*Unstageable pressure injury: obscured full-thickness skin and tissue loss*

Full-thickness skin and tissue loss in which the extent of tissue damage
  within the ulcer cannot be confirmed because it is obscured by slough
  or eschar. If slough or eschar is removed, a stage 3 or stage 4 pressure
  injury will be revealed. Stable eschar (i.e., dry, adherent, intact
  without erythema, or fluctuance) on the heel or ischemic limb should
  not be softened or removed

*Deep tissue pressure injury: persistent non-blanchable deep red,
  maroon, or purple discoloration*

Intact or non-intact skin with localized area of persistent non-blanchable
  deep red, maroon, purple discoloration, or epidermal separation
  revealing a dark wound bed or blood-filled blister. Pain and
  temperature change often precede skin color changes. Discoloration
  may appear differently in darkly pigmented skin. This injury results
  from intense and/or prolonged pressure and shear forces at the
  bone-muscle interface. The wound may evolve rapidly to reveal the
  actual extent of tissue injury, or may resolve without tissue loss. If
  necrotic tissue, subcutaneous tissue, granulation tissue, fascia,
  muscle, or other underlying structures are visible, this indicates a full
  thickness pressure injury (unstageable, stage 3 or stage 4). Do not use
  DTPI should not be used to describe vascular, traumatic, neuropathic
  or dermatologic conditions

## 5.3.2   Epidemiology

Elderly and ICU patients are the populations most affected by
PIs. These dimensions are important both for the number of
patients involved and for time and resources required to treat it.
As concomitant comorbidity, PIs, in fact, negatively influence
the quality of life and drastically worsen the prognosis [18–20].

A review carried out in this area showed that among IV° stage injuries the incidence of osteomyelitis was around 32%, while another study has reported that severe stage infections evolved very often in severe sepsis with mortality rates at 6 months, up to 68% [21].

Only a few studies investigated PIs' prevalence in ICU. Some researches showed that over 15% of ICU patients developed a PI during their stay, while the elderly was the highest-risk population of patients. In general, from 34% to 81% of the PIs arise within the first 10 days of hospitalization [22–24].

## 5.3.3   Physiopathology and Main Risk Factors

Most PIs develop when compression of soft tissues occurs for a prolonged time, as for tissues placed between a bony protuberance and a surface, such as the bed mattress. When the constrictive force between body surface and mattress is more intense than blood pressure relative to the compressed arteriolar capillary, it determines a condition of permanent ischemia [25]. Among the main risk factors, there are nurses' workload, patient's gender, albumin blood level, and hemodynamic instability during positioning, vasopressor administration, and previous surgery [15].

## 5.3.4   Risk Assessment

An accurate clinical evaluation is crucial to identify the patients at risk for PIs' development [26], particularly for those with previous PIs' history, who are considered at risk irrespective of the assessment score [27]. PIs' risk is established combining the clinical judgment with the use of a reliable scale. The use of assessment tools to predict individual patient risk factors for

PIs' development is routinely recommended in PIs' prevention guidelines [15]. Studies suggest the adoption of the Braden scale that has been tested and validated in various settings of care (including ICUs) [28, 29]. The Braden scale takes into account six items scored from 1 to 4 points (sensory perception, moisture, activity, mobility) and is identified as the scale with the best combined sensitivity and specificity in predicting risk of PIs in general wards.

The lowest the score, the highest is the PIs' risk, with a risk cutoff $\leq 16$ points [30]. Despite its wide validation, a case-control study [31] suggested a low implementation rate in ICU (only 11.26% of hospital days), also highlighting a low to moderate positive predicting performance. Interestingly, a lower-risk cutoff ($\leq 13$) balanced the highest sensitivity and specificity (0.75 and 0.47, respectively). Similar results were found a few years later [32] in a large retrospective study, indicating a poor accuracy of the Braden scale in predicting PIs, mainly related to the lack of consideration for ICU-specific risk factors such as MV, hypotension, cardiovascular instability, and ICU-LOS.

The Braden scale does not identify hemodynamic instability as a risk factor for PIs' development. This kind of clinical condition is common in the ICU. One consequence of hemodynamic instability that may contribute to PIs' development is the impossibility to accomplish patient repositioning [15].

Another available tool for PIs' assessment is the Cubbin-Jackson scale, originally introduced in 1991 [33]. The first version of this scale was composed of ten items (age, weight, skin conditions, mental conditions, mobility, hemodynamics, respiration, nutrition, incontinence, and hygiene) [33]. Each item was scored from 1 to 4, and highest scores were associated with lower risk. Further improvements introduced oxygen requirements, past medical history, and detrimental factors (surgery, transport for diagnostic imaging, need for hemotransfusion, or hypothermia) [34]. The risk cutoff, previously stated at 24 points, was moved on to 29. As for other tools, the Cubbin-Jackson scale showed an unsatisfactory performance in ICU populations, reaffirming the importance to use clinical judgment together with stratification tools [35] (Fig. 5.3).

| Age (years) | Score point | Hemodynamics | Score point |
|---|---|---|---|
| <40 | 4 | Stable without inotropes | 4 |
| 40-54 | 3 | Stable with inotropes | 3 |
| 55-70 | 2 | Unstable without inotropes | 2 |
| >70 | 1 | Unstable with inotropes | 1 |
| **Weight/tissue viability** | | **Respiration** | |
| Average weight BMI 18-25.9 kg/m$^2$ | 4 | Spontaneous | 4 |
| Obese 26-39.9 kg/m$^2$ | 3 | Non-nvasive, CPAP/BiPAP | 3 |
| Cachectic <18 kg/m$^2$ | 2 | Mechanical ventilation | 2 |
| Any of the above plus severe edema or >40 kg/m$^2$ | 1 | Mechanical ventilation. **No spontaneous breathing** | 1 |
| **Past medical history** | | **Oxygen requirements** | |
| None | 4 | Requires <40% $O_2$, stable on movement | 4 |
| Mild | 3 | Requires 40%-60% $O_2$, stable on movement | 3 |
| Severe | 2 | Requires 40%-60% $O_2$, stable ABGs but desaturates on movement | 2 |
| Very Severe | 1 | Requires 60% $O_2$ or above.Inability to maintain ABGs/desaturates at rest | 1 |
| **General skin condition** | | **Nutrition** | |
| Intact | 4 | Full diet + fluids | 4 |
| Red skin affecting areas prone to pressure | 3 | Clear IV fluids only | 3 |
| Grazed/excoriated superficial skin areas | 2 | Light diet, oral fluids, enteral feeding | 2 |
| Deep wounds, necrotized or heavily exudating wounds | 1 | Parenteral feeding | 1 |
| **Mental condition** | | **Incontinence** | |
| Awake and alert | 4 | None/anuric/catheterized (urine **and/or feces catheter)** | 4 |
| Agitated/restless/confused | 3 | Urine/profound sweating | 3 |
| Apathic/sedated but responsive | 2 | Feces/occassional diarrhea | 2 |
| Coma/unresponsive/paralyzed and sedated | 1 | Urine and feces/prologed diarrhea (≥3 times/day) | 1 |
| **Mobility** | | **Hygiene** | |
| Walks with help | 4 | Independent | 4 |
| Very limited, chairbound | 3 | Needs assistance | 3 |
| Immobile but tolerates change of position | 2 | Needs much assistance | 2 |
| Unable to tolerate moverment, nursed prone | 1 | Fully dependent | 1 |
| **Deduct points** | | | |
| Deduct 1 point, if patient has been in surgery or transported to CT, MRI or **HBOT during the last 48 hours** | | | |
| Deduct 1 point, if patient has required blood or clotting factors **during last 24 hours** | | | |
| Deduct 1 point, if patient has hypothermia of **35°C or under (core temperature)** | | | |

*Revised sections (marked as bolded) of the Jackson/Cubbin risk scale[14] Utilized in this program to improve the clarity and reproducibility of the scale. The maximum score is 48 (low risk) and the minimum score 9 points signifying high risk.*
*BMI = body mass index; CPAP= continuous positive airway pressure; BiPAP = bilevel positive airway pressure; ABGs = arterial blood gases; CT = computerized tomography; MRI = magnetic resonance imaging; HBOT = hyperbaric oxygen therapy*

**Fig. 5.3** Cubbin-Jackson pressure ulcer risk scale [35] "used with permission"

Recently, the development and implementation of the COHMON (conscious level, mobility, hemodynamics, oxygenation, nutrition) index opened a new opportunity in the evaluation of PIs' risk. This tool includes five items (level of consciousness, mobility, hemodynamic, oxygenation, and nutrition) scored from 1 to 4 points (the higher is the score, the higher is the risk). When compared with traditional scoring systems, the COHMON index showed a better sensitivity and specificity, positive and negative predictive values, and very good reliability both for single items and the global index [36]. When compared with Braden, Norton, and Waterlow scales, this index also showed the highest interrater reliability and agreement [37].

Irrespective of the chosen PIs' risk assessment tool, use of vasopressors (vasopressin and norepinephrine), mean arterial pressure <60 mmHg, cardiac arrest, and prolonged MV (>72 h) has been associated with PIs' development [38], thus suggesting the need for a higher vigilance in patients with those clinical and treatment features.

Currently, there is no strong evidence regarding optimal PIs' risk reassessment intervals. Widely accepted and published clinical standards suggest a weekly revaluation. However, in certain clinical situations, risk assessment scales may have limits, since they don't consider PIs' risk associated with the use of devices.

## 5.4   Conclusions

The intensive care unit-acquired weakness is an important adverse effect due to bed rest in critically ill patients. This kind of complication is a hindrance to implement a fast recovery of patients. For these reasons, nurses during their clinical practice should keep in mind the eventuality of its emergence and early activate the search of its clinical signs. Moreover, one of the new aims to pursue is to implement the ICU-AW prevention through an active collaboration in early patients' positioning, progressive mobilization, and active collaboration during physiotherapy interventions. These activities should become nursing priorities in the ICUs' dynamic frameworks, since there are scarce contraindications to start progressive mobility programs during acuity conditions. These are hemodynamic instability, intracranial hypertension, and severe multiple bone injuries. Another major positive consequence of early mobilization is the pressure ulcers (pressure injuries—PIs) prevention in ICU.

Currently the use of Braden scale for PIs' risk assessment in critical care patients seems not to be further recommended because it has a poor accuracy in predicting PIs, mainly related to the lack of consideration for ICU-specific risk factors such as MV, hypotension, cardiovascular instability, and ICU-LOS. Even the Cubbin-Jackson scale seems to have important limitations in some ICU populations. Recently, a new scale, called COHMON (conscious level, mobility, hemodynamics, oxygenation, nutrition) index for PIs' risk assessment in ICU, seems to be promising.

## Take-Home Messages

- ICU-AW is one of the most underrated complications in ICU patients.
- Early mobilization programs and optimal nutritional support are the main interventions to prevent the development of ICU-AW.
- Prevention of PIs is an established nursing quality indicator.
- Multidisciplinary approaches to reduce the risk of ICU-AW and HAPU are needed.

# References

1. Truong AD, Fan E, Brower RG, Needham DM. Bench-to-bedside review: mobilizing patients in the intensive care unit—from pathophysiology to clinical trials. Crit Care. 2009;13:216. https://doi.org/10.1186/cc7885.

 2. Allen C, Glasziou P, Del Mar C. Bed rest: a potentially harmful treatment needing more careful evaluation. Lancet. 1999;354:1229–33. https://doi.org/10.1016/S0140-6736(98)10063-6.
 3. McPeake J, Quasim T. Quality of life in intensive care survivors. Br J Nurs. 2015;24:1016. 10.12968/bjon.2015.24.20.1016.
 4. Gillespie BM, Chaboyer WP, McInnes E, Kent B, Whitty JA, Thalib L. Repositioning for pressure ulcer prevention in adults. Cochrane Database Syst Rev. 2014;4:Cd009958. https://doi.org/10.1002/14651858.CD009958.pub2.
 5. Fletcher SN, Kennedy DD, Ghosh IR, Misra VP, Kiff K, Coakley JH, et al. Persistent neuromuscular and neurophysiologic abnormalities in long-term survivors of prolonged critical illness. Crit Care Med. 2003;31:1012–6. https://doi.org/10.1097/01.CCM.0000053651.38421.D9.
 6. Asfour HI. Contributing factors for acquired muscle weakness in the intensive care unit. J Nurs Educ Pract. 2016;6:102–11. https://doi.org/10.5430/jnep.V6n8p102.
 7. Rukstele CD, Gagnon MM. Making strides in preventing ICU-acquired weakness involving family in early progressive mobility. Crit Care Nurs Q. 2013;36:141–7. https://doi.org/10.1097/CNQ.0b013e31827539cc.
 8. Fan E. Critical illness neuromyopathy and the role of physical therapy and rehabilitation in critically ill patients. Respir Care. 2012;57:933–44. https://doi.org/10.4187/respcare.01634.
 9. SE H, Kannus P, Natri A, Latvala K, Järvinen MJ. Isokinetic performance of the thigh muscles after tibial plateau fractures. Int Orthop. 1997;21:323–6.
10. Hollander JM, Mechanick JI. Nutrition support and the chronic critical illness syndrome. Nutr Clin Pract. 2006;21:587–604. https://doi.org/10.1177/0115426506021006587.
11. Hermans G, De Jonghe B, Bruyninckx F, Van den Berghe G. Interventions for preventing critical illness polyneuropathy and critical illness myopathy. Cochrane Database Syst Rev. 2014;30:CD006832. https://doi.org/10.1002/14651858.CD006832.pub3.
12. Morris PE, Goad A, Thompson C, Taylor K, Harry B, Passmore L, et al. Early intensive care unit mobility therapy in the treatment of acute respiratory failure. Crit Care Med. 2008;36:2238–43. https://doi.org/10.1097/CCM.0b013e318180b90e.
13. Foster J. Complications of sedation in critical illness: an update. Crit Care Nurs Clin North Am. 2016;28:227–39. https://doi.org/10.1016/j.cnc.2016.02.003.

14. Gosselink R, Bott J, Johnson M, Dean E, Nava S, Norrenberg M, et al. Physiotherapy for adult patients with critical illness: recommendations of the European Respiratory Society and European Society of Intensive Care Medicine Task Force on physiotherapy for critically ill patients. Intensive Care Med. 2008;34:1188–99. https://doi.org/10.1007/s00134-008-1026-7.

15. Krupp AE, Monfre J. Pressure ulcers in the ICU patient: an update on prevention and treatment. Curr Infect Dis Rep. 2015;17:468. https://doi.org/10.1007/s11908-015-0468-7.

16. National Pressure Ulcer Advisory Panel, European Pressure Ulcer Advisory Panel and Pan Pacific Pressure Injury Alliance. Prevention and Treatment of Pressure Ulcers: Quick Reference Guide. Emily Haesler (Ed.). Cambridge Media: Osborne Park; 2014.

17. National Pressure Ulcer Advisory Panel (NPUAP). Announcement of change in terminology from pressure ulcer to pressure injury. 2016. http://www.npuap.org/national-pressure-ulcer-advisory-panel-npuap-announces-a-change-in-terminology-from-pressure-ulcer-to-pressure-injury-and-updates-the-stages-of-pressure-injury/. Accessed 7 Apr 2017.

18. Jugun K, Richard JC, Lipsky BA, Kressmann B, Pittet-Cuenod B, Suvà D, et al. Factors associated with treatment failure of infected pressure sores. Ann Surg. 2016;264:399–403. https://doi.org/10.1097/SLA.0000000000001497.

19. Rennert R, Golinko M, Yan A, Flattau A, Tomic-Canic M, Brem H. Developing and evaluating outcomes of an evidence-based protocol for the treatment of osteomyelitis in Stage IV pressure ulcers: literature and wound electronic medical record database review. Ostomy Wound Manage. 2009;55:42–53.

20. Brunel AS, Lamy B, Cyteval C, Perrochia H, Téot L, Masson R, et al. OSTEAR Study Group. Diagnosing pelvic osteomyelitis beneath pressure ulcers in spinal cord injured patients: a prospective study. Clin Microbiol Infect. 2016;22:267.E1–8. https://doi.org/10.1016/j.cmi.2015.11.005.

21. Schiffman J, Golinko MS, Yan A, Flattau A, Tomic-Canic M, Brem H. Operational debridement of pressure ulcers. World J Surg. 2009;33:1396–402. https://doi.org/10.1007/s00268-009-0024-4.

22. Behrendt R, Ghaznavi AM, Mahan M, Craft S, Siddiqui A. Continuous bedside pressure mapping and rates of hospital-associated pressure ulcers in a medical intensive care unit. Am J Crit Care. 2014;23:127–33. https://doi.org/10.4037/ajcc2014192.

23. Cremasco MF, Wenzel F, Zanei SS, Whitaker IY. Pressure ulcers in the intensive care unit: the relationship between nursing workload, illness

severity and pressure ulcer risk. J Clin Nurs. 2013;22:2183–91. https://doi.org/10.1111/j.1365-2702.2012.04216.x.

24. Barrois B, Labalette C, Rousseau P, Corbin A, Colin D, Allaert F, et al. A national prevalence study of pressure ulcers in the French hospital inpatients. J Wound Care. 2008;17:373–6, 378–9. 10.12968/jowc.2008.17.9.30934.

25. Martin E. Concise medical dictionary. 9th ed. Oxford: Oxford University Press; 2015. Market House Books

26. National Institute for Health and Care Excellence (NICE). Pressure ulcers. https://www.nice.org.uk/guidance/qs89 . Accessed 7 Apr 2017.

27. Bredesen IM, Bjøro K, Gunningberg L, Hofoss D. Effect of e-learning program on risk assessment and pressure ulcer classification—a randomized study. Nurse Educ Today. 2016;40:191–7. https://doi.org/10.1016/j.nedt.2016.03.008.

28. Bergstrom N, Braden BJ, Laguzza A, Holman V. The Braden Scale for predicting pressure sore risk. Nurs Res. 1987;36:205–10.

29. Swafford K, Culpepper R, Dunn C. Use of a comprehensive program to reduce the incidence of hospital-acquired pressure ulcers in an intensive care unit. Am J Crit Care. 2016;25:152–5. https://doi.org/10.4037/ajcc2016963.

30. Serpa LF, Santos VL, Campanili TC, Queiroz M. Predictive validity of the Braden scale for pressure ulcer risk in critical care patients. Rev Lat Am Enfermagem. 2011;19:50–7.

31. Cho I, Noh M. Braden Scale: evaluation of clinical usefulness in an intensive care unit. J Adv Nurs. 2010;66:293–302. https://doi.org/10.1111/j.1365-2648.2009.05153.x.

32. Hyun S, Vermillion B, Newton C, Fall M, Li X, Kaewprag P, et al. Predictive validity of the Braden scale for patients in intensive care units. Am J Crit Care. 2013;22:514–20. https://doi.org/10.4037/ajcc2013991.

33. Jackson C. The revised Jackson/Cubbin pressure area risk calculator. Intensive Crit Care Nurs. 1999;15:169–75.

34. Wheeler H. Positioning: one good turn after another? Nurs Crit Care. 1997;2:129–31.

35. Ahtiala MH, Soppi E, Kivimäki R. Critical evaluation of the Jackson/Cubbin pressure ulcer risk scale—a secondary analysis of a retrospective cohort study population of intensive care patients. Ostomy Wound Manage. 2016;62:24–33.

36. Cobos Vargas A, Garofano Jerez JR, Guardia Mesa MF, Carrasco Muriel C, Lopez Perez F, Gonzalez Ramırez AR, et al. Design and validation of a new rating scale (COMHON Index) to estimate the risk of

pressure ulcer in patients attended in critical care units. Connect: The World of Critical Care. Nursing. 2011;8:41.
37. Fulbrook P, Anderson A. Pressure injury risk assessment in intensive care: comparison of inter-rater reliability of the COMHON (Conscious level, Mobility, Haemodynamics, Oxygenation, Nutrition) Index with three scales. J Adv Nurs. 2016;72:680–92. https://doi.org/10.1111/jan.12825.
38. Cox J, Roche S. Vasopressors and development of pressure ulcers in adult critical care patients. Am J Crit Care. 2015;24:501–10. https://doi.org/10.4037/ajcc2015123.

# Part II
# Basic Care in ICU

# Chapter 6
# Interventional Patient Hygiene Model: New Insights in Critical Care Nursing, Starting from the Basics of Care

Stefano Bambi

## 6.1 Introduction

The modern ICUs are widely diffused from the 1970s, with the introduction of the positive-pressure mechanical ventilators to support the respiratory function and the advanced hemodynamic monitoring performed with pulmonary artery catheters [1].

After a first phase characterized for the healthcare professionals' attention focused on the technologies supporting and monitoring the vital function and the organs/systems of patients, the appearance of evidence-based medicine and nursing, about 20 years ago, has deeply modified the approach to the patients and environments. The evidence-based practice (EBP), together with other tools of clinical governance as clinical risk management and health technology assessment, has shifted critical care medicine toward a more proactive patient-centered approach. Moreover, we have assisted to the introduction of critical thinking about the risk-benefit balancing related to the employment of vital support technologies, the medical humanities movement, and the liberalizing of the visiting policies in the ICUs [2]. Lastly, ethical issues related to the limitations of care delivering

© Springer International Publishing AG, part of Springer Nature 2018    157
I. Comisso et al., *Nursing in Critical Care Setting*,
https://doi.org/10.1007/978-3-319-50559-6_6

and to the availability of resources are exerting an important influence on the choices made by the ICU teams [2].

At present, the new mantra of healthcare is "to ensure safety, be proactive." Behind this simple rule, there is the professionals' attention focused to reach patients' health outcomes while preventing iatrogenic complications.

Hospital-acquired conditions (HAC) are a set of unanticipated complications occurring during patients' stay in hospital [3]. These are air embolism, blood incompatibility, catheter-acquired urinary tract infection (CAUTI), pressure ulcers (PUs), vascular catheter-associated infections, surgical site infections (SSI), falls and trauma, and objects left during surgery [3]. A special subset of HAC is the hospital-acquired infections (HAIs), defined as infections that are acquired by a patient during a hospitalization [3]. HAC and HAI determine an increasing of hospital LOS, mortality, and costs. It's esteemed that every year 1.7 million of HAIs contribute to 99,000 patients' deaths [3].

Nursing care is strongly involved in the development and, so, in the prevention of HAC and HAI [3]. Lots of nursing-sensitive outcomes showed how this statement is true, and it's mainly related to the quality of delivered basic nursing care (e.g., incidence rates of PU, failure to rescue rate, HAP, ventilator-associated pneumonia (VAP), CAUTI, CLABSI, patients falls, patients restraints) [4].

## 6.2 From Evidence-Based Nursing to Interventional Patient Hygiene Model: The Conceptual Framework

About 10 years ago, some authors introduced a new school of nursing thought called "get back to the basics" or "get back to the fundamentals of care." This movement is centered on the concept of "patient's safety—do not to harm", focusing on the prevention of errors during the delivering of critical care nursing [5]. Most nursing interventions that produce patients outcomes are basic, as mobilization and hygiene [5]. According to some authors, nurses seem to have missed their attention to the basic of nursing in favor of advanced competences and delegate the basic care interventions to nursing aids or non-licensed staff [3]. Actually these two approaches are not mutually exclusive, and the value of nursing basic interventions needs to be rediscovered [3].

Evidence-based (basic) nursing intervention can heavily affect patients' outcomes (also when included in bundle of care) [6] contributing to the prevention of HAC and HAI. In Table 6.1 there are some examples of evidence of basic care interventions related to patients' sensitive outcomes. Currently, a simple saving life action as hand hygiene has a poor compliance by healthcare personnel (almost 40%) [8].

Kathleen Vollman, a nurse with large experience in critical care and a great spirit of professional innovation, has made critical reflections about the link between safety, patients outcomes, and basic nursing care. On this basis, she has designed a new model for critical care nursing: the Interventional Patient Hygiene Model (IPHM) [5]. Vollman used the term hygiene in its wider meaning, that is, "the science of establishing and maintaining health" [5].

This model considers a systematic approach to implement evidence-based basic nursing intervention on patients hygiene (bioburden reduction) and mobility strategies to proactively prevent HAI and skin injuries [5]. The components of IPHM were originally bed bathing management, oral care, wound dressing, mobilization, incontinence management, and urinary catheter care [27]. Later, hand hygiene and skin antisepsis have been included in the model [28] (Fig. 6.1).

**Table 6.1** Interventional Patient Hygiene Model issues and evidence-based nursing basic care interventions

| Issue | Intervention | References |
|---|---|---|
| Hand hygiene | Hand hygiene technique<br>Surgical hand preparation<br>Selection and handling of hand hygiene agents<br>Skin care<br>Use of gloves | CDC guidelines [7]<br>WHO guidelines [8] |
| VAP | HOB elevation 30°–45°<br>Sedation daily interruptions and weaning readiness evaluation<br>Peptic ulcers prevention<br>DVT prevention<br>Chlorhexidine rinse for oral care<br>Endotracheal tubes with subglottic drainage lumen | Wip and Napolitano, 2009 [9]<br>Bouadma et al., 2012 [10] |
| CAUTI | Appropriateness of urinary catheter insertion criteria (indications)<br>Early removal of urinary catheters<br>Use of urinary catheter in perioperative period, only if there is a real need (not routine insertion)<br>Insertion of urinary catheter through aseptic technique, when performed in hospital setting<br>Adequate fixation of the catheter to prevent urethral traction and movement<br>Use of urinary closed systems<br>The urine collection bag should not lay on the floor<br>Change of the urinary catheter and collection bag only in presence of clear clinical indication (not routine changes)<br>Routine hygiene of periurethral area without antiseptic solutions | NHS epic3 guidelines [11]<br>HICPAC guidelines [12] |

**Table 6.1**  (continued)

| Issue | Intervention | References |
|-------|-------------|-----------|
| CLABSI | Early removal of intravascular catheters that are no longer needed<br>Hand hygiene technique<br>Surveillance on aseptic technique maintenance<br>Adoption of alcohol-based chlorhexidine solutions >0.5%<br>Wound dressing<br>Infusion set and transducers' interval of change<br>Daily patient bath with chlorhexidine 2% solutions | NHS epic3 guidelines [11]<br>CDC guidelines [13]<br>Shah et al., 2016 [14] |
| SSI | Preoperative bath or showering<br>No routine preoperative hair removal<br>If hair removal is necessary, use clipping<br>No routine mechanical bowel preparation unless mandatory<br>Aseptic technique/no touch for wound dressing change<br>Normal saline for cleaning the surgical wound<br>Postoperative bath or showering | SHEA/IDSA practice recommendations [15]<br>NICE guidelines [16, 17]<br>Dayton et al., 2013 [18]<br>Karki et al., 2012 [19]<br>Cochrane systematic review [20] |

(continued)

**Table 6.1**  (continued)

| Issue | Intervention | References |
|-------|-------------|------------|
| Skin injury | Incontinence-associated dermatitis<br>    Use skin cleanser with<br>adequate pH instead of water and<br>soap<br>    Skin protectant agents<br>    Polymer diaper or underpads<br>are better than non-polymer tools<br>to prevent dermatitis<br>Pressure ulcer bundle<br>    Comprehensive skin<br>assessment<br>    Pressure ulcers risk<br>standardized assessment<br>    Nursing planning and<br>implementation on skin areas at<br>risk of ulcer<br>Skin care/hygiene<br>    The kind of cleanser or soap<br>affects the skin pH<br>    Alkaline cleanser determines a<br>significant increasing of skin pH<br>    Cleanser agents with pH > 5.5<br>should not be employed in ICU<br>Bed bathing<br>    98% of basin for patients<br>hygiene with soap and water are<br>prone to develop biofilm<br>    Hygiene performed through<br>chlorhexidine reduces the<br>contamination of the basins | Beeckman et al.,<br>    2009 [21]<br>Sullivan and<br>    Schoelles, 2013<br>    [22]<br>AHRQ PU bundle<br>    [23]<br>Duncan et al., 2013<br>    [24]<br>Powers et al., 2012<br>    [25]<br>Johnson et al., 2009<br>    [26] |

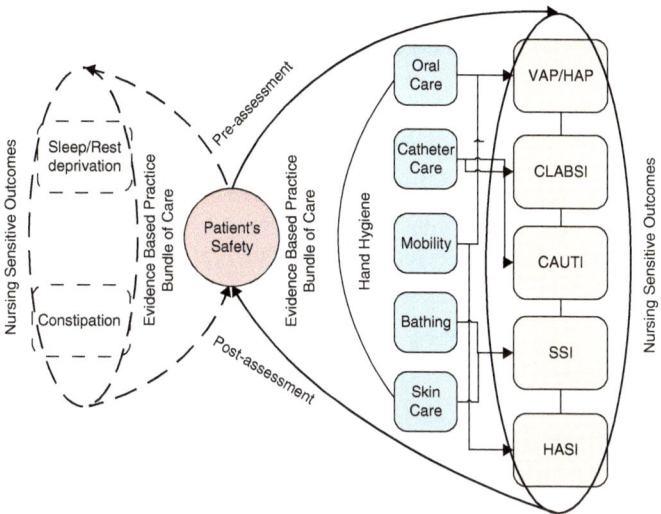

**Fig. 6.1** Interventional Patient Hygiene Model [5, 28]. *Dot line:* potential development of the model. *CAUTI* catheter-associated urinary tract infection, *CLABSI* central line-associated bloodstream infection, *HAP* hospital-acquired pneumonia, *HASI* hospital-acquired skin injury, *SSI* surgical site infection, *VAP* ventilator-associated pneumonia

Vollman suggests the implementation of IPHM according to the Deming Cycle (PDCA–plan–do–check–act) [5]:

- Assessment about the level of evidence of routine nursing practices should be first performed.
- Devise of a bundle of nursing intervention to implement the IPHM.
- Pre-intervention measure of nursing-sensitive outcomes.
- Selection of processes and products to ease the changing, with a shared decision-making approach.
- Implementation of the bundle.

- Post-intervention measure of nursing-sensitive outcomes and comparison with the baseline data.
- Celebration of the obtained improvement.
- Trimestral assessment of the compliance levels to the bundle till it will be routinely implemented.

The support to the changing of nursing practices is based on three main cornerstones: knowledge and skills, attitude and accountability, and resources and system [5].

## 6.3    The Priorities of Intensive Care Nursing

The implementation of a nursing model is based on the basics of care as the IPHM needs to be matched with a deep reflection about the nursing priorities in the critical care setting. The reason is that the hygiene process is active and needs high-level priority among the tasks routinely performed by critical care nurses [3]. Traditionally, the concept of priorities in the healthcare framework is related to the well-known lifesaving ABCDE resuscitation approach, deriving from the advanced trauma life support guidelines and education courses, since the 1980s [29]. The ABCDE is a vertical-order approach to the evaluation and resolution of lifesaving problems applied in all kinds of emergency codes inside and outside the hospital. This simple and mnemonic method is very useful and effective to establish the priorities of medical and nursing interventions [30].

In ICU the concept of priority takes on a wider meaning than in the emergency settings and involves all the team of care and all the nursing care activities [31]. In fact, the nursing care plans can be frequently modified by the changes of the patients' clinical conditions and the sudden emergence of new diagnostic or therapeutic needs. These variations can considerably affect the sequence in which the medical and nursing activities are accomplished [31]. Therefore, some nursing care interventions should be delayed, or even deleted from the scheduling in the work-shift. The multitasking nature of the nurses' work in ICU is characterized for a mix of basic and advanced assessments and interventions continuously rearranged [31]. For example, the sudden medical order of a computed tomography scan can over-come the scheduled oral care and wound dressing of a patient. As a result, the referral nurse for that patient has immediately to prepare him for in-hospital transfer to radiological department, rearranging the plan of care [31]. This way to perform the tasks is beyond the question. Nevertheless, the real strength of nurs-ing basic care interventions lies in their continuity. Lots of nurs-ing interventions as oral hygiene, HOB elevation, controlling the cuff pressure of endotracheal tubes, regular repositioning, and scrubbing the vascular catheters' hubs before access, affect positively the patients' outcomes only if carefully performed and frequently repeated [31]. The task-time imperatives tradi-tionally featuring the work shifts [32], together with the current increasing in workloads and the lack of resources [33], induce critical care nurses to make "triage" decision about their sched-uled activities, even if based on effectiveness evidence coming from clinical research. A large multicenter cross-sectional study performed on 33,659 medical and surgical nurses from 488 hospitals in 12 European countries, has revealed that the nursing tasks left undone due to lack of time were mainly "comfort talk to patients" (median 47.5%, range 36%–81%), "educating patients and family" (median 47%, range 24%–61%), "oral hygiene" (median 30.5%, range 23%–62%), and "patient sur-veillance" (median 25.5%, range 15%–56%) [33]. Observational studies have showed that the missed nursing care is significantly lower if the number of hours per patient day is higher [34]. Nevertheless, critical care nurses recognize high priorities to the basic nursing care. A survey, performed in two ICUs in the UK, asked nurses to rate the priority given to basic nursing care on a scale from 1 (lowest) to 10 (highest). "Eye care," "oral care," "bowel care," and "personal hygiene" obtained mean scores from 7.81 to 8.61, compared to the score of 9.76 given to the "care related to the reason for admission" [35].

The driving force to maintain high levels of priority for basic nursing care should rely upon outcomes measuring systems. Nurses should be informed about the incidence and trends of the major and minor complications that they contribute to prevent through their basic care interventions. In a survey performed by American Association of Critical Care, 80% of respondent nurses stated that they didn't know the VAP incidence rate in their institution [36]. In the same study, only 47% of nurses rated oral care as high priority, and only 48% have sufficient time to perform oral hygiene to patients every 4 h [36].

## 6.4    Experiences About the IPHM Implementation

Despite a strong rationale coming from evidence-based nursing interventions, at the present there are few published studies about the implementation of IPHM in clinical practice.

McGuckin et al., in a survey performed to determine the knowledge about the components of IPHM on nurses who attended at the Association of Critical Care Nurses Annual Meetings and Association of Professionals in Infection Control and Epidemiology Annual Meetings (in years 2004–2006), found high percentages of knowledge base: hand hygiene (96%), oral hygiene (95%), early preoperative skin preparation (70%), bathing/skin care (94%), and incontinence care (93%)  [28]. However, the survey revealed that nurses were much less informed about the outcomes related to the IPHM and about the presence of IPH policies in their institutions (less than 50%) [28]. Nurses should be aware about the economic impact of IPHM implementation, beyond the "lonely" healthcare outcome affected by the model. McGuckin et al. reported that the removal of prepackaged bath towel product from an ICU, in favor of the adoption of standard basins and towels for daily bathing of patients, produced the increasing of UTI rates from 9 infections per 1000 device days to 15 infections per 1000 device days, during 9 months of surveillance [28]. A projection about the costs determined by these changes, taking in account the increased LOS due to the higher rates of UTIs, showed a redoubled healthcare expense if compared with the "prepackaged bath towel" product period [28].

After only 2 years from the introduction of the "daily bathing with an antibacterial soap" practice in a US hospital, the incidence rates of MRSA, VRE, *Klebsiella*, and quinolone-resistant *Escherichia coli* were lowered nearly to 0%, saving over 2 millions of dollars [37].

Carr and Benoit implemented an IPH program integrating patients' bathing and incontinence protocols in a surgical ICU in the USA [38]. The aims of this evidence-based program were to reduce the incidence of PUs, improve the clinical knowledge in non-licensed staff, and enhance their communication with the ICU nurses. The improvement program was performed through six areas: staff empowerment, early identification of skin changes, assessment of patient risk, implementation of quality improvement initiatives, task delegation to non-licensed staff, and communication among staff members [38]. The program was successfully implemented: PUs' incidence decreased from 7.14% to 0%. The knowledge of non-licensed staff improved completely in all areas, and a better communication with nurses was reached [38].

Mahanes et al. described the implementation of the advanced practice nurse-led nursing rounds in a Neurosciences ICU in the USA, with the aim to sustain the IPHM and the introduction of evidence-based nursing practices, maintaining the view on nursing care multiple priorities [39]. The core concept behind the implementation of the rounds was "to highlight nursing indicators for each patient and provide a time for sharing of ideas to improve outcomes." Nurses discussion focused mainly around the patients' vulnerability, management of constipation, incontinence care, pain management, and mobility [39]. Even if, at present, there are no available data about their effectiveness, the APN-led nursing rounds were found "extremely valuable" by over 60% of surveyed nurses, finding an extensive implementation in other hospital's acute care areas [39].

## 6.5  Potential Developments of HPIM

Initially the IPHM included oral care, patients' mobility, wound dressing, bathing, catheters' management, and incontinence management [27]. Later, skin care and hand hygiene were introduced into the model, giving it a wider spectrum of view in terms of complication prevention through the implementation of nursing basic care [28]. Given that HPIM turns around the central concepts of patients' safety and outcomes, we hypothesize that bowel constipation management, and sleep and rest promotion, could be gathered in the model. Currently, nursing interventions to manage these two kinds of problems need more evidences from researches, pointing at a potential weakness for the model. Nonetheless the care about these kinds of patients' needs can heavily affect the outcomes in critical care settings, and we think that these issues should be addressed in the IPHM.

Constipation, defined as failure of the bowel to open from 3 to 9 days [40, 41] affects up to 83% of ICU patients [41]. Despite its high prevalence, only 3.5% of ICU seems to have dedicated protocols to identify and manage the problem. Constipation impacts both on minor (nausea, vomiting, abdominal pain) and major (ICU-LOS, MV duration) outcomes for ICU patients [42, 43].

Moreover, constipation is an independent risk factor for mortality in critically ill patients [43]. Data from observational studies revealed the significant increasing of 12% ($p < 0.001$) in mortality, and of 32% ($p < 0.001$) in acquired bacterial infections between mechanical ventilated patients with late opening of bowel (after the fifth day of ICU stay) [44].

At present, constipation in critically ill patients remains an open issue due to the lack of studies evaluating the efficacy of bowel management protocols implementation, and the important limitations of the published research, often related to small samples or to inclusion criteria [45]. Furthermore, some authors speculated that bowel management protocol failure could be due to the lack of adherence clinicians [46]. Hence, this issue assumes a high value in term of nursing outcomes and interventions, requiring energies to spend in the research and in clinical practice improvement.

Currently, as for bowel management, there are no evidence-based practice guidelines to optimize the conditions of sleep and rest for patients in ICUs [47]. Nevertheless, promoting sleep and rest for patients remains an open issue for ICU nurses because of the important consequences and complications caused by sleep deprivation [48], and it should have a place in the IPHM. The sleep in critically ill patients is mainly characterized by severe fragmentation, equally distributed between day and night, increased time in stage 1 sleep, decreased time in stages 2, 3, 4, REM stage, and increased arousals and awakenings [49]. From an epidemiologic point of view, sleep disturbance in critically ill patients is difficult to estimate, due to the variation in its definition provided in literature. However, studies from literature suggest that high percentages of ICU patients are affected by poor sleep quality, prolonged sleep latency, and frequent arousals/awakenings [50]. Some authors report that 38% of ICU patients had difficulties to fall asleep, and almost 70% of cancer patients admitted in ICU had serious sleep disturbances [50].

Factors affecting the architecture and quality of sleep in ICU patients are [48, 49, 51, 52]:

- Environmental noise, i.e., staff conversations and monitoring alarms
- Prolonged exposure to low levels of artificial light, lighting practices
- Pain or illness and consequent psychosocial stress
- Anxiety
- Psychosis
- Patient care activities, i.e., vital signs, medication administration, and diagnostic testing
- Dyssynchrony with mechanical ventilation
- Inflammatory mediators
- Pharmacological agents, i.e., sedative, opioids, benzodiazepines, and inotropes
- Increased cortisol release
- Decreased endogenous melatonin levels
- Preexisting sleep disorders

At present there is no clear evidence about the relationship between sleep deprivation and mortality in ICU. Researches performed on animals showed that lack of sleep was associated with increasing in mortality rates, offering the basis to hypothesize an association to be proved by large observational studies [51].

However, sleep deprivation produces multisystem consequences in critically ill patients, summarized in Table 6.2.

The approach to prevention of sleep disturbance in ICU is clearly multi-professional and needs a strong contribution from nurses, with simple basic interventions [53].

Some authors have developed a clinical practice guideline (CPG) to promote sleep and rest in ICU patients, using the consultation with healthcare personnel to overcome the lack of evidence from research [47]. The CPG leading principles were provide optimal conditions for nighttime sleep, optimize circadian rhythm, manage pain well, and provide a daytime rest period [47]. The components of rest and sleep CPG were

**Table 6.2** Consequences of sleep disturbance on ICU patients [53]

| System | Consequences |
| --- | --- |
| Neurological | Agitation |
| | Delirium |
| | Post-traumatic stress disorder |
| | Continued sleep disruption |
| | Reduced tolerance of pain |
| | Neurocognitive disfunction |
| Respiratory | Weakness of upper airway muscles |
| | Delayed ventilator weaning |
| | Apnea and hypopneas |
| | Decreased hypercapnic and hypoxic responsiveness |
| Cardiovascular | Arrhythmias |
| | Nocturnal hypertension |
| | Worsening heart failure |
| | Death |
| Immune | Delayed healing |
| | Reduced ability to fight infections |
| | Altered tissue repair |

"optimize the environment," "rest and sleep interventions," and, only at last, "consider sleep-promoting medication" [47]. The nursing interventions provided for the "optimize the environment" were [47]:

- Report faulty equipment and fittings.
- Quiet shoe rule.
- Environmental cleaning during daylight hours only.
- Quiet conversation.
- Lightings appropriate for the time of day.

The "rest and sleep interventions" were [47]:

- Manage pain well.
- Optimize normal circadian rhythm.
- Rest period during daytime hours.
- Provide optimal conditions for nighttime sleep.

The keyword emerging from this project was "sleep hygiene" [47]. Therefore, this issue seems naturally to claim the right to enter in the Interventional Patient Hygiene Model.

Take Home Messages
- Basic nursing care interventions, if constantly performed, can exert a positive influence on patients outcomes and prevent complications.
- At present, the components of IPHM are bathing and incontinence management, patient mobility, oral care, dressing change, surgical site infection care, hand hygiene, skin antisepsis, and urinary catheter care.
- HPIM provides for evidence-based nursing interventions and nursing-sensitive outcomes assessment.
- HPIM gives a conceptual framework to strengthen the nursing priorities.

# References

1. Vincent JL. Critical care - where have we been and where are we going? Crit Care. 2013;17:S2. https://doi.org/10.1186/cc11500.
2. Bambi S, Lucchini A, Solaro M, Lumini E, Rasero L. Interventional Patient Hygiene Model. A critical reflection on basic nursing care in intensive care units. Assist Inferm Ric. 2014;33:90–6. https://doi.org/10.1702/1539.16815.
3. Burns SM, Day T. A return to the basics: "Interventional Patient Hygiene" (a call for papers). Intensive Crit Care Nurs. 2012;28:193–6. https://doi.org/10.1016/j.iccn.2012.05.004.
4. Savitz LA, Jones CB, Bernard S. Quality Indicators Sensitive to Nurse Staffing in Acute Care Settings. In: Henriksen K, Battles JB, Marks ES, et al., editors. Advances in Patient Safety: From Research to Implementation (Volume 4: Programs, Tools, and Products). Rockville (MD): Agency for Healthcare Research and Quality (US); 2005. http://www.ncbi.nlm.nih.gov/books/NBK20600/. Accessed 05 Dec 2015.
5. Vollman KM. Interventional patient hygiene: discussion of the issues and a proposed model for implementation of the nursing care basics. Intensive Crit Care Nurs. 2013;29:250. https://doi.org/10.1016/j.iccn.2013.04.004.

6. Camporota L, Brett S. Care bundles: implementing evidence or common sense? Crit Care. 2011;15:159. https://doi.org/10.1186/cc10232.

7. Boyce JM, Pittet D, Healthcare Infection Control Practices Advisory Committee; HICPAC/SHEA/APIC/IDSA Hand Hygiene Task Force. Guideline for Hand Hygiene in Health-Care Settings. Recommendations of the Healthcare Infection Control Practices Advisory Committee and the HICPAC/SHEA/APIC/IDSA Hand Hygiene Task Force. Society for Healthcare Epidemiology of America/Association for Professionals in Infection Control/Infectious Diseases Society of America. MMWR Recomm Rep. 2002;51(RR-16):1–45.

8. World Health Organization. WHO Guidelines on Hand Hygiene in Health Care. First Global Patient Safety Challenge Clean Care Is Safer Care. Geneva: World Health Organization; 2009. http://apps.who.int/iris/bitstream/10665/44102/1/9789241597906_eng.pdf. Accessed 5 Dec 2015.

9. Wip C, Napolitano L. Bundles to prevent ventilator-associated pneumonia: how valuable are they? Curr Opin Infect Dis. 2009;22:159–66. https://doi.org/10.1097/QCO.0b013e3283295e7b.

10. Bouadma L, Wolff M, Lucet JC. Ventilator-associated pneumonia and its prevention. Curr Opin Infect Dis. 2012;25:395–404. https://doi.org/10.1097/QCO.0b013e328355a835.

11. Loveday HP, Wilson JA, Pratt RJ, Golsorkhi M, Tingle A, Bak A, et al. epic3: national evidence-based guidelines for preventing healthcare-associated infections in NHS hospitals in England. J Hosp Infect. 2014;86:S1–70. https://doi.org/10.1016/S0195-6701(13)60012-2.

12. Gould CV, Umscheid CA, Agarwal RK, Kuntz G, Pegues DA, Healthcare Infection Control Practices Advisory Committee. Guideline for prevention of catheter-associated urinary tract infections 2009. Infect Control Hosp Epidemiol. 2010;31:319–26. https://doi.org/10.1086/651091.

13. O'Grady NP, Alexander M, Burns LA, Dellinger EP, Garland J, Heard SO, et al. Summary of Recommendations: Guidelines for the Prevention of Intravascular Catheter-related Infections. Clin Infect Dis. 2011;52:1087–99. https://doi.org/10.1093/cid/cir138.

14. Shah HN, Schwartz JL, Gaye L, Cullen DL. Bathing with 2% chlorhexidine gluconate. evidence and costs associated with central line–associated bloodstream infections. Crit Care Nurs Q. 2016;39:42–50. https://doi.org/10.1097/CNQ.0000000000000096.

15. Anderson DJ, Podgorny K, Berríos-Torres SI, Bratzler DW, Dellinger EP, Greene L, et al. Strategies to prevent surgical site infections in acute care hospitals: 2014 update. Infect Control Hosp Epidemiol. 2014;35:605–27. https://doi.org/10.1086/676022.

16. National Collaborating Centre for Women's and Children's Health (UK). Prevention and treatment of surgical site infection. NICE Clinical Guidelines. London: RCOG Press; 2008. https://www.nice.org.uk/guidance/cg74/evidence/full-guideline-242005933. Accessed 3 Oct 2016.

17. National Institute for Health and Care Excellence. Surgical site infection. Evidence Update June 2013. A summary of selected new evidence relevant to NICE Clinical Guideline 74 'Prevention and treatment of surgical site infection' (2008). Evidence Update 43. Manchester: National Institute for Health and Care; 2013. https://www.nice.org.uk/guidance/cg74/evidence/evidence-update-241969645. Accessed 3 Oct 2016.

18. Dayton P, Feilmeier M, Sedberry S. Does postoperative showering or bathing of a surgical site increase the incidence of infection? A systematic review of the literature. J Foot Ankle Surg. 2013;52:612–4. https://doi.org/10.1053/j.jfas.2013.02.016.

19. Karki S, Cheng AC. Impact of non-rinse skin cleansing with chlorhexidine gluconate on prevention of healthcare-associated infections and colonization with multi-resistant organisms: a systematic review. J Hosp Infect. 2012;82:71–84. https://doi.org/10.1016/j.jhin.2012.07.005.

20. Webster J, Osborne S. Preoperative bathing or showering with skin antiseptics to prevent surgical site infection. Cochrane Database Syst Rev. 2006;2:CD004985. https://doi.org/10.1002/14651858.CD004985.pub2.

21. Beeckman D, Schoonhoven L, Verhaeghe S, Heyneman A, Defloor T. Prevention and treatment of incontinence-associated dermatitis: literature review. J Adv Nurs. 2009;65:1141–54. https://doi.org/10.1111/j.1365-2648.2009.04986.x.

22. Sullivan N, Schoelles KM. Preventing in-facility pressure ulcers as a patient safety strategy: a systematic review. Ann Intern Med. 2013;158:410–6. https://doi.org/10.7326/0003-4819-158-5-201303051-00008.

23. Agency for Healthcare Research and Quality's (AHRQ). Preventing pressure ulcers in hospitals. A Toolkit for improving quality of care. http://www.ahrq.gov/sites/default/files/publications/files/putoolkit.pdf. Accessed 3 Dec 2015.

24. Duncan CN, Riley TV, Carson KC, Budgeon CA, Siffleet J. The effect of an acidic cleanser versus soap on the skin pH and micro-flora of adult patients: a non-randomised two group crossover study in an intensive care unit. Intensive Crit Care Nurs. 2013;29:291–6. https://doi.org/10.1016/j.iccn.2013.03.005.

25. Powers J, Peed J, Burns L, Ziemba-Davis M. Chlorhexidine bathing and microbial contamination in patients' bath basins. Am J Crit Care. 2012;21:338–42. https://doi.org/10.4037/ajcc2012242.

26. Johnson D, Lineweaver L, Maze LM. Patients' bath basins as potential sources of infection: a multicenter sampling study. Am J Crit Care. 2009;18:31–8. https://doi.org/10.4037/ajcc2009968.

27. Vollman K. Back to the fundamentals of care: why now, why us! Aust Crit Care. 2009;22:152. https://doi.org/10.1016/j.aucc.2009.09.001.

28. McGuckin M, Shubin A, Hujcs M. Interventional patient hygiene model: Infection control and nursing share responsibility for patient safety. Am J Infect Control. 2008;36:59–62. https://doi.org/10.1016/j.ajic.2007.01.010.

29. Kool DR, Blickman JG. Advanced Trauma Life Support®. ABCDE from a radiological point of view. Emerg Radiol. 2007;14:135–41. https://doi.org/10.1007/s10140-007-0633-x.

30. Monsieurs KG, Nolan JP, Bossaert LL, Greif R, Maconochie IK, Nikolaou NI, et al. European Resuscitation Council Guidelines for Resuscitation 2015: Section 1. Executive summary. Resuscitation. 2015;95:1–80. https://doi.org/10.1016/j.resuscitation.2015.07.038.

31. Bambi S. Nursing clinical practice in intensive care unit (ICU) settings. Dimens Crit Care Nurs. 2012;31:212–3. https://doi.org/10.1097/DCC.0b013e318253e61f.

32. Farrell GA. From tall poppies to squashed weeds*: why don't nurses pull together more? J Adv Nurs. 2001;35:26–33.

33. Aiken LH, Sloane DM, Bruyneel L, Van den Heede K, Sermeus W, RN4CAST Consortium. Nurses' reports of working conditions and hospital quality of care in 12 countries in Europe. Int J Nurs Stud. 2013;50:143–53. https://doi.org/10.1016/j.ijnurstu.2012.11.009.

34. Kalisch BJ, Tschannen D, Lee KH. Do staffing levels predict missed nursing care? Int J Qual Health Care. 2011;23:302–8. https://doi.org/10.1093/intqhc/mzr009.

35. Jones H, Newton JT, Bower EJ. A survey of the oral care practices of intensive care nurses. Intensive Crit Care Nurs. 2004;20:69–76. https://doi.org/10.1016/j.iccn.2004.01.004.

36. Feider LL, Mitchell P, Bridges E. Oral care practices for orally intubated critically ill adults. Am J Crit Care. 2010;19:175–83. https://doi.org/10.4037/ajcc2010816.

37. McGuckin M, Torress-Cook A. Interventional patient hygiene for the wound care professional. Adv Skin Wound Care. 2009;22:416–20. https://doi.org/10.1097/01.ASW.0000360257.38099.68.

38. Carr D, Benoit R. The role of interventional patient hygiene in improving clinical and economic outcomes. Adv Skin Wound Care. 2009;22:74–8. https://doi.org/10.1097/01.ASW.0000345281.97908.24.

39. Mahanes D, Quatrara BD, Shaw KD. APN-led nursing rounds: an emphasis on evidence-based nursing care. Intensive Crit Care Nurs. 2013;29:256–60. https://doi.org/10.1016/j.iccn.2013.03.004.

40. Mostafa SM, Bhandari S, Ritchie G, Gratton N, Wenstone R. Constipation and its implications in the critically ill patient. Br J Anaesth. 2003;91:815–9.

41. Nassar AP Jr, da Silva FM, de Cleva R. Constipation in intensive care unit: incidence and risk factors. J Crit Care. 2009;24:630.e9–12. https://doi.org/10.1016/j.jcrc.2009.03.007.

42. McPeake J, Gilmour H, Macintosh G. The implementation of a bowel management protocol in an adult intensive care unit. Nurs Crit Care. 2011;16:235–42. https://doi.org/10.1111/j.1478-5153.2011.00451.

43. de Azevedo RP, Rezende Freitas FG, Ferreira EM, Ribeiro MF. Intestinal constipation in intensive care units. Rev Bras Ter Intensiva. 2009;21:324–31.

44. Gacouin A, Camus C, Gros A, Isslame S, Marque S, Lavoué S, et al. Constipation in long-term ventilated patients: associated factors and impact on intensive care unit outcomes. Crit Care Med. 2010;38:1933–8. https://doi.org/10.1097/CCM.0b013e3181eb9236.

45. Bambi S, Lumini E. "Back to basic": starting again from the "basics" of nursing to improve patient outcomes. Scenario. 2012;29:5–7.

46. Knowles S, McInnes E, Elliott D, Hardy J, Middleton S. Evaluation of the implementation of a bowel management protocol in intensive care: effect on clinician practices and patient outcomes. J Clin Nurs. 2014;23:716–30. https://doi.org/10.1111/jocn.12448.

47. Elliott R, McKinley S. The development of a clinical practice guideline to improve sleep in intensive care patients: a solution focused approach. Intensive Crit Care Nurs. 2014;30:246–56. https://doi.org/10.1016/j.iccn.2014.04.003.

48. Pisani MA, Friese RS, Gehlbach BK, Schwab RJ, Weinhouse GL, Jones SF. Sleep in the intensive care unit. Am J Respir Crit Care Med. 2015;191:731–8. https://doi.org/10.1164/rccm.201411-2099CI.

49. Weinhouse GL, Schwab RJ. Sleep in the critically ill patient. Sleep. 2006;29:707–16. https://doi.org/10.1164/rccm.201411-2099CI.

50. Matthews EE. Sleep disturbances and fatigue in critically ill patients. AACN Adv Crit Care. 2011;22:204–24. https://doi.org/10.1097/NCI.0b013e31822052cb.

51. Delaney LJ, Van Haren F, Lopez V. Sleeping on a problem: the impact of sleep disturbance on intensive care patients - a clinical review. Ann Intensive Care. 2015;5:3. https://doi.org/10.1186/s13613-015-0043-2.

52. Friese RS. Sleep and recovery from critical illness and injury: a review of theory, current practice, and future directions. Crit Care Med. 2008;36:697–705. https://doi.org/10.1097/CCM.0B013E3181643F29.

53. Tembo AC, Parker V. Factors that impact on sleep in intensive care patients. Intensive Crit Care Nurs. 2009;25:314–22. https://doi.org/10.1016/j.iccn.2009.07.002.

# Chapter 7
# Eye, Mouth, Skin Care, and Bed Bath

**Gian Domenico Giusti, Irene Comisso, and Alberto Lucchini**

## 7.1 Introduction

The basic care involves all those activities performed in each context of care and in intensive care units that characterize the nurses' job, drawing attention to sensitive outcomes such as infection prevention and patients' safety. For this reason, primary care in this context becomes really important to prevent infections and to safely manage the patients [1].

The study of the importance of basic nursing care has created a school of thought called interventional patient hygiene model (IPHM), extensively treated in Chap. 6, which highlights the patient safety importance, by drawing critical care nurses on the prevention of errors and risks associated with nursing care activities [2].

In this chapter, we will discuss how the basic nursing care to the person in the intensive care unit (ICU) is widely different if compared to other departments, and, especially, the eye, mouth, and skin care management and the bed bath will be highlighted.

© Springer International Publishing AG, part of Springer Nature 2018    177
I. Comisso et al., *Nursing in Critical Care Setting*,
https://doi.org/10.1007/978-3-319-50559-6_7

## 7.2  The Eye Care in ICU

In the past, ICU medical and nursing staff concentrated the majority of their efforts on life-threatening problems, lacking attention to other serious issues [3].

Considering this activity with a low level of priority can lead to complications to the eye level in ICU patients. This situation is promoted by a treatment focused on the organ failure management while delivering a marginal attention to the ocular surface [3–5].

The nursing team should deliver holistic patient care, paying attention to possible factors that may trigger related risk factors or the aggravation of pathologies resulting from ICU hospitalization. Nurses must predict complications and prevent risk factors from advancing to actual problems whenever possible by promoting health within the ICU environment [6].

Ocular disorders in ICU depend on the damage of systemic and ocular protection systems caused by metabolic impairment, multiorgan dysfunctions, invasive and noninvasive mechanical ventilation (MV), reduced level of consciousness, hypotension, and high volemic filling [7–10].

In a healthy individual, the eyelids act as a mechanical barrier that protects the eyes from trauma, dehydration, and adhesion of microorganisms. The cornea's reflex is needed for an adequate distribution of tears on the ocular surface. Corneal moistness is maintained by a lipid film, also when eyes are closed during sleep. Tears contribute to maintain the integrity of ocular surface and to remove noxious and potentially pathogenic stimuli due to their antibacterial properties, being the vehicle for the transit of leucocytes.

The corneal and conjunctival epithelium enhances the maintenance of tears in the eyes. Their constant evaporation allows the conjunctival sac to preserve an adequate temperature to avoid bacterial proliferation. The conjunctival epithelium also furnishes a physical barrier that protects from physical damages and microorganisms. Corneal reflex is a defense from physical menaces, and the REM (rapid eye movements) are essential during sleep to ensure the distribution of the watery humor behind the closed eyelids, thus preventing anoxia corneal epithelium and breakage [5].

The incidence of eye problems is significantly related with intensive care unit length of stay (ICU-LOS), concurrent diseases, and gastrointestinal or respiratory problems ($p \leq 0.01$) [11]. Furthermore, it significantly relates with the patient's level of consciousness, use of artificial airway, tracheostomy, positive end-expiratory pressure (PEEP), presence of bronchial secretions, and use of sedatives and muscle relaxants ($p \leq 0.01$) [11, 12]. The risk of developing eye problems increased 2.8-fold in patients with ICU-LOS longer than 7 days, 7.0-fold in patients with state of depressed consciousness, 10.8-fold in comatose patients, 2.9-fold in patients with PEEP, 4.2 times in sedated patients, and 2.3 times in patients treated with myorelaxants [5, 11, 12].

## 7.2.1 Main Ocular Complications in ICU

Exposure keratopathy (3.6%–60%), conjunctival chemosis (9%–80%), and bacterial keratitis (unknown incidence) are the major ocular complications in ICU [8, 9], while the abrasions reach their peak incidence between the 2nd and 7th day of hospitalization [13].

The exposure keratopathy is caused by the lack of physiological mechanisms of corneal protection (as the wink), depending on the underlying disease, use of sedatives, and myorelaxants. Among the risk factors, there are the use of noninvasive ventilation masks, prone position, and lagophthalmos (incomplete eyelid closure). The exposure keratopathy causes microlesions that can evolve from major lesions up to the complete loss of sight [14, 15].

The conjunctival chemosis is a common complication mainly related to MV. The positive pressure during MV and the endotracheal tube (ETT) fixing clamps can compress the jugular vein, affecting the venous return to the eye structures, causing the *ventilator eye* [16].

The bacterial keratitis has unknown incidence, also because the prevention of infections in ICU is focused on ventilator-associated pneumonia (VAP), catheter-associated urinary tract infection (CAUTI), and central line-associated bloodstream infection (CLABSI), disregarding the study of eye infections. The exposure keratopathy increases the risk of microbial infections.

About 20 years ago, some practices were identified as leading to an increased infectious risk [17]:

- Using the same applicator for ocular instillation (artificial tears and/or drugs) for both eyes.
- Touching the surface of the eye with the applicator.
- Using the patches on the open or partially open eyes.
- Apply patches on the eyes with the presence of secretions.
- Proceed to the tracheal suction without adequate coverage of the eyes.
- Contact lenses not removed.

With the name "red eye" is meant a recurring complication, including local edema, conjunctival hyperemia, subconjunctival bleeding, and local corneal opacities [18], if not adequately treated it can affect the sight.

## 7.2.2   *Prevention and Treatment*

Sight is a very important aspect of the quality of life; therefore, this should never be neglected. Sedated or unconscious patients are at high risk to develop eye complications. Attempts to standardize eye care in ICU through staff education, utilization and implementation of eye care algorithms, and development of general guidelines for eye care should be performed [16].

Literature recommendations for eyes' complication prevention include:

- Assess each patient to identify risk factors for iatrogenic ophthalmologic complications.
- Perform daily assessment of the patient's ability to maintain eyelids closed.
- Run at least once a week the evaluation of ocular micro-epithelium complications (e.g., using the instillation of fluorescein and a pen with a blue light).
- Close eyelids for all patients unable to keep them closed.
- When necessary, maintain the closure of the eyelids with mechanical methods.
- In patients not able to close the eyelids, unconscious or heavily sedated, perform eye care every 2 h (with gauze soaked in physiological solution or specific lubricants) [13].

Figure 7.1 shows a protocolized eye care approach.

Complications management and treatment include instillation of ointments and/or ophthalmic drops, more effective in preventing corneal abrasions then saline solutions drops, and the application of a polyethylene films to prevent corneal lesions, when available [16]. Polyethylene film is transparent and thin and adheres easily to the surfaces. It is very resistant to water and other solutions. Once applied by the upper eyelid up to cheek, it forms a humid chamber resulting from the lacrimal fluid that preserves the integrity of the cornea [6, 20].

The ointments have a prolonged effect compared to topical treatments, protecting the cornea for long periods; if the staff is properly trained, ointments may be replaced by *polyacrylamide hydrogels* dressings. Made of 96% of water, their main use is directed to the treatment of cutaneous lesions but not the eyepiece. To be safely used, the eye should not present lagophthalmos [21, 22].

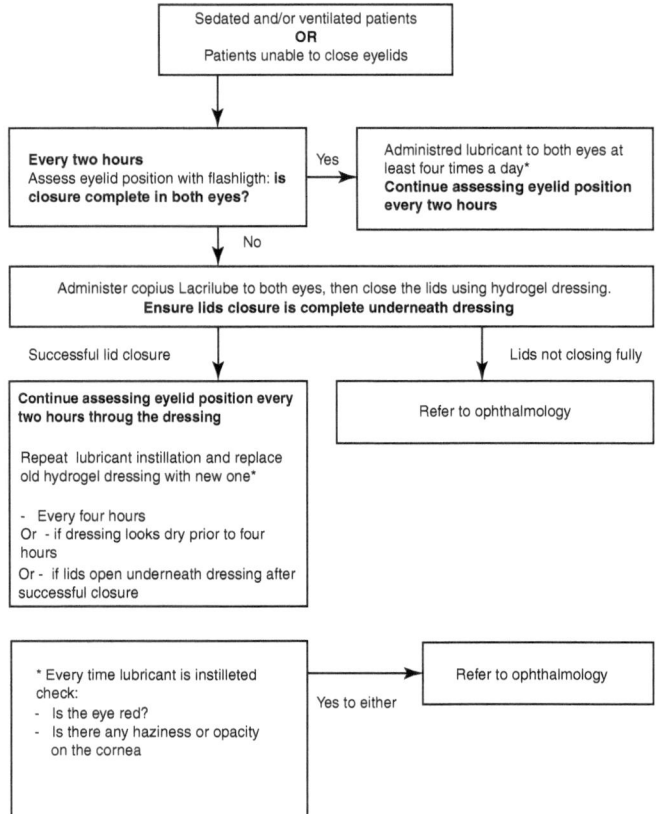

**Fig. 7.1** Proposed universal protocol for prevention of eye complications in critically ill patients [19]. Adapted with permission

## 7.3   Oral Care in ICU

The role of oral hygiene in the ICU is unquestionable both because most patients cannot perform it by themselves and because intubated and sedated patients have an alteration of the physiological mechanisms such as hydration, salivation, chewing, and tongue movements, necessary to maintain the oral cavity intact [23]. However, the importance of oral hygiene relates to the general concept of health, since the oropharyngeal colonization is associated with cardiovascular and respiratory diseases and bacteremia [24, 25].

About 48 h after ICU admission, the oropharynx bacterial flora significantly changes, and Gram-negative bacteria begin to proliferate and can migrate to the respiratory tract causing pneumonia.

Coughing reflex is often inhibited in intubated patients. Furthermore, the ETT obliges the person to keep the mouth open with a decreased salivation (xerostomia), also worsened by several drugs.

In ICU, the interest for oral hygiene arises as preventive intervention for VAP. "Oral health, which includes accumulation of dental plaque, oral microbial flora, and local oral immunity, influences the number of organisms, including pathogens that may cause VAP, in the oral cavity. Thus, oral care interventions that prevent the accumulation of plaque and stimulate local oral immunity during the early period of hospitalization may reduce development of VAP" [26].

Oropharynx colonization is one of the main factors in VAP development. The growth of potentially pathogenic bacteria in dental plaque is seen as a source of infection. Dental plaque gives to other microorganisms the possibility to adhere and move toward pharyngeal portion. Dental plaque can be removed by toothbrushing [27].

A proper oral hygiene management requires mouth, mucosa, and gum assessment to be performed at early stage in ICU and daily after to plan care. It is suggested to use a tongue depressor and a light source and remove oropharyngeal cannulas, bites, and dental prostheses, if present.

Several assessment tools are available (Oral Assessment Tool and Oral Assessment Checklist, Mouth Care Assessment Tool,

Beck Oral Assessment Scale) but none validated. It is recommended to choose the most simple and easy to apply, properly translated, and culturally adapted.

## 7.3.1 Management of Oral Hygiene

Several oral hygiene procedures are described in the available literature, with protocols often contradicting each other [28]. To date, optimal oral care frequency has not been determined, but the implementation of programs for its systematic application improves the mouth care [23].

The mechanical interventions are directed to remove plaque and clean the oral cavity. Toothbrush and toothpaste are the most suitable tools. These should be used to brush teeth, tongue, and gums at least twice a day, possibly using a soft brush with pediatric bristles [27]. Swabs are ineffective in removing debris between teeth and gum [29].

Patients with coagulative disorders or undergoing the administration of anticoagulant medications (e.g., in presence of continuous renal replacement therapy, extracorporeal membrane oxygenation, or intra-aortic balloon pump supports) require special attention during oral care procedures to prevent accidental bleeding. Toothbrush requires mandatory extra-soft bristles, and, if disposable kit of suctioning cannula plus sponge is adopted, nurses should pay attention to avoid direct contact between the suction tip and the oral tissues.

Before performing the procedure, nurses should inform the patient, if aware, to obtain the maximum collaboration by valorizing the autonomy. Once controlled the ETT cuff pressure or tracheostomy cannula, if not contraindicated by underlying disease, patient should assume semi-Fowler or a supine position (in anti-Trendelenburg), with head rotated sideways to facilitate the removal of saliva and liquid used for the hygiene [23].

Great importance is given to mouthwashes and their use in VAP prevention: chlorhexidine gluconate (CHG) mouthwash is an antiplaque agent with potent antimicrobial activity that is effective at low concentrations (0.12%) without causing increased resistance of oral bacteria. CHG mouth rinse or gel has been used in many clinical trials, primarily in cardiac surgery patients, to improve gingival health and to treat oral infections [28–30]. Routine use of CHG in ICU patients is not recommended [31]. Some studies show that using CHG at least three times a day decreases the frequency of VAP, but there are no differences with those who used a placebo in terms of mortality and survival [32]. Furthermore there are low efficacy trials related to combined use of CHG and toothbrush, compared to only use of mouthwash in reduction of VAP [32]. Using toothbrush and mouthwash together decreases the oral cavity lesions and ulcers [33].

Sodium bicarbonate rinse can dissolve mucus and loosen oral debris, but no trial confirmed this theory nor demonstrated its superiority toward the CHG mouthwash [29].

Hydrogen peroxide was used in the past to clean the oral cavity, but when not properly diluted, it can cause mouth burns, and sometimes patients have reported a bad taste and refused to use it [29].

Saline solution (NaCl 0.9%) may cause dry mouth, and for this reason, patients consider it unpleasant, while tap water, although readily available and free, can be a source of nosocomial infections in hospitals [29].

There is some weak evidence that povidone-iodine mouth rinse is more effective than saline in reducing VAP [32].

Factors influencing quality in oral care can be organized in "rejecting" and "facilitating." Rejecting factors refer to the working organization (little time available due to the many activities, excessive workload) and the absence of adequate equipment. Also, a number of physical barriers, such as ETT fastening devices, temperature probes, and enteral feeding tubes, can decrease oral care quality. Inadequate equipment includes toothbrushes with bristles for adults, too large to proper brush teeth and tongue. Facilitating factors are adequate trained staff and experience in ICU [34, 35].

Oral care in ICU plays a great deal of interest among the staff because of the attention required (use of time and resources) [36]. Despite numerous guidelines refer to it as a VAP prevention method, there is not yet a common procedure. There is also a low adherence to standards from those indicated, if they are not disseminated and implemented on institutional base [37, 38].

Oral care effectiveness not only relates with mortality or VAP rates. It should be considered a standard to increase patient's comfort.

## 7.4    Body Care and Hygiene in the ICU

During ICU stay body care and hygiene are generally fully supported by nurses and nurses' aides.

The skin is normally colonized by a permanent and transitory bacterial flora. The first mainly consists in cocci bacteria, Gram-positive bacilli, and lyophil yeasts; the second includes germs accidentally on the skin or for contiguity (periorificial zone). Skin flora changes depend on the level of personal hygiene and activity, mental state and underlying disease, and environment.

ICU patients acquire within a few hours environmental microorganisms, some of which represent a risk for infection. Moreover, despite skin defensive mechanisms against the multiplication of resident microorganisms (integrity of the corneal stratum, physiological hydro-lipid film, immunological defense system), it must be pointed out that these mechanisms may be altered and the person may be more exposed to the attack of saprophytes/pathogens microorganisms.

Bedridden patients' skin undergoes several complications such as ulcers and colonization by pathogens with the subsequent skin (e.g., mycosis) and/or systemic infections.

## 7.4.1   The Hygiene of the Person

The basic hygiene care is an integral part of the nursing plan and represents a valuable opportunity for an overall assessment of the patient.

The first programming phase provides the assessment for hygiene need through consultation of clinical documentation and the evaluation of the general conditions to define times and way to perform hygiene program.

It is necessary to perform daily observation of integrity, complexion, skin temperature and color, and nail integrity (e.g., inflammation, injuries, seborrheic or dehydrated skin) also to prevent skin lesions and PUs.

The daily evaluation allows to plan the more suitable hygiene care for the clinical conditions of the singular patient. However, the general hygienic principles should always be guaranteed despite the critical conditions and the intensive care environment [39].

Besides increasing the general comfort, body hygiene must be focused on the skin colonization that can lead to hospital infections, on the correct use of the materials, and any complications that can arise during the nursing activities.

## 7.4.2   Issues Related to the Bowel Incontinence

Bowel management, probably due to its "low technology" nature, seems to be a little neglected compared to other nursing aspects with greater technical and technological content [40]. Constipation and diarrhea (see Chap. 15) are very frequent and require a careful management [41]; especially liquid feces may be related to problems linked to the skin, with increased risk of PUs, infection, morbidity, and LOS [42].

Diarrhea is associated with dehydration, impaired electrolyte balance, bedsores, and catheter-related infections, and increases the burden of nursing care and related investigations. In the daily clinical practice, the onset of diarrhea frequently leads to discontinuation of enteral nutrition (EN), with consequent energy and protein deficit, resulting in undernutrition and poor clinical outcome [43, 44].

The perianal area is most at risk of PU and irritative dermatitis development. Contact between feces and ulcer increases the risk of infections, thus complicating the care and causing pain. It would be therefore appropriate to implement interventions in order to reduce fecal incontinence and consider the use of devices to avoid the contact between skin and feces (Fecal Management Systems) [45].

## 7.4.3   *Dermatitis Associated to Incontinence*

Incontinence often leads to a skin integrity damage, with the onset of lesions of the perineal skin (IAD, incontinence-associated dermatitis). IAD can be defined as the appearance of erythema and edema, sometimes with blisters, exudate, erosion, or infection of the skin area in the perineal zone. Generally, in the past, IAD were underestimated or confused with superficial pressure ulcers. IAD is secondary to prolonged skin exposure to humidity due to stools or urine, when the skin is not adequately protected [46].

IAD represents the damage extending from skin surface toward the underlying layers. IAD risk is enhanced by tissue alterations related to age, inadequate feeding, and exposure to fecal material. In acute care settings, fecal incontinence affects up to 33% of the patients [47].

A recent systematic review and meta-analysis confirmed incontinence (and humidity in general) and the IAD as major risk factors for PU development [48].

Perineal skin cleansing must be carried out with products complying with the acid pH (5.4–5.9) of healthy skin. Increased skin pH may lead to colonization by microorganisms potentially pathogenic, which can block the skin barrier function and expose it to the aggression of external agents. It should be recalled that the pH of a normal soap is alkaline and varies from 9.5 to 11.0.

Cutaneous detergents provide an alternative to water and soap when washing perineal area and the peri-genital skin. They can reduce the negative effects of the soap and help to maintain an adequate pH. Many detergents without rinsing have a "balanced pH" to ensure that their pH is closer to that of healthy skin.

Many products are indicated for hydration, protection, and safety of skin barrier function. Many skin protectors contain occlusive substances, as for Vaseline and oils, but no evidence supports their use. Protective agent currently used includes ointments based on petroleum jelly, dimethicone, creams, oils, and oxides. Products based on zinc oxide showed a good protection against irritant substances but poor hydration of skin and poor barrier properties to prevent maceration [2].

## 7.4.4   Hemodynamic Alterations and Hygiene Care

Hygiene care in critical patient represents a particularly intense and important moment of nursing care. These maneuvers can cause problems such as accidental extubation, disconnection from ventilator, or alteration of vital signs due to stimulation, manipulation, and postural changes [49].

The most critical maneuver is the side rotation to change bed sheets, also, as a result of possible interruptions in the administration of drugs determined by the accidental kinking of vascular catheter or the mobilization of bronchial secretions induced by postural variation [49].

Sponging may cause modifications in vital signs, due to the changes of body temperature despite the control of water temperature.

Systolic blood pressure is more influenced by bedpan positioning to perform the perineal hygiene and by side rotations [50]. Also, respiratory rate significantly alters, since an effort might be requested to lift the pelvis and the perineal hygiene may have psychological implications that can exacerbate anxiety.

Tidal volume is substantially stable, with significant alterations after moving the endotracheal tube from one side of the mouth to the other, probably due to the induced airways irritation [50, 51] .

## 7.5   Bed Bath in Intensive Care

Bathing is both a nursing ritual and fundamental therapeutic nursing intervention [51]. For bedridden patients that are unable to perform personal hygiene because of acute illness or chronic debilitation, bed bath improves hygiene and comfort [52]. The bath of the critical patient requires proper planning because of its characteristics and peculiarities.

### 7.5.1   Procedure for the Bed Bath

All areas of the body must be cleaned with the aim to remove microorganisms, dirt, and sweat. Particular attention should be given to patient face, oral cavity, hands, armpits, and perineum to prevent PUs, bad smell, and patient discomfort.

Prior to bathing the patient, it is important to consider the clinical conditions, the presence of dressings, plasters, and/or external fixation.

The bath can be performed with wet wipes impregnated with detergent or antiseptic, which contain a solution that evaporates quickly (no need to rinse), or with soap-containing knobs that must be wet with water or detergent solution and used for cleansing and massaging the affected area.

To reduce contamination, it is suggested to use disposable material and trays instead of reusable ones [52, 53].

## 7.5.2   Hygiene Care in Patients Undergoing ECMO

Daily routine basic nursing care in critically ill, as hygiene, could markedly affect the vital signs of patients [54, 55]. Specific interventions like mouth care, bed bathing, and management of airway's fixation devices are recognized as the most influencing factors [49, 56]. Nevertheless, cardiovascular alterations are not the only potential side effects of nursing care: even vascular lines displacement and unplanned extubation are described [57]. Changing the patient's body positions (alongside, flat, etc.) could also modify the intravenous delivery of vasoactive drugs [58]. As an external source of stimuli, during nursing care, patients' sedation level may become lighter. All these mentioned issues are potential adverse events, and the ECMO support could only amplify these side effects [59].

Daily nursing care activities in these fragile patients distinguished by poor oxygenation, high dependence from ECMO's blood flow, and continuous anticoagulation treatment are challenging the nurse staff to deliver the care at its best.

Basically two nursing care goals seem to be crucial:

• Avoid any alterations in the BF.
• Avoid any risks of maneuver-related bleeding.

Blood flow itself sometimes on VV-ECMO approach may represent the only prime factor providing patient's oxygenation. On low BF values, a portion of the entire amount of oxygenation is performed via mechanical ventilation. However, a loss equal to 0.5 Lt/min (BF = 2 Lt/min) due to a repositioning on the side of the patient results in a reduction of 25% of total amount.

In case of higher BF range (4–5 Lt/min), the loss of flow (0.5 Lt/min) will cause a reduction in the total amount of BF from 1/6 to 1/8.

Higher blood flow range (i.e., 4–5 L/min) usually requires a higher volume status to ensure an adequate venous drainage without hemolysis. Thus, patients with higher blood flow had fewer episodes of dropping in BF and, consequently, fewer desaturation events and reduction in $SvO_2$ values. Veno-venous ECMO improves arterial oxygenation through elevation in mixed venous saturation. Thus, BF level and SvO2 and SpO2 are strictly dependent. So despite the patient's BF value, it is paramount to minimize manual handling, especially logroll on sides and hip's lifting (e.g., bedpan positioning). While experiencing a BF drop, a slight reduction in RPM could be tested as a technique to stabilize it. Lately, Redaelli et al. have performed a prospective observational study about BF's alterations during nursing care [59]. According to protocol, to avoid any rolling on sides, daily nursing was carried out using a combination of hoister plus a stiff board [59]. Despite the aim of lifting approach as strategy for manual handling, it has appeared unsuitable: data have shown to be the main factor affecting the BF. Then authors' suggestion was to perform manual handling and rolling of patient through a less invasive and minimal rolling plus a shifting of the body inside the bed [59].

A second main issue affecting BF was the sponge bath patient's hygiene.

Sponge bath, the first step usually performed, was mostly associated with hypertensive and tachycardic events, probably due to an inadequate level of sedation [59]. Despite the use of warm water during the sponge bath, the average increase in systolic pressure was 31% of baseline, which lasted for slightly less than half an hour [59]. Indeed, in spite of a good sedation plan before nursing, additional bolus was often required [59]. Thus, the sedation status should be carefully assessed before and during nursing care and deepened if necessary. In VV-ECMO patients, an inadequate sedation plan may lead also to oxygen consumption increase, elevation in cardiac output (CO), and subsequent arterial desaturation. In spontaneous breathing patients, mobilization and painful stimulation may increase their work of breathing, leading to a critical elevation in minute ventilation.

The exit site of cannulae requires a daily-based monitoring, like any other vascular access, to early detect and prevent any signs of infections and bleeding.

In the absence of bleeding, semipermeable transparent film dressing represents the first-line option with a length of stay in situ until 7 days would be the better option (as highlighted in Chap. 11). In the process of choosing the most suitable dressing, two aspects should be ruled out: blood clot presence and ability to keep the cannula in place.

In case of blood clots, before to commence any interventions, a chat with the ECMO consultant in charge and a proper coagulation assessment of patient is mandatory. Regarding antiseptic wound treatment, please see Chap. 11.

Daily care of ECMO dressing (check or change) should be also focused and accurate about the cannulae distance from their exit site, because even minimal alterations from the original placement site will bring into a potential increasing of recirculation or air embolism.

## 7.6   Hygiene Care and Infections Preventions

ICU patients are extremely prone to infections, including those caused by antimicrobial-resistant bacteria (AMRB). Main infections are caused by MRSA, VRE, and *Acinetobacter baumannii*.

Nosocomial infections with AMRB are associated with a delay in administration of appropriate medication, failure in the therapeutic approach, and increased LOS with consequent increase of mortality [60], since this kind of infections often require a long and complex treatment period. The Center for Disease Control and Prevention (CDC) recommends hand washing and isolation precautions, but these strategies are not easy to achieve, because a lots of healthcare workers should be consistently adherent to them and continuously sustaining them [61].

CHG is a cationic biguanide developed in the UK around 1950. It is a water-soluble antiseptic preparation with broad activity against Gram-negative and Gram-positive organisms, facultative anaerobes, aerobes, and yeasts [62]. Its bactericidal action is based on drastic increase of bacterial cell membrane permeability by altering the protein structure. This causes the precipitation of various cytoplasmic macromolecules and subsequent cell death for lysis. In recent years this antiseptic obtained a renewed success in the prevention of infections, and its use has been tested both for the disinfection of the intact skin, oral, and body hygiene. CHG is available in different concentrations and presentations (alcoholic/aqueous, rinse/non-rinse solutions and impregnated cloths). It is indicated to prevent infections from AMRB in ICU patients. It is available in a variety of formulations, such as bulk solution that can be diluted in water or alcohol, and with prepackaged, 2% aqueous CHG-impregnated wipes.

Bathing with wipes soaked in CHG 2% solution is more effective in preventing bloodstream infections caused by MRSA and VRE compared to traditional bath. Lower effectiveness in reducing Gram-negative antibiotic-resistant bacteria infections (ARGNB) has been reported [53]. Wipes soaked in CHG compared to traditional bath in two recent RCT [63, 64] showed no difference as regards to the infections incidence. Nonetheless, they are disposable and charge a constant CHG amount, may not be rinsed, and can be used by disabled or patients with bathing contraindications (e.g., external fixation or surgical dressing)

[65, 66]. According to manufacturer's instructions, they cannot be used to wash mucous membranes.

The effectiveness of body hygiene with CHG has been studied in adults ($\geq$18 years) hospitalized in various types of ICU. To date, no severe adverse events have been reported when bathing with CHG. Cutaneous rush or skin reactions not well specified may occur [67]. The comparison between products (e.g., CHG vs. traditional bath) highlighted that all hospitalized patients should be bathed with CHG to prevent and reduce infections' transmission [68], while it is not possible to have the same efficacy trials for children.

Although body hygiene with CHG has no influence on ICU-LOS [62], comparison between studies is complicated by lack of standardized protocols and different approaches concerning timing of interventions, patients' illness and comfort needs, available time, number of dedicated staff, and the typology of ICU [65].

Take-Home Messages
- Development and implementation of oral care assessments and evidence-based oral care protocols help prevent infections or complications during intensive care treatment.
- The importance to constantly monitor vital signs during all maneuvers is highlighted because they were identified critical factors relating to individual maneuvers of hygiene care.
- Using CHG for body hygiene allows to reduce the transmission of infections, but it is still debated if it contributes completely to the reduction in infections in ICU.

# References

1. Leslie GD. Nursing sensitive outcomes for intensive care - the push back to basics. Aust Crit Care. 2009;22:149–50. https://doi.org/10.1016/j.aucc.2009.10.003.

2. Bambi S, Lucchini A, Solaro M, Lumini E, Rasero L. Interventional patient hygiene model. A critical reflection on basic nursing care in intensive care units. Assist Inferm Ric. 2014;33:90–6. https://doi.org/10.1702/1539.16815.

3. Rosenberg JB, Eisen LA. Eye care in the intensive care unit: narrative review and meta-analysis. Crit Care Med. 2008;36:3151–5. https://doi.org/10.1097/CCM.0b013e31818F0ee7.

4. Grixti A, Sadri M, Datta AV. Uncommon ophthalmologic disorders in intensive care unit patients. J Crit Care. 2012;27:746.E9–22. https://doi.org/10.1016/j.jcrc.2012.07.013.

5. Coiz F, Peressoni L. Preventive care and treatment of ophthalmologic complications in critical patients. A bibliographic review. Scenario. 2014;31:5–22.

6. Werli-Alvarenga A, Ercole FF, Herdman TH, Chianca TC. Nursing Interventions for adult intensive care patients with risk for corneal injury: a systematic review. Int J Nurs Knowl. 2013;24:25–9. https://doi.org/10.1111/j.2047-3095.2012.01218.x.

7. Hughes EH, Graham EM, Wyncoll DL. Hypotension and anaemia-a blinding combination. Anaesth Intensive Care. 2007;35:773–5.

8. Grixti A, Sadri M, Edgar J, Datta AV. Common ocular surface disorders in patients in intensive care units. Ocul Surf. 2012;10:26–42. https://doi.org/10.1016/j.jtos.2011.10.001.

9. Saritas TB, Bozkurt B, Simsek B, Cakmak Z, Ozdemir M, Yosunkaya A. Ocular surface disorders in intensive care unit patients. Sci World J. 2013;2013:182038. https://doi.org/10.1155/2013/182038. eCollection 2013

10. Alansari but Hijazi MH, Maghrabi KA. Making a difference in eye care of the critically ill patients. J Intensive Care Med. 2015;30:311–7. https://doi.org/10.1177/0885066613510674.

11. Oh EG, Lee WH, Yoo JS, Kim SS, Ko IS, Chu SH, Song EK, Kang SW. Factors related to incidence of eye disorders in Korean patients at intensive care units. J Clin Nurs. 2009;18:29–35. https://doi.org/10.1111/j.1365-2702.2008.02388.x.

12. Werli-Alvarenga A, Ercole FF, Botoni ago Oliveira JA, Chianca TC. Corneal injuries: incidence and risk factors in the Intensive Care Unit. Rev Lat Am Enfermagem. 2011;19:1088–95.

13. Marshall AP, Elliott R, Rolls K, Schacht S, Boyle M. Eyecare in the critically ill: clinical practice guidelines. Aust Crit Care. 2008;21:97–109. https://doi.org/10.1016/j.aucc.2007.10.002.

14. Demirel S, Cumurcu T, Firat P, Aydogan MS, Doganay S. Effective management of exposure keratopathy developed in intensive care units: the impact of an evidence-based eye care education program. Intensive

Crit Care Nurs. 2014;30:38–44. https://doi.org/10.1016/j.iccn.2013.08. 001.
15. Kuruvilla S, Peter J, David S, Premkumar PS, Ramakrishna K, Thomas L, et al. Incidence and Risk factor evaluation of exposure keratopathy in critically ill patients: a cohort studies. J Crit Care. 2015;30:400–4. https://doi.org/10.1016/j.jcrc.2014.10.009.
16. The Joanna Briggs Institute for Evidence Based Nursing and Midwifery. Eye care for intensive care patients. Best practice, 2002;6(1):1-6. http:// graphics.ovid.com/db/cinahl/pdfs/2002044923.pdf. Accessed on 16 Sep 2016.
17. Dua HS. Bacterial keratitis in the critically ill and coma patient. Lancet. 1998;351:387–8. https://doi.org/10.1016/S0140-6736(05)78351-3.
18. Van der Wekken RJ, Torn E, Ros FE, Haas LE. A red eye on the intensive care unit. Exposure keratopathy with corneal abrasion secondary to lagophthalmos two to chemosis. Neth J Med. 2013;71:204–7.
19. Kam KYR, Haldar S, Papamichael E, Pearce KCS, Hayes M, Joshi N. Eye Care in the critically ill: A National Survey and Protocol. J Intensive Care Soc. 2013;14:150–4. https://doi.org/10.1177/175114371301400213.
20. Azfar MF, Khan MF, Alzeer AH. Protocolized eye care prevents corneal complications in ventilated patients in a medical intensive care unit. Saudi J Anaesth. 2013;7:33–6. https://doi.org/10.4103/1658-354X.109805.
21. Ezra DG, Chan MP, Solebo L, Malik AP, Crane E, Coombes A, et al. Randomised trial comparing ocular lubricants and polyacrylamide hydrogel dressings in the prevention of exposure keratopathy in the critically ill. Intensive Care Med. 2009;35:455–61. https://doi.org/10.1 007/S-1284-400134-008.
22. Jammal H, Khader Y, Shihadeh W, Ababneh L, Aljizawi G, Al Qasem A. Exposure keratopathy in sedated and ventilated patients. J Crit Care. 2012;27:537–41. https://doi.org/10.1016/j.jcrc.2012.02.005.
23. Lint G, Ciucur M, Giacovelli M, Lucchini A, Luongo M. The hygiene of the oral cavity. Scenario. 2013;30(3Sup):23–34.
24. Li X, Kolltveit KM, Tronstad L, Olsen I. Systemic diseases caused by oral infection. Clin Microbiol Rev. 2000;13:547–58.
25. Kholy KE, Genco RJ, Van Dyke TE. Oral infections and cardiovascular disease. Trends Endocrinol Metab. 2015;26:315–21. https://doi. org/10.1016/j.tem.2015.03.001.
26. Munro CL, Grap Overgrip MJ. Oral health and care in the intensive care unit: state of the science. Am J Crit Care. 2004;13:25–33.
27. American Association Critical Care nurses. Oral care for patients at risk for Ventilator-Associated Pneumonia. http://www.aacn.org/wd/ practice/docs/practicealerts/oral-care-patients-at-risk-vap.pdf?menu= aboutus. Accessed on 30 Mar 2016.

28. Rello J, Koulenti D, Blot S, Sierra R, Diaz E, De Waele JJ, Macor A, Agbaht K, Rodriguez A. Oral care practices in intensive care units: a survey of 59 European ICUs. Intensive Care Med. 2007;33:1066–70. https://doi.org/10.1007/s00134-007-0605-3.

29. Berry AM, Davidson PM, Masters J, Rolls K. Systematic literature review of oral hygiene practices for intensive care patients receiving mechanical ventilation. Am J Crit Care. 2007;16:552–62.

30. Plantinga NL, Wittekamp BHJ, Leleu K, Depuydt P, Van den Abeele AM, Brun-Buisson C, Bonten MJM. Oral mucosal adverse events with chlorhexidine 2% mouthwash in ICU. Intensive Care Med. 2016;42:620–1. https://doi.org/10.1007/S-4217-700134-016.

31. Feider LL, Mitchell P, Bridges E. Oral care practices for orally intubated critically ill adults. Am J Crit Care. 2010;19:175–83. https://doi.org/10.4037/ajcc2010816.

32. Shi Z, Xie H, Wang P, Zhang Q, Wu Y, Chen E, et al. Oral hygiene care for critically ill patients to prevent ventilator-associated pneumonia. Cochrane Database Syst Rev. 2013;8:CD008367. https://doi.org/10.1002/14651858.CD008367.pub2.

33. Estaji Z, Alinejad M, Hassan Rakhshani M, Rad M. The comparison of chlorhexidine solution and swab with toothbrush and toothpaste effect on preventing oral lesions in hospitalized patients in intensive care unit. Glob J Health Sci. 2015;8:54266. https://doi.org/10.5539/gjhs.V8n5p211.

34. Allen Furr L, Binkley CJ, McCurren C, Carrico R. Factors affecting quality of oral care in intensive care units. J Adv Nurs. 2004;48:454–62. https://doi.org/10.1111/j.1365-2648.2004.03228.x.

35. Lin HL, Yang LY, Lai CC. Factors related to compliance among critical care nurses with performing oral care protocols for mechanically ventilated patients in the intensive care unit. Am J Infect Control. 2014;42(5):533. https://doi.org/10.1016/j.ajic.2014.01.023.

36. Munro CL. Oral health: something to smile about! Am J Crit Care. 2014;23:282–8. https://doi.org/10.4037/ajcc2014440.

37. Kiyoshi-Teo H, Blegen M. Influence of institutional guidelines on oral hygiene practices in Intensive Care Units. Am J Crit Care. 2015;24:309–18. https://doi.org/10.4037/ajcc2015920.

38. Kiyoshi-Teo H, Cabana MD, Froelicher ES, Blegen MA. Adherence to institution-specific ventilator-associated pneumonia prevention guidelines. Am J Crit Care. 2014;23:201–14. https://doi.org/10.4037/ajcc2014837.

39. Lint G, Luongo M, Giacovelli M, Ciucur M, Lucchini A. The body hygiene. Scenario. 2013;30(3Sup):11–22.

40. Dorman BP, Hill C, McGrath M, Mansour A, Dobson D, Pearse T, et al. Bowel management in the intensive care unit. Intensive Crit Care Nurs. 2004;20:320–9. https://doi.org/10.1016/j.iccn.2004.09.004.

41. Mcpeake J, Gilmour H, MacIntosh G. The implementation of a bowel management protocol in an adult intensive care unit. Nurs Crit Care. 2011;16:235–42. https://doi.org/10.1111/j.1478-5153.2011.00451.x.

42. Ferrie S, East V. Managing diarrhea in intensive care. Aust Crit Care. 2007;20:7–13.

43. Thibault R, Graf S, Clerc A, Delieuvin N, Heidegger CP, Pichard C. Diarrhea in the ICU: respective contribution of feeding and antibiotics. Crit Care. 2013;17:R153. https://doi.org/10.1186/CC12832.

44. Reintam A, Parm P, Kitus R, Kern H, Starkopf J. Gastrointestinal symptoms in intensive care patients. Acta Anaesthesiol Scand. 2009;17:318–24. https://doi.org/10.1111/j.1399-6576.2008.01860.x.

45. Benoit RA Jr, Watts C. The effect of a pressure ulcer prevention program and the bowel management system in reducing pressure ulcer prevalence in an ICU setting. J Wound Ostomy Continence Nurs. 2007;34:163–75. https://doi.org/10.1097/01.WON.0000264830.26355.64.

46. Gray M, Bliss DZ, Doughty DB, Ermer-Seltun J, Kennedy-Evans KL, Palmer MH. Incontinence-associated dermatitis: a consensus. J Wound Ostomy Continence Nurs. 2007;34:45–54.

47. Kottner J, Blume-Peytavi U, Lohrmann C, Halfens R. Associations between individual characteristics and incontinence-associated dermatitis: a secondary data analysis of a Multicenter Prevalence Study. Int J Nurs Stud. 2014;51:1373–80. https://doi.org/10.1016/j.ijnurstu.2014.02.012.

48. Beeckman D, Van Lancker A, Van Hecke A, Verhaeghe S. A systematic review and meta-analysis of incontinence associated dermatitis, incontinence, and moisture as risk factors for pressure ulcer development. Res Nurs Health. 2014;37:204–18. https://doi.org/10.1002/nur.21593.

49. Elli S, Lucchini A, Minotti D, Giacovelli M, Coppolecchia G, Bertin A, et al. Level of sedation level and modifications of vital signs during hygienic care in patients admitted to an intensive care unit. Assist Inferm Ric. 2014;33:7–14. https://doi.org/10.1702/1443.15973.

50. Lucchini A, Paganini D, Amoretti C, Bordoli D. Changes in vital signs and oxygenation before and after hygienic care in critically ill patients. Scenario. 2012;29:7–14.

51. Happ MB, Tate JA, Swigart VA, Di Virgilio-Thomas D, Hoffman LA. Wash and wean: bathing patients undergoing weaning trials during prolonged mechanical ventilation. Heart Lung. 2010;39(6 Suppl):S47–56. https://doi.org/10.1016/j.hrtlng.2010.03.002.

52. Larson EL, Ciliberti T, Chantler C, Abraham J, Lazaro EM, Venturanza M, Pancholi P. Comparison of traditional and disposable bed baths in critically ill patients. Am J Crit Care. 2004;13:235–41.

53. Derde LPG, Dautzenberg MJD, Bonten MJM. Chlorhexidine body washing to control antimicrobial-resistent bacteria in intensive care

units: a systematic review. Intensive Care Med. 2012;38:931–9. https://doi.org/10.1007/s00134-012-2542-z.

54. Lewis P, Nichols E, Mackey G, Fadol A, Sloane L, Villagomez E. The effect of turning and backrub on mixed venous oxygen saturation in critically ill patients. Am J Crit Care. 1997;6:132–40.

55. Vollman KM. Understanding critically ill patients hemodynamic response to mobilization: using the evidence to make it safe and feasible. Crit Care Nurs Q. 2013;36:17–27. https://doi.org/10.1097/CNQ.0b013e3182750767.

56. Lucchini A, Giacovelli M, Elli S, Gariboldi R, Pelucchi G, Bondi H, et al. Modifications of vital signs during hygiene care in intensive care patients: an explorative study. Assist Inferm Ric. 2009;28:131–7.

57. Kiekkas P, Aretha D, Panteli E, Baltopoulos GI, Filos KS. Unplanned extubation in critically ill adults: clinical review. Nurs Crit Care. 2013;18:123–34. https://doi.org/10.1111/j.1478-5153.2012.00542.

58. Morrice A, Jackson E, Farnell S. Practical considerations in the administration of intravenous vasoactive drugs in the critical care setting. Part II—how safe is our practice? Intensive Crit Care Nurs. 2004;20:183–9. https://doi.org/10.1016/j.iccn.2004.04.008.

59. Redaelli S, Zanella A, Milan M, Isgrò S, Lucchini A, Pesenti A, et al. Daily nursing care on patients undergoing venous-venous extracorporeal membrane oxygenation: a challenging procedure! J Artif Organs. 2016;19:343–9. https://doi.org/10.1007/s10047-016-0912-y.

60. Powers J, Peed J, Burns L, Ziemba-Davis M. Chlorhexidine bathing and microbial contamination in patients' bath basins. Am J Crit Care. 2012;21:338–42. https://doi.org/10.4037/ajcc2012242.

61. Choi EY, Park by Kim HJ, Park J. Efficacy of chlorhexidine bathing for reducing healthcare associated bloodstream infections: a meta-analysis. Ann Intensive Care. 2015;5:31. https://doi.org/10.1186/s13613-015-0073-9.

62. Weinstein RA, Milstone AM, Passaretti CL, Perl TM. Chlorhexidine: expanding the armamentarium for infection control and prevention. Clin Infect Dis. 2008;46:274–81. https://doi.org/10.1086/524736.

63. Boonyasiri A, Thaisiam P, Permpikul C, Judaeng T, Suiwongsa B, Apiradeewajeset N, et al. Effectiveness of chlorhexidine wipes for the prevention of multidrug-resistant bacterial colonization and hospital-acquired infections in intensive care unit patients: a randomized trial in Thailand. Infect Control Hosp Epidemiol. 2016;37:245–53. https://doi.org/10.1017/ice.2015.285.

64. Noto MJ, Domenico HJ, Byrne DW, Talbot T, Rice TW, Bernard GR, et al. Chlorhexidine bathing and health care-associated infections: a

randomized clinical trial. JAMA. 2015;313:369–78. https://doi.
org/10.1001/jama.2014.18400.

65. Ottawa (ON)–Canadian Agency for drugs and technologies in health.
Chlorhexidine gluconate wipes for infection prevention in acute and
critical care: A review of clinical effectiveness and cost-effectiveness.
2016. https://www.ncbi.nlm.nih.gov/books/NBK362245. Accessed on
24 Nov 2016.

66. Raines K, Rosen K. The effect of chlorhexidine bathing on rates of nosocomial infections among the critically ill population: an analysis of current clinical research and recommendations for practice. Dimens Crit Care
Nurs. 2016;35:84–91. https://doi.org/10.1097/DCC.0000000000000165.

67. O'Horo JC, Silva GL, Munoz-Price LS, Safdar N. The efficacy of daily
bathing with chlorhexidine for reducing healthcare-associated bloodstream infections: a meta-analysis. Infect Control Hosp Epidemiol.
2012;33:257–67. https://doi.org/10.1086/664496.

68. Bonten MJ, Slaughter S, Ambergen AW, Hayden MK, Voorhis J,
Nathan C, et al. The role of "colonization pressure" in the spread of
vancomycin-resistant enterococci: an important infection control variable. Arch Intern Med. 1998;158:1127–32. https://doi.org/10.1001/
archinte.158.10.1127.

# Chapter 8
# Positioning the Critically Ill Patient: Evidence and Impact on Nursing Clinical Practice

Stefano Bambi and Stefano Elli

## 8.1  Introduction

Changing position during bedrest is a basic daily life activity for every human being. This action allows to maintain the human body in a permanent condition of comfort and prevention of a large number of complications ranging from pressure ulcers to venous thromboembolism. During sleep, healthy persons change their position on average every 11.6 min [1].

Critically ill patients lay in bed since the beginning of the acute clinical condition. Often they are forced to bedrest for long periods, due to lifesaving treatments and technologies supporting organ/system failures. Both for the presence of sedation and neuromuscular blocking agents and for their clinical conditions affecting the cognitive and neuromuscular status, patients lose their ability to reposition by themselves, meeting the risk of complications reported in Table 8.1. Consequently, patient repositioning represents the umpteenth high-priority task for critical care nurses.

Patient repositioning in critical care is strongly linked to the interventional patient hygiene model (IPHM) concerning

© Springer International Publishing AG, part of Springer Nature 2018    203
I. Comisso et al., *Nursing in Critical Care Setting*,
https://doi.org/10.1007/978-3-319-50559-6_8

**Table 8.1** Complications of prolonged bed rest [2–5]

| Organ/system | Complications |
|---|---|
| Cognitive | Depression |
| | Anxiety |
| | Delirium |
| | Disorientation |
| | Psychosis |
| Respiratory | Hypoxemia |
| | Atelectasis |
| | Pneumonia |
| | Impaired pulmonary maximal volumes and capacities |
| Circulatory | Venous thromboembolism |
| | Reduced venous compliance in the lower extremities |
| | Reduced cardiac size |
| | Impaired tolerance to orthostatic positioning, syncope |
| | Deconditioning |
| | Reduced cardiac output and peripheral vascular resistance |
| | Reduced response to carotid sinus stimulation |
| Hematological | Anemia |
| Gastrointestinal | Hospital-acquired malnutrition |
| | Anorexia |
| | Constipation |
| | Fecal impaction |
| Urinary | Infections |
| | Calculosis |
| | Nephritis |
| Endocrine | Reduced insulin sensitivity |
| | Reduced activity of aldosterone and renin |
| | Augmented levels of atrial natriuretic peptide |
| Metabolical | Negative nitrogen balance |

**Table 8.1**  (continued)

| Organ/system | Complications |
|---|---|
| Musculoskeletal | Reduced bone density; osteoporosis |
|  | Muscle atrophy and loss of lean muscular mass |
|  | Reduced muscular strength |
|  | Reduced exercise capacity and resistance |
|  | Shortening of connective tissue |
|  | Joint contractures; loss of normal range of motion |
| Skin | Pressure ulcers |

pressure ulcer (PU), ventilator-associated pneumonia (VAP), and immobilization syndrome prevention. At the same time, patient positioning is the antecedent of patient mobilization and early physiotherapy, which are part of the ABCDE bundle, discussed in Chap. 17. So, repositioning becomes an important link between a nursing model and a nursing outcomes-oriented bundle of care. Finally, the answer to this basic human need, beyond being an active part in patients respiratory treatment and increasing the level of comfort and sleep, involves important ergonomic issues for the healthcare workers. The conceptual framework is shown in Fig. 8.1.

This chapter will discuss the rationale and evidence for patient positioning in critical care units. Moreover, the therapeutic advantages and limits for every position will be showed (Table 8.2, Fig. 8.2). Lastly, this chapter will provide some suggestions for the repositioning of hemodynamically unstable patients.

## 8.2   Overview About Patients' Turning Frequency in Intensive Care Setting

In the view of critical care nurses, the main targets of patients position changing are to prevent PUs and VAP and improve comfort and oxygenation, secretion mobilization, and postural drainage [6].

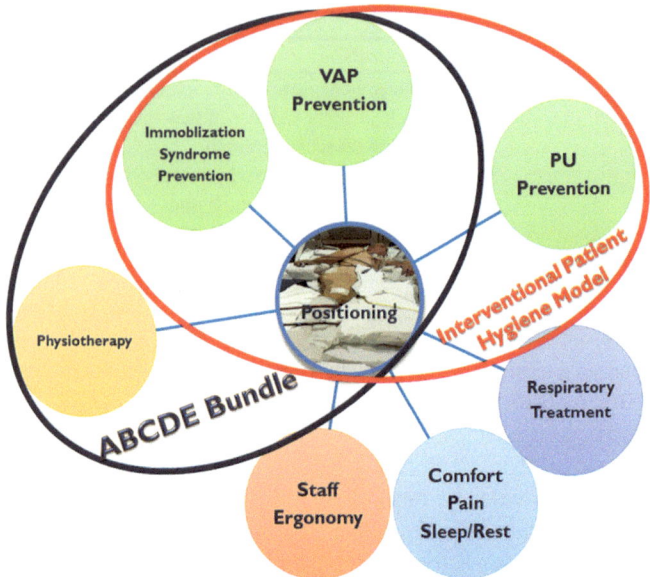

**Fig. 8.1** Conceptual framework for patient positioning in critical care settings

**Table 8.2** Patient positions in critical care settings and key points

| Position | Main key points |
|----------|-----------------|
| Head of bed elevation | • HOB elevation can influence hemodynamic parameters and their measurement<br>• 45° HOB can improve the respiratory muscles unloading<br>• HOB in patients with cerebral vascular issues does not alter the CBF<br>• Tissue-interface pressure increases with the increasing of the HOB elevation degrees<br>• There is a lack of nurses' compliance to the prescription of HOB elevation maintenance |

**Table 8.2** (continued)

| Position | Main key points |
|---|---|
| Lateral position | • The "good lung down" generally produces increases in $PaO_2$ when implemented in patients affected by mono-pulmonary diseases<br>• In ARDS right lateral position determines light improvements in $PaO_2$ in the presence of pulmonary infiltrates mainly in the left lung or bilaterally<br>• Lateral positioning does not cause hemodynamic effects compared to supine positioning<br>• Lateral horizontal position is associated with higher rates of ventilator-free days than HOB elevation position<br>• Some reported adverse events associated with lateral positioning are agitation, reduced $SpO_2$, and increased pressure in dialysis catheter placed in the subclavian vein |
| Prone position | • $PaO_2$ in V-V ECMO can be improved till 6 h after patient supination<br>• Recruitment maneuvers performed in prone position through pressures of $50\ cmH_2O$ maintained for 30 seconds produce sustained increase of $PaO_2$<br>• Prone position is feasible even in patients with open abdomen<br>• Air mattresses limit the increase of endoabdominal pressure in prone position<br>• Prone position combined with HOB elevation and 20° lowering of the foot end of the bed determines increase of $PaO_2/FiO_2$ at least for 8 h<br>• Prone position combined with anti-Trendelenburg 25° and administration per NGT of erythromycin 250 mg every 6 h allows higher volumes of administered EN<br>• Prolonged prone position (mean > 48 h) is associated with better gas exchanges and no major complications<br>• Prone position in patients with intracranial pressure issues can determine increase of $PaO_2$ and ICP and reduction of CPP if MAP is not adequate<br>In head-injured patients, prone position is associated with more frequent events of ICP ≥ 20 mmHg and PPC ≤ 70 mmHg, compared to supine position |

| Kind of position | Image |
| --- | --- |
| Supine 0° | 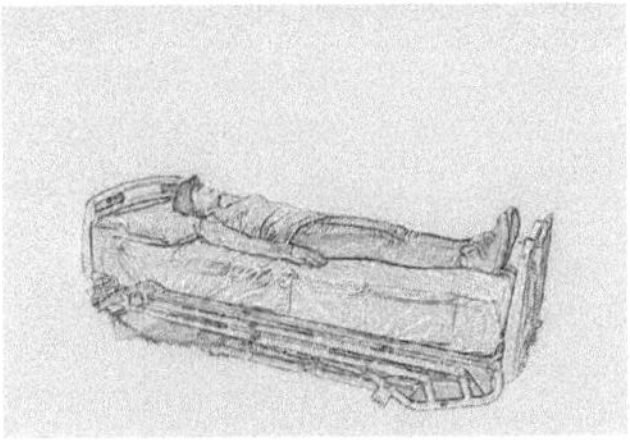 |
| Semirecumbent 30° (supine 30°) | 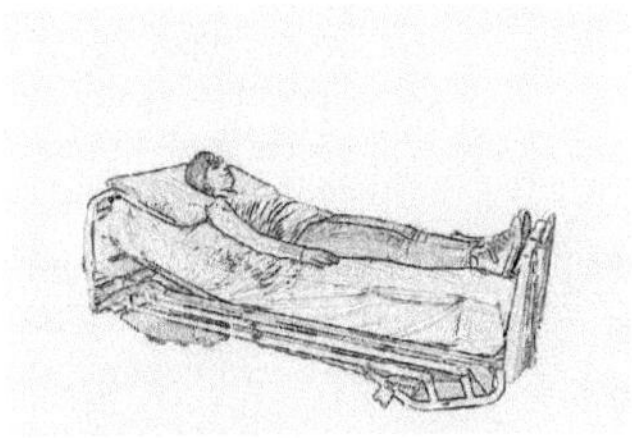 |
| Semirecumbent 45° | 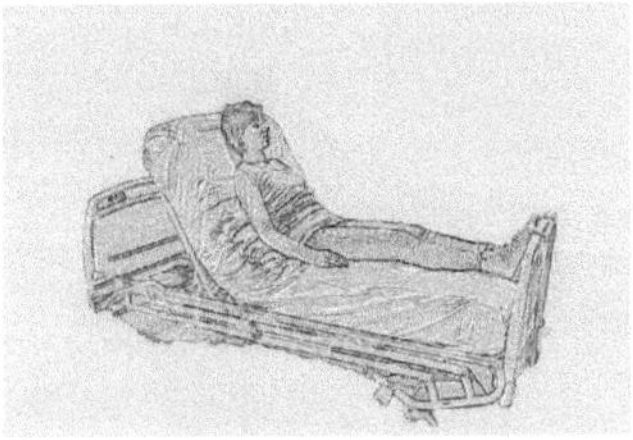 |

**Fig. 8.2** Most common critically ill patient positions

| Kind of position | Image |
|---|---|
| Semi Fowler 30° | 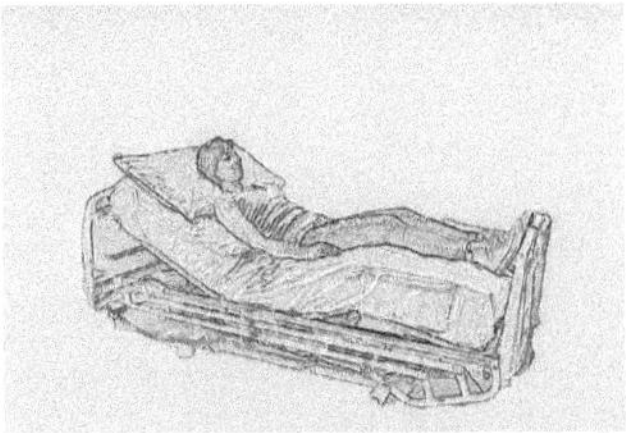 |
| Lateral position with 30° rotation | 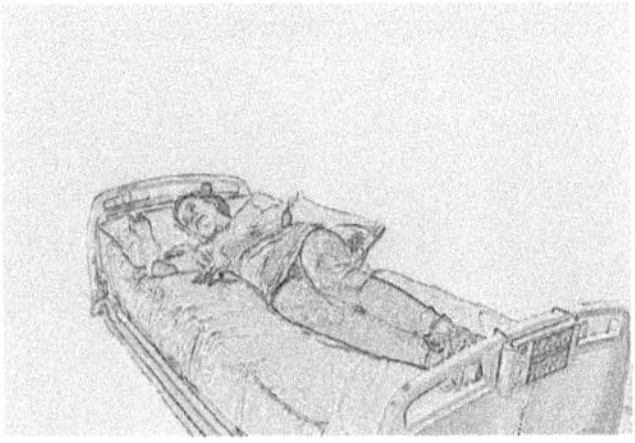 |
| Lateral position with 90° rotation not lying on the shoulders | 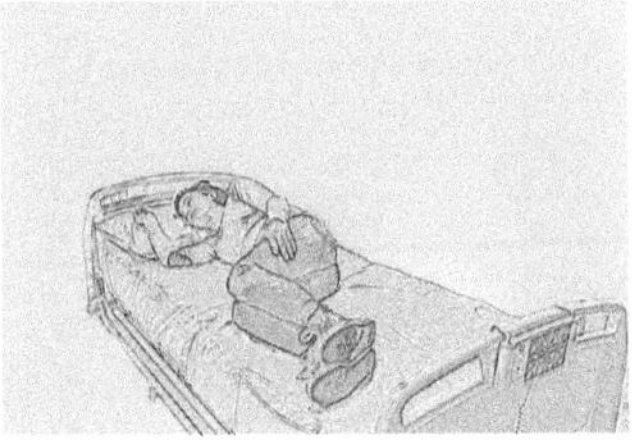 |

**Fig. 8.2**  (continued)

| Kind of position | Image |
|---|---|
| Lateral position with 90° rotation lying on the shoulders | 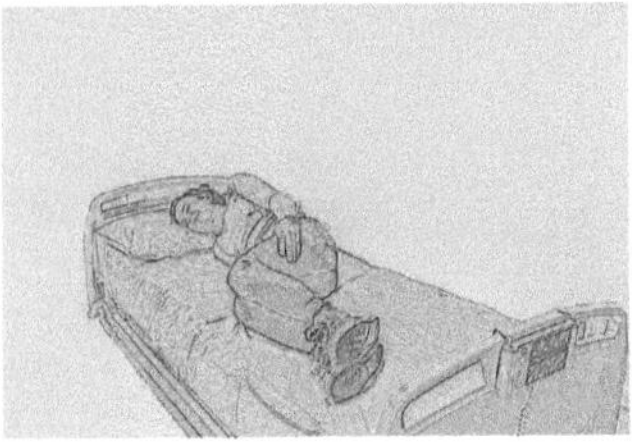 |
| Prone position (hands under forehead) | 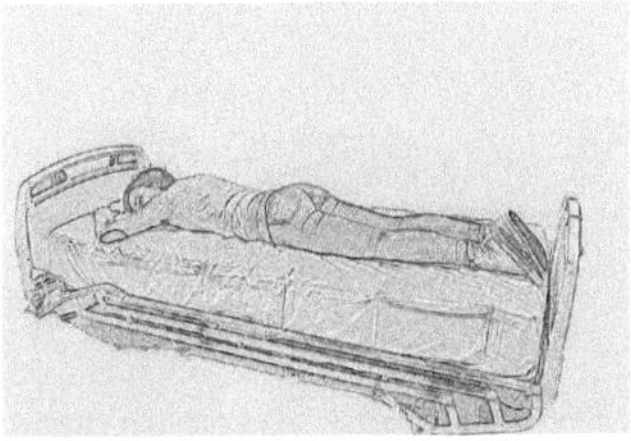 |
| Prone position (arms next to the body) | 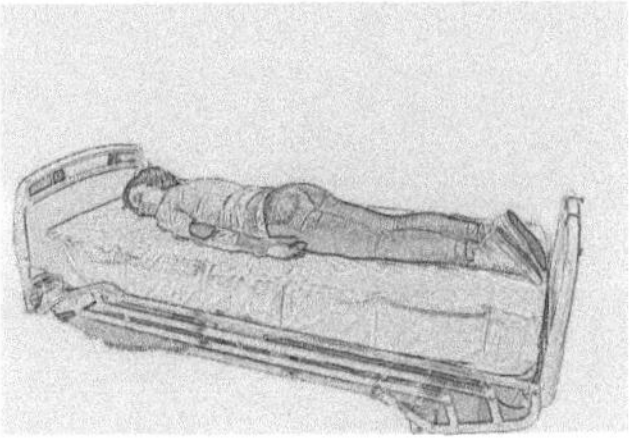 |

**Fig. 8.2** (continued)

| Kind of position | Image |
|---|---|
| Prone with anti-Trendelenburg | 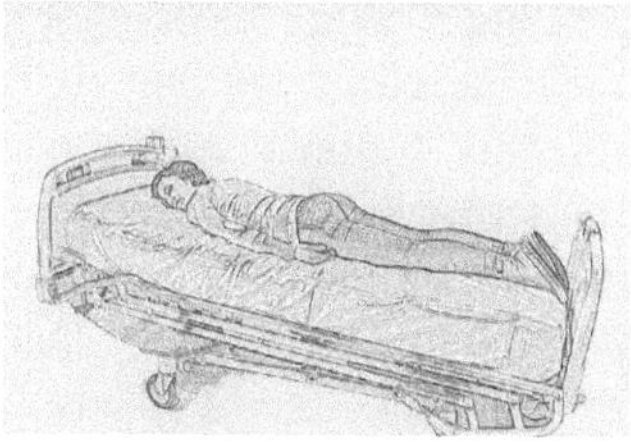 |

**Fig. 8.2** (continued)

One of the most critical issues related to patient positioning is the optimal turning frequency, in order to prevent PUs. Currently, the standard time interval accepted by all the nursing community is 2 h. However, at this moment, there is no strong scientific evidence to support this indication [7].

A 4 h turning frequency combined with viscoelastic foam mattress in geriatric patients staying in nursing home showed a significant reduction of PU occurrence when compared to standard institutional mattress combined with a turning interval of 2 h [8]. Nonetheless, a systematic review published in 2008 revealed only limited evidence about the equivalence between a 4 h turning regimen combined with appropriate pressure redistribution mattresses and the standard 2 h turning frequency in preventing PUs [8].This lack of clarity deserves more research to identify which is the best approach in the clinical setting and particularly in critical care units.

Some studies have investigated the different behaviors adopted by critical care nurses among the world toward the patient repositioning issue. The results show a wide variability of working habits.

Data from a longitudinal study performed in the USA showed that only 2.7% of patients were repositioned every 2 h, while only 57% nurses thought that this standard was observed in their intensive care unit (ICU) [9]. Another survey from a community hospital in Idaho (USA) reported that 64% of patients at risk of PU underwent a 2–3 h interval repositioning schedule [10]. A descriptive study conducted on a large number of Australian ICUs revealed that about 50–60% of nurses usually repositioned their patients every 2–4 h for all the kinds of positions, except for supine (46%) and prone (maintained ≥4 h by 44% of respondents) [6]. The frequency of patient repositioning in a Saudi ICU was every 2 h in 41.6% and every 3 h in 38.4% [11]. Lastly, a prospective study performed in the UK found that 42% of ICU patients underwent a change in their position within 2 h from the last time [12].

## 8.3    Effects of Different Positions in Critically Ill Patients

Although no absolute contraindication for specific positions in ICU patients exists, supine and Trendelenburg position should be used only in limited exceptions. The first, producing an important decrease in function residual capacity, should be required only in cases of elevated hemodynamic instability and merely for the time required to improve patient's vital signs. The positive effects of Trendelenburg position on arterial systemic pressures in patients with hypovolemic shock have been questioned since 15 years ago, being a maneuver with potential complication, especially in obese patients and those affected by intracranial hypertension [13]. Moreover, a recent review highlighted the brevity of its effect on patients' cardiac output (CO) (about only 1 minute), versus the passive leg-raising maneuvers, which seem to have a more sustained effect [14].

Currently, the trend characterizing the positioning of patients in ICU is to maintain the head of the bed (HOB) with some degrees of elevation for all kinds of achieved position.

## 8.3.1   Semi-recumbent Position and Head of Bed Elevation

HOB elevation higher than 30° has become a modern mantra in ICUs, since it has been recognized as a low-cost intervention to prevent VAP. The underlying rationale is to prevent micro-inhalation of gastric content. This problem can be more easily triggered by the presence of a gastric tube for enteral nutrition (EN) administration. In fact, gastric tubes alter the functionality of the low esophageal sphincter, making easier the occurrence of gastroesophageal reflux.

Nevertheless, a descriptive study showed how nurses' compliance to HOB ≥ 30° is generally scarce and does not depend on EN administration. Seventy percent of ICU patients is maintained in supine position, with intubated patients in higher rates than those not intubated [15]. Given that nurses tend to underestimate the degree of HOB elevation [16], angle monitoring systems, either inside the critical care bed structure or through the suitable adaptation of a pressure transducer, can be solutions to a better achievement of the target [17]. Moreover, educative programs alone seem not to be sufficient to increase nurses' compliance toward accomplishing of semi-recumbent position with HOB ≥ 30° [18].

A 45° semi-recumbent position can help to unload respiratory muscles, it produces some reduction of intrinsic positive end-expiratory pressure (PEEPi), and it is comfortable for patients during difficult weaning from mechanical ventilation (MV) [19]. Other authors showed that this position does not negatively affect gas exchange and hemodynamic parameters after 30 min in patients ventilated more than 48 h, during weaning phase [20].

However, the research results about the hemodynamic impact of HOB elevation are rather various. Seventy percent of CO measurements performed with pulmonary artery catheter in 45° semi-recumbent position provides lower values by a mean of 11%, than in supine position [21].

HOB elevation of 45° is associated to a diminishing mean arterial pressure (MAP) and central venous oxygen saturation ($ScvO_2$), especially in patients treated with pressure-controlled ventilation [22]. In septic patients maintained with HOB at 30°, an increase in stroke volume variation (SVV) values and, contemporarily, a reduction in cardiac index (CI), stroke volume index, and global end-diastolic volume values have been recorded [23]. Concerning vascular brain issues, the elevation of HOB from 0° to 45° does not produce dangerous alterations of cerebral blood flow in patients with cerebral vasospasm [24].

Tissue-interface pressures (TIP) increase with increasing HOB elevation, especially in the sacral area [24]. Since HOB elevation at 45° causes the higher sacral TIP, combining a 30° HOB elevation with a slight reverse Trendelenburg position and air loss mattresses allows to obtain the desired HOB target, limiting the values of TIP, even if shear forces due to progressive sliding in the bed cannot be completely avoided [25]. A descriptive study performed in the UK reported that ICU patients stayed with their heads up for the 97.4% of the observations [12].

Currently a great concern inside the scientific community remains unresolved, since the guidelines on PU prevention indicate the need to limit shear forces, maintaining HOB $\leq$ 30°, while recommendations for prevention of VAP require HOB elevation at 30°, even if this intervention is not evidence based [26, 27]. Therefore, authors recommend to use semi-recumbent position in MV patients if it is not in conflict with nursing or medical tasks, or with the patients' will [28].

## 8.3.2 Lateral Position

The rationale underlying the change of patient position from one side to the other is based on some physiology assumptions [29]:

- In patients with healthy lungs, different positions seem not to significantly affect gas exchanges.
- When positioning aims to improve gas exchanges, the ventilation/perfusion (V/Q) mismatch is the central element.
- Patients with healthy condition or bilateral lung pathologic processes can take advantage from right lateral position, improving the V/Q ratio, because the right lung is heavier and more vascularized than the left one,
- The "good lung down theory" can be adequate for unilateral lung pathologies, except for hemothorax, interstitial emphysema, and pulmonary abscess.

Concerning major outcomes, ICU patients in horizontal lateral position showed higher numbers of ventilator-free days than those in semi-recumbent position, whereas the rate of gastric content aspiration was equal [30].

One study reported the occurrence of adverse events associated to lateral position in 21% of cases: oxygen desaturation, agitation, and increase of pressure inside the dialysis catheter placed in the subclavian vein [31].

There is a large amount of scientific literature with contradictory results about the respiratory, hemodynamic, and skin effects of lateral repositioning. A recent systematic review concludes that there are no clear evidence about the risk-benefit balance related to the use of lateral repositioning in critically ill patients. So, more methodologically strong researches are needed to explore the effects on major outcomes (mortality, morbidity, clinical adverse events) [32].

The "good lung down" position showed better partial pressure of oxygen ($PaO_2$) values in unilateral right or left pathologies in one study [33], while other authors found no differences in $PaO_2/FiO_2$ measurements between lateral and supine position [31]. Another study performed on acute respiratory distress syndrome (ARDS) patients with main left or bilateral infiltrates revealed slight increases of mean $PaO_2$ in right lateral than in supine position [34].

Concerning the hemodynamic effects, as above, there are not univocal results: while some studies highlighted some increasing in CI and arterial blood pressure (ABP) in left and right lateral positions if compared with supine position [31], other researches have revealed no significant differences between supine and lateral positions of critically ill patients in terms of respiratory rate, heart rate, peripheral oxygen saturation, CO, arterial oxygen content, lactate levels [35], and stroke volume and SVV [23]. In healthy patients, heart rate, ABP, and oxygen consumption were found lesser in lateral than in sitting and supine positions [36].

Even lateral positioning involves an important risk of PU development. Lateral position combined with 30° HOB elevation significantly increases the TIP ≥32 mmHg [37]. This condition is present even if air loss mattresses are employed [37]. Moreover, the use of wedge in place of pillows to achieve lateral position worsens these effects [37].

### 8.3.3 Prone Position

Prone position is a rescue therapy employed in ARDS patients with hypoxemia refractory to high levels of $FiO_2$ and positive end-expiratory pressure (PEEP).

The physiologic effects of prone position on pulmonary ventilation and gas exchanges have still to be completely explained. However, the ventilation improvement provided by prone posi-

tioning is due to the fact that the heart and other anterior anatomical structures do not compress the lungs [38]. Moreover, in
prone patients, the abdominal content does not compress the
posterior-inferior portion of lungs region, and there is a reduction of the vertical gradient of pleural pressure. These factors
determine higher parts of obtained recruited lungs than in
supine position [38]. In ARDS the V/Q is matching, since the
flow distribution seems not to change between supine and prone
position. Therefore, in prone position, the oxygenation is
improved [38].

There are some conditions that increase the probability on
oxygenation improvement [38]:

- Early increase of oxygenation after initiation of prone posi-
  tion ($PaO_2 > 10$ mmHg, within 30 min)
- Lower patient's thoracic compliance in prone position than
  supine
- Increase in intra-abdominal pressure
- Diffuse pulmonary edema
- Collapsed of alveoli in lung-dependent regions
- Extrapulmonary causes of ARDS.

Prone position should be early started in patients with $PaO_2/$
$FiO_2 \leq 150$, $FiO_2 \geq 0.6$, and PEEP $\geq 5$ cm $H_2O$ [39]. Reported
contraindications to this position are high intracranial pressure
(ICP), decreased cerebral perfusion pressure (CPP), immediate
need of surgical treatment, recent thoracic surgery, recent tracheostomy, presence of pacemaker, hemodynamic instability,
maxillofacial injury or surgery, pregnancy, abdominal compartment syndrome, and unstable fractures of pelvis, femur, or vertebral column [39]. Probably such conditions do not represent
an absolute contraindication but require an accurate evaluation
before definitively deciding if implement or not the pronation.

A recent systematic review about the effectiveness of prone
position in ARDS patients showed a short-term relative risk
(RR) of mortality of 0.84 (95% CI 0.69–1.02) if compared with

supine position and for the long-term a RR of mortality of 0.86 (95% CI 0.72–1.03), even if these results were both not statistically significant [40].

The patients' subgroups that most benefit from prone position were patients enrolled within 48 h from the presence of inclusion criteria (RR of 0.75; 95% CI 0.59–94), patients more hypoxemic at the moment of pronation (RR 0.77; 95% CI 0.65–0.92), and patients maintained ≥16 hours/day in prone position (RR 0.77; 95% CI 0.61–0.99) [40].

Prone position is affected by some kind of complications: PU (RR 1.37; 95% CI 1.05–1.79) and endotracheal tube obstruction (RR 1.78; 95% CI 1.22–2.60) [40].

Moreover, loss of venous access displacement of endotracheal tube or thoracotomy tube occur in more than 30% of patients' repositioning [41].

Concerning the prevention of traditional and device-related PUs, beyond the standard precautions to limit the contact areas at risk, currently, there is the need to conduct more research to say a definitive word about the employ (or not) of advanced wound dressing to prevent PU.

Prone position can be safely performed through manual repositioning or special kinetic beds able to completely rotate the patient, maintained aligned and secured by the presence of special foam pillows and belt [42].

Optimal number of healthcare workers needed to accomplish the task can vary according to patient's clinical condition, weight, number and typologies of invasive devices (especially extracorporeal supports), and the availability of local resources. However, a minimum of five persons should take part in the procedure.

Even if a large part of published studies was performed on limited numerical samples, some findings deserve to be deepened through better designed researches.

During prone position in septic patients, some hemodynamic changes can occur, as an increase in SVV and reduction of CI [23].

Prone positioning has a good feasibility even in patients with open abdomen, treated with continuous renal replacement therapy (CRRT), [43] and in patients with post-cardiac surgery ARDS without reported complications [44]. Using air mattresses instead of traditional foam mattresses limits the increase of endoabdominal pressure during prone position [45].

Some authors found improvements of $PaO_2/FiO_2$ in patients enduring at least 8 hours of combined prone position with 20° HOB elevation and lowering of the foot end of the bed [46].

The enhancement of gas exchange without complications has been also found in patients maintained in prone position for prolonged time (mean 78.5, SD ± 61.2 h) [47].

After 6 h from the beginning of pronation, performing a recruitment maneuver using pressure of 50 cm $H_2O$ for 30 s can induce an improvement of oxygenation in patient affected by extrapulmonary ARDS [48].

A recent pilot study has shown the potential benefit for oxygenation of prone position in non-intubated ARDS patients treated with helmet CPAP [49]. The median prone position cycle duration was 3 h (IQR 2–4 h), and the patients' tolerance was very good: only 2 on 43 (4.6%) procedures were interrupted for discomfort [49].

Since prone position is usually maintained for several consecutive hours, the problem of safe EN management arises. While higher gastric residual volume and vomit episodes are present in the first 4 days with consequent smaller volume of administered EN [50], the combination of 25° anti-Trendelenburg position with erythromycin 250 mg every 6 h allows the administration of higher EN volumes without complications [51].

Concerning one of the most apparently controversial issues in prone position, which is performing it in patients affected by intracranial hypertension patients, gas exchanges are improved even if ICP values significantly rise, but CPP remains strictly dependent on the mean arterial pressure [52, 53]. However, as expected, in head-injured patients, prone position, if compared to supine position, is associated with a larger number of episodes of ICP $\geq$ 20 mmHg and CPP $\leq$ 70 mmHg [54].

## 8.3.4 Tissue-Interface Pressure Induced by Different Positions

The threshold value of TIP to develop PUs is widely accepted as 32 mmHg, even if some authors have distrusted it [55].

Research results showed that semi-Fowler's and prone positions provide lower levels of TIP. In healthy human subjects, the 30° inclined lateral position produces less TIP levels than 90° lateral position (both lying and not on shoulder), since this position recorded the highest values of TIP [55].

Sacral TIP increases with increasing of HOB elevation. 30° HOB position is a compromise between the need to reduce the PU risk in the sacral area and the need to prevent VAP occurrence [56].

Usually anti-Trendelenburg position decreases the levels of TIP [56], even if it determines some risk of shear forces exertion due to the natural patient gliding in the bed. Likewise, air loss mattresses reduce the sacral TIP in all the positions [56].

Some recent studied interventions to prevent PU in ICU settings, beyond the usual implementation of interval turning and air-mattresses, are:

- A PU prevention bundle of care, including the scheduled patient turning frequency every 3 h alternating right lateral, supine, and left lateral positions [56]
- Special electronic mapping system incorporated in a cover put over a mattress, even if this system can interfere with the air loss of the mattress [25]
- Implementation of PU prevention team, to ensure on-time patient turning every 2 h [57]

## 8.4  Special Issues About Patient Positioning in Critical Care Setting

### 8.4.1  Positioning the Morbidly Obese Patients

Morbidly obese patients (body mass index $\geq$40 Kg/m$^2$) are a population with particular physiopathological features, requiring special precaution in their repositioning management.

Obese patients maintained in supine position undergo hypoxemia, due to the reduction of pulmonary volume induced by the increasing of endoabdominal pressure [58].

Extreme consequences are reported in literature, such as some cases of death during the supine positioning of obese patients with acute respiratory failure needing to perform radiological examinations [59]. Under this rationale basis, the anti-Trendelenburg should be completely avoided in this category of patients [58].

Lateral positioning should be performed but with frequent alternation between the right and left sides, for the risk of atelectasis in the dependent lung and/or unilateral pulmonary edema [58].

The "beach chair" sitting position and, in alternative, 45° anti-Trendelenburg are the best positions to achieve an optimal breathing condition in obese patients [60]. The sitting position diminishes airflow limitations and the auto-PEEP levels, providing a drastic lowering of alveolar pressures and improving the respiratory mechanics [61].

Concerning prone positioning in patients with morbid obesity affected by ARDS, a recent case control study showed its feasibility and safety, in terms of invasive device displacement, pressure ulcers, and cardiac arrests, when compared with non-obese patients [62].

A typical limitation to the movement of morbidly obese patients is provided by the inadequacy of hospital beds and lifting devices for these patients. Bariatric bed, holding up till about 400 kg, should be used, instead of standard bed, capable to hold a maximum weight of 150–170 kg [63].

Moreover, a consistent number of healthcare operators should be employed during patient repositioning, to prevent workplace accidents. Some authors have proposed to use the Trendelenburg position with the aim to aid nurses during obese patient repositioning and prevent some degree of occupational risks. A 6° Trendelenburg can reduce 49% of work while a 12° reaches a reduction of 67%. Unfortunately, at least for critically ill obese patients, this kind of position constitutes a danger, as previously showed, which is the reason why it should be avoided [64].

## 8.4.2 Positioning Spinal Cord-Injured Patients

A recent systematic review about PU prevention in spinal cord-injured patients showed that [65]:

- A 30° semi-recumbent position, with raised feet, can diminish the interface pressure on the heels, but the effects on the sacrum are still not clear.
- A 90° lateral position is associated with higher pressures on the trochanter.
- During tilting and sitting positions, the pressures are linearly redistributed.
- In reclined sitting positions, shearing forces are exerted on tissues.
- There is lack of evidence about optimal turning interval time.

Concerning the respiratory effects of positioning, the use of thoracic optimization with physiokinesitherapy during

Trendelenburg position in patients affected by low cervical spine injuries seems to have positive effect on ventilation and weaning through spontaneous breathing trials [66].

### 8.4.3    Positioning the Patient with Extracorporeal Membrane Oxygenation (ECMO)

Currently, there is not much published literature about the repositioning of patients during venous-artery (V-A) or venous-venous (V-V) ECMO.

The use of prone position in ARDS patient with V-V ECMO is associated with an improvement of gas exchange lasting $\geq 6$ h after the return to supine position [67]. Rare occurrence of complications, among which are bleeding from cannula site, hemodynamic instability [68], and the need of V-V ECMO cannula reposition, is reported [43].

However, there are no particular contraindications to the repositioning of V-V ECMO patients for any kind of position, except for the limitation imposed by the cannula site of insertions (femoro-jugular, femoro-femoral, double-lumen cannula in the jugular vein) and by the possibility to bend some parts of the body. The availability of adequate aids or pillows to achieve a stable position with sufficient comfort for the patients is important. Particular care should be adopted in the assessment of the cannula sites for the risk of dislodgment and/or bleeding, the influence of the achieved position on the ECMO blood flow, and the sufficient level of sedation to guarantee the patient compliance to the procedure. The presence of cannulas increases the risk of device-related pressure ulcer; therefore, special precautions should be employed to their prevention in the points of contact between devices and the skin determined by the change of position (see Chap. 14). Once the position has been changed, ECMO performance, vital signs, and arterial blood gas analysis should be performed simultaneously, to evaluate the influence on the gas exchange and the clinical conditions of the patient.

## 8.4.4   Treatment and Care Conditions Affected by Patient Repositioning

Patient positions can affect patient monitoring, mechanical ventilation modes, hemodynamic invasive supports, and nursing care, requiring some precautions during bedside activities.

Patient position can widely affect intra-abdominal pressure (IAP) measurement, with the risk of misleading in the treatment decisions about the critically ill patients. IAP biases vary with the degrees of HOB elevation: mean bias between 0° and 15° is 1.5 mmHg (1.3–1.7), and mean bias between 0° and 30° is 3.7 mmHg (3.4–4.0) [69]. More importantly, a study revealed that the differences in mean IAP can largely change from almost normal condition (9.84 ± 3.581) at 0° of HOB elevation to the point of intra-abdominal hypertension "erroneous diagnosis" at 30° of HOB elevation (13.95 ± 3.600) and at 45° of HOB elevation (16.56 ± 3.862), almost reaching the values of a "fake" abdominal compartment syndrome [70].

Neurally adjusted ventilatory assist (NAVA) is a promising new mode of ventilation, based on the synchronization between the ventilator and the patient's diaphragmatic electrical activity (EAdi), detected through a special nasogastric (NG) tube equipped with electrodes. During NAVA, EAdi detection is affected by the lateral-45° semi-recumbent patient position, but the numerous electrodes compensate the alteration in signal reading, as long as NG tube is adequately placed [71].

In patients supported through intra-aortic balloon pump, during 30° semi-recumbent position, the aortic MAP is lowered by 10% and blood flow toward the left ascending coronary by 15% [72].

Some studies showed that Trendelenburg and anti-Trendelenburg positions do not produce significant changes in patients' gas exchanges [73] and hemodynamic status [74].

Critical care nurses have to manage accurately the cuff pressure of endotracheal device, especially after patient change of position. In particular, median values of cuff pressure drop below the threshold of 30 cmH$_2$O during (left or right) lateral flexion of the head, (left or right) lateral rotation of the head, supine position, semi-recumbent position at 10° or 30°, and Trendelenburg position at 10° [75]. Moreover, it is advisable to suction the patient's oral cavity before his/her repositioning, since this intervention produces a RR reduction of 0.32 (95% CI 0.11–0.92) for VAP [76].

Finally, the effectiveness of music therapy before and during repositioning in reducing patients' discomfort and anxiety currently has not still been proven [77].

## 8.4.5  Kinetic Beds

Currently, there is no full clarity about the concept of bed for kinetic therapy (KT) and continuous lateral rotation therapy (CLRT). Some authors refer to beds for KT, those which rotate in a turn of at least 40° and for CLRT lesser than 40° [78], while others state that CLRT beds can rotate up to 60°, with setting varying in speed, degree, and duration [79]. However, the implementation of CRLT and KT aims to prevent and treat respiratory complications due to immobility and bed rest in ICU [4].

There is a wide variability in literature about the employ modes of kinetic beds: rotation degrees ranging from 30° to 72°, rotation intervals ranging from 2 to 8 rotations per hour, and duration till 16–24 h per day [4].

Even if CLRT and KT were studied in order to identify their effects on prevention of pneumonia, transport of airways secretions, hemodynamic consequences, intrapulmonary shunt, urine output, and ICP, the meta-analysis showed their effect on lowering the incidence of pneumonia but not on hospital deaths, duration of ICU stay, and mechanical ventilation days [4, 80]. Moreover, there is no clarity regarding the most effective therapy parameters to set [4]. Complications reported with the use of KT and CLRT beds are intolerance, increasing ICP, intravascular catheter disconnections, and arrhythmias [4].

Recently, some authors performed laboratory tests on cadavers, to explore the safety of KT implementation in patients with unstable cervical spinal cord injuries (with cervical collar in place) [81]. When compared with manual log rolling, KT produces less motion in flexion-extension, lateral bending, and axial dislocation [81].

The main indications and mode of use of KT and CLRT beds are [82, 83]:

- Manual lateral repositioning, differently to automated repositioning, produces changes in MAP, pulse pressure, and HR, sustained up to 45 minutes after the maneuvers.
- Suggested thresholds to start with automated therapies are $PaO_2/FiO_2 < 300$, increasing level of PEEP, atelectasis, and infiltrates showed by chest X-rays.
- Consistent implementation of CLRT using the same degrees obtained with pillows in manual turning, till the maximum level of patient's tolerance and at least 18 h per day.
- Use of progressive mode.
- In the occurrence of hemodynamic or oxygenation instability, stop the automated therapies just for the time required to resolve the problems.
- CLRT does not eliminate the need for respiratory and skin assessments and manual repositioning every 2 h.

## 8.5 Implementing Early Repositioning in Critically Ill Patients

The correct approach to be held in ICU is to try the repositioning in all patients as early as possible, leaving the patient's clinical response to pose the limitation to the maneuver, in place of the healthcare staff dread that patient could be excessively unstable [84].

Recently, a consensus paper has been published, with some meaningful recommendations about the management of early repositioning in clinically unstable patients [84]. The key points are listed below [84]:

- The first assumption is that there is no shared set of vital signs defining hemodynamic instability, but, undoubtedly, hemodynamic instability produces change and/or impairment in neurological, respiratory, and cardiovascular systems.
- Every positioning should be preceded by vital signs recording and the first reevaluation performed after 10 min from the baseline.
- In the presence of instability, do not position the patient if there is a life-threatening arrhythmia, actual volemic resuscitation, and active bleeding, vital signs do not return to baseline values within 10 min, or there is no expected outcome related to patient's clinical diagnosis.
- Do not reposition patients with unstable vertebral injuries or pelvic fractures with active bleeding.
- Do not reposition patient in presence of supraglottic airways.
- Use CLRT and/or prone position in presence of oxygenation instability.
- CLRT should be deserved in all patients that do not tolerate the 30° lateral manual repositioning.

- Patients with ARDS, chest injuries, and pulmonary contusions should be reassessed after 20 min from the baseline, before deciding if the procedure has failed or not.
- CLRT in unstable patients should be performed 18 h per day, with interruptions every 2 h and manual repositioning on right and left side, each one lasting 30 min.
- In patients who cannot tolerate lateralization, it is necessary to begin with 15° and then reevaluate before going to 30° (target).
- The frequency of position changing in stable patients that tolerate the reposition varies from 1 to 4 h, depending on the kind of bed mattresses and on individual basis.
- If a patient cannot tolerate any change of position due to his/her instability, perform a new repositioning trial at least every 8 h; in the meantime, passive mobilization strategies should be implemented in any case.

## Take-Home Messages

- There is a lack of evidence for the "2-hourly turning" of patients lying in beds.
- Literature suggests that a "4-hourly turning" regimen associated with a pressure-relieving surface can be as effective as 2-hourly turning to prevent pressure ulcers.
- Trendelenburg position in critically ill obese patients can be deadly.
- Prone positioning in severe ARDS patients reduces the overall mortality rates and produces better effects if prolonged beyond 10 h per session.
- Rotational bed therapy can prevent pneumonia but has no influence on mortality, length of stay, and duration of mechanical ventilation.
- Critically ill patients too unstable to be repositioned should be reviewed at least every 8 h for a positioning trial.

# References

1. Hawkins S, Stone K, Plummer L. An holistic approach to turning patients. Nurs Stand. 1999;6-12:51–6. https://doi.org/10.7748/ns1999.10.14.3.51.c2689.
2. Truong AD, Fan E, Brower RG, Needham DM. Bench-to-bedside review: mobilizing patients in the intensive care unit-from pathophysiology to clinical trials. Crit Care. 2009;13:216. https://doi.org/10.1186/cc7885.
3. Johnson KL, Meyenburg T. Physiological rationale and current evidence for therapeutic positioning of critically ill patients. AACN Adv Crit Care. 2009;20:228–40. https://doi.org/10.1097/NCI.0b013e3181add8db.
4. Goldhill DR, Imhoff M, McLean B, Waldmann C. Rotational bed therapy to prevent and treat respiratory complications: a review and meta-analysis. Am J Crit Care. 2007;16:50–61.
5. Corcoran PJ. Use it or lose it-the hazards of bed rest and inactivity. West J Med. 1991;154:536–8.
6. Thomas PJ, Paratz JD, Stanton WR, Deans R, Lipman J. Positioning practices for ventilated intensive care patients: current practice, indications and contraindications. Aust Crit Care. 2006;19:122–6, 128, 130-2.
7. Hagisawa S, Ferguson-Pell M. Evidence supporting the use of two-hourly turning for pressure ulcer prevention. J Tissue Viability. 2008;17:76–81. https://doi.org/10.1016/j.jtv.2007.10.001.
8. Defloor T, De Bacquer D, Grypdonck MH. The effect of various combinations of turning and pressure reducing devices on the incidence of pressure ulcers. Int J Nurs Stud. 2005;42:37–46. https://doi.org/10.1016/j.ijnurstu.2004.05.013.
9. Krishnagopalan S, Johnson EW, Low LL, Kaufman LJ. Body positioning of intensive care patients: clinical practice versus standards. Crit Care Med. 2002;30:2588–92. https://doi.org/10.1097/01.CCM.0000034455.71412.8C.
10. Voz A, Williams C, Wilson M. Who is turning the patients? A survey study. J Wound Ostomy Continence Nurs. 2011;38:413–8. https://doi.org/10.1097/WON.0b013e318220b6ec.
11. Tayyib N, Lewis PA, Coyer FM. A prospective observational study of patient positioning in a Saudi intensive care unit. MEJN. 2013;7:26–34.
12. Goldhill DR, Badacsonyi A, Goldhill AA, Waldmann C. A prospective observational study of ICU patient position and frequency of turning. Anaesthesia. 2008;63:509–15. https://doi.org/10.1111/j.1365-2044.2007.05431.x.

13. Fink KC. Is Trendelenburg a wise choice? J Emerg Nurs. 1999;25:60–2.

14. Geerts BF, van den Bergh L, Stijnen T, Aarts LP, Jansen JR. Comprehensive review: is it better to use the Trendelenburg position or passive leg raising for the initial treatment of hypovolemia? J Clin Anesth. 2012;24:668–74. https://doi.org/10.1016/j.jclinane.2012.06.003.

15. Grap MJ, Munro CL, Bryant S, Ashtiani B. Predictors of backrest elevation in critical care. Intensive Crit Care Nurs. 2003;19:68–74.

16. Hiner C, Kasuya T, Cottingham C, Whitney J. Clinicians' perception of head-of-bed elevation. Am J Crit Care. 2010;19:164–7. https://doi.org/10.4037/ajcc2010917.

17. Wolken RF, Woodruff RJ, Smith J, Albert RK, Douglas IS. Observational study of head of bed elevation adherence using a continuous monitoring system in a medical intensive care unit. Respir Care. 2012;57:537–43. https://doi.org/10.4187/respcare.01453.

18. Rose L, Baldwin I, Crawford T. The use of bed-dials to maintain recumbent positioning for critically ill mechanically ventilated patients (The RECUMBENT study): multicentre before and after observational study. Int J Nurs Stud. 2010;47:1425–31. https://doi.org/10.1016/j.ijnurstu.2010.04.002.

19. Deye N, Lellouche F, Maggiore SM, Taillé S, Demoule A, L'Her E, et al. The semi-seated position slightly reduces the effort to breathe during difficult weaning. Intensive Care Med. 2013;39:85–92. https://doi.org/10.1007/s00134-012-2727-5.

20. Thomas P, Paratz J, Lipman J. Seated and semi-recumbent positioning of the ventilated intensive care patient - effect on gas exchange, respiratory mechanics and hemodynamics. Heart Lung. 2014;43:105–11. https://doi.org/10.1016/j.hrtlng.2013.11.011.

21. Driscoll A, Shanahan A, Crommy L, Foong S, Gleeson A. The effect of patient position on the reproducibility of cardiac output measurements. Heart Lung. 1995;24:38–44.

22. Göcze I, Strenge F, Zeman F, Creutzenberg M, Graf BM, Schlitt HJ, et al. The effects of the semirecumbent position on hemodynamic status in patients on invasive mechanical ventilation: prospective randomized multivariable analysis. Crit Care. 2013;17:R80. https://doi.org/10.1186/cc12694.

23. Daihua Y, Wei C, Xude S, Linong Y, Changjun G, Hui Z. The effect of body position changes on stroke volume variation in 66 mechanically ventilated patients with sepsis. J Crit Care. 2012;27:416.e7–12. https://doi.org/10.1016/j.jcrc.2012.02.009.

24. Peterson M, Schwab W, McCutcheon K, van Oostrom JH, Gravenstein N, Caruso L. Effects of elevating the head of bed on interface pressure in volunteers. Crit Care Med. 2008;36:3038–42. https://doi.org/10.1097/CCM.0b013e31818b8dbd.

25. Behrendt R, Ghaznavi AM, Mahan M, Craft S, Siddiqui A. Continuous bedside pressure mapping and rates of hospital-associated pressure ulcers in a medical intensive care unit. Am J Crit Care. 2014;23:127–33. https://doi.org/10.4037/ajcc2014192.

26. Reilly ER, Karakousis GC, Schrag SP, Stawicki SP. Pressure ulcers in the intensive care unit: the 'forgotten' enemy. OPUS 12. Scientist. 2007;1:17–30.

27. Burk RS, Grap MJ. Backrest position in prevention of pressure ulcers and ventilator-associated pneumonia: conflicting recommendations. Heart Lung. 2012;41:536–45. https://doi.org/10.1016/j.hrtlng.2012.05.008.

28. Niël-Weise BS, Gastmeier P, Kola A, Vonberg RP, Wille JC, van den Broek PJ, et al. An evidence-based recommendation on bed head elevation for mechanically ventilated patients. Crit Care. 2011;15:R111. https://doi.org/10.1186/cc10135.

29. Marklew A. Body positioning and its effect on oxygenation--a literature review. Nurs Crit Care. 2006;11:16–22.

30. Mauri T, Berra L, Kumwilaisak K, Pivi S, Ufberg JW, Kueppers F, et al. Lateral-horizontal patient position and horizontal orientation of the endotracheal tube to prevent aspiration in adult surgical intensive care unit patients: a feasibility study. Respir Care. 2010;55:294–302.

31. Thomas PJ, Paratz JD, Lipman J, Stanton WR. Lateral positioning of ventilated intensive care patients: a study of oxygenation, respiratory mechanics, hemodynamics, and adverse events. Heart Lung. 2007;36:277–86. https://doi.org/10.1016/j.hrtlng.2006.10.008.

32. Hewitt N, Bucknall T, Faraone NM. Lateral positioning for critically ill adult patients. Cochrane Database Syst Rev 2016, Issue 5. Art. No.: CD007205. DOI:https://doi.org/10.1002/14651858.CD007205.pub2.

33. Kim MJ, Hwang HJ, Song HH. A randomized trial on the effects of body positions on lung function with acute respiratory failure patients. Int J Nurs Stud. 2002;39:549–55.

34. Tongyoo S, Vilaichone W, Ratanarat R, Permpikul C. The effect of lateral position on oxygenation in ARDS patients: a pilot study. J Med Assoc Thail. 2006;89:S55–61.

35. Banasik JL, Emerson RJ. Effect of lateral positions on tissue oxygenation in the critically ill. Heart Lung. 2001;30:269–7895. https://doi.org/10.1067/mhl.2001.116012.

36. Jones AY, Dean E. Body position change and its effect on hemodynamic and metabolic status. Heart Lung. 2004;33:281–90.
37. Peterson MJ, Schwab W, van Oostrom JH, Gravenstein N, Caruso LJ. Effects of turning on skin-bed interface pressures in healthy adults. J Adv Nurs. 2010;66:1556–64. https://doi.org/10.1111/j.1365-2648.2010.05292.x.
38. Henderson WR, Griesdale DE, Dominelli P, Ronco JJ. Does prone positioning improve oxygenation and reduce mortality in patients with acute respiratory distress syndrome? Can Respir J. 2014;21:213–5.
39. Senecal PA. Prone position for Acute Respiratory Distress Syndrome. Crit Care Nurse. 2015;35:72. https://doi.org/10.4037/ccn2015990.
40. Bloomfield R, Noble DW, Sudlow A. Prone position for acute respiratory failure in adults. Cochrane Database Syst Rev 2015, Issue 11. Art. No.: CD008095. DOI:https://doi.org/10.1002/14651858.CD008095.pub2.
41. Taccone P, Pesenti A, Latini R, Polli F, Vagginelli F, Mietto C, et al. Prone positioning in patients with moderate and severe acute respiratory distress syndrome: a randomized controlled trial. JAMA. 2009;302:1977–84. https://doi.org/10.1001/jama.2009.1614.
42. Lucchini A, Pelucchi G, Gariboldi R, Vimercati S, Brambilla D, Elli S, et al. Prone position in patients with acute lung injury. Scenario. 2010;27:23–8.
43. Goettler CE, Pryor JP, Hoey BA, Phillips JK, Balas MC, Shapiro MB. Prone positioning does not affect cannula function during extracorporeal membrane oxygenation or continuous renal replacement therapy. Crit Care. 2002;6:452–5.
44. Maillet JM, Thierry S, Brodaty D. Prone positioning and acute respiratory distress syndrome after cardiac surgery: a feasibility study. J Cardiothorac Vasc Anesth. 2008;22:414–7. https://doi.org/10.1053/j.jvca.2007.10.013.
45. Michelet P, Roch A, Gainnier M, Sainty JM, Auffray JP, Papazian L. Influence of support on intra-abdominal pressure, hepatic kinetics of indocyanine green and extravascular lung water during prone positioning in patients with ARDS: a randomized crossover study. Crit Care. 2005 Jun;9:R251–7. https://doi.org/10.1186/cc3513.
46. Robak O, Schellongowski P, Bojic A, Laczika K, Locker GJ, Staudinger T. Short-term effects of combining upright and prone positions in patients with ARDS: a prospective randomized study. Crit Care. 2011;15:R230. https://doi.org/10.1186/cc10471.
47. Romero CM, Cornejo RA, Gálvez LR, Llanos OP, Tobar EA, Berasaín MA, et al. Extended prone position ventilation in severe acute respiratory distress syndrome: a pilot feasibility study. J Crit Care. 2009;24:81–8. https://doi.org/10.1016/j.jcrc.2008.02.005.

48. Oczenski W, Hörmann C, Keller C, Lorenzl N, Kepka A, Schwarz S, et al. Recruitment maneuvers during prone positioning in patients with acute respiratory distress syndrome. Crit Care Med. 2005;33:54–61.
49. Scaravilli V, Grasselli G, Castagna L, Zanella A, Isgrò S, Lucchini A, et al. Prone positioning improves oxygenation in spontaneously breathing nonintubated patients with hypoxemic acute respiratory failure: A retrospective study. J Crit Care. 2015;30:1390–4. https://doi.org/10.1016/j.jcrc.2015.07.008.
50. Reignier J, Thenoz-Jost N, Fiancette M, Legendre E, Lebert C, Bontemps F, et al. Early enteral nutrition in mechanically ventilated patients in the prone position. Crit Care Med. 2004;32:94–9. https://doi.org/10.1097/01.CCM.0000104208.23542.A8.
51. Reignier J, Dimet J, Martin-Lefevre L, Bontemps F, Fiancette M, Clementi E, et al. Before-after study of a standardized ICU protocol for early enteral feeding in patients turned in the prone position. Clin Nutr. 2010;29:210–6. https://doi.org/10.1016/j.clnu.2009.08.004.
52. Reinprecht A, Greher M, Wolfsberger S, Dietrich W, Illievich UM, Gruber A. Prone position in subarachnoid hemorrhage patients with acute respiratory distress syndrome: effects on cerebral tissue oxygenation and intracranial pressure. Crit Care Med. 2003;31:1831–8. https://doi.org/10.1097/01.CCM.0000063453.93855.0A.
53. Nekludov M, Bellander BM, Mure M. Oxygenation and cerebral perfusion pressure improved in the prone position. Acta Anaesthesiol Scand. 2006;50:932–6. https://doi.org/10.1111/j.1399-6576.2006.01099.x.
54. Roth C, Ferbert A, Deinsberger W, Kleffmann J, Kästner S, Godau J, et al. Does prone positioning increase intracranial pressure? A retrospective analysis of patients with acute brain injury and acute respiratory failure. Neurocrit Care. 2014;21:186–91. https://doi.org/10.1007/s12028-014-0004-x.
55. Defloor T. The effect of position and mattress on interface pressure. Appl Nurs Res. 2000;13:2–11.
56. Lippoldt J, Pernicka E, Staudinger T. Interface pressure at different degrees of backrest elevation with various types of pressure-redistribution surfaces. Am J Crit Care. 2014;23:119–26. https://doi.org/10.4037/ajcc2014670.
57. Still MD, Cross LC, Dunlap M, Rencher R, Larkins ER, Carpenter DL, et al. The turn team: a novel strategy for reducing pressure ulcers in the surgical intensive care unit. J Am Coll Surg. 2013;216:373–9. https://doi.org/10.1016/j.jamcollsurg.2012.12.001.
58. Lewandowski L, Lewandowski M. Intensive care in the obese. Best Pract Res Clin Anaesthesiol. 2011;25:95–108.

59. Tsueda K, Debrand M, Zeok SS, Wright BD, Griffin WO. Obesity supine death syndrome: reports of two morbidly obese patients. Anesth Analg. 1979;58:345–7.
60. Charlebois D, Wilmoth D. Critical Care of Patients With Obesity. Crit Care Nurse. 2004;24:19–27.
61. Lemyze M, Mallat J, Duhamel A, Pepy F, Gasan G, Barrailler S, et al. Effects of sitting position and applied positive end-expiratory pressure on respiratory mechanics of critically ill obese patients receiving mechanical ventilation*. Crit Care Med. 2013;41:2592–9. https://doi.org/10.1097/CCM.0b013e318298637f.
62. De Jong A, Molinari N, Sebbane M, Prades A, Futier E, Jung B, et al. Feasibility and effectiveness of prone position in morbidly obese patients with ARDS: a case-control clinical study. Chest. 2013;143:1554–61. https://doi.org/10.1378/chest.12-2115.
63. Bambi S, Ruggeri M, Becattini G, Lumini E. Bariatric patients in emergency department: a challenge for nursing care. Scenario. 2013;30:4–15.
64. Fragala G. Facilitating repositioning in bed. AAOHN J. 2011;59:63–8. https://doi.org/10.3928/08910162-20110117-01.
65. Groah SL, Schladen M, Pineda CG, Hsieh CH. Prevention of pressure ulcers among people with spinal cord injury: a systematic review. PMR. 2015;7:613–36. https://doi.org/10.1016/j.pmrj.2014.11.014.
66. Gutierrez CJ, Stevens C, Merritt J, Pope C, Tanasescu M, Curtiss G. Trendelenburg chest optimization prolongs spontaneous breathing trials in ventilator-dependent patients with low cervical spinal cord injury. J Rehabil Res Dev. 2010;47:261–72.
67. Guervilly C, Hraiech S, Gariboldi V, Xeridat F, Dizier S, Toesca R, et al. Prone positioning during veno-venous extracorporeal membrane oxygenation for severe acute respiratory distress syndrome in adults. Minerva Anestesiol. 2014;80:307–13.
68. Culbreth RE, Goodfellow LT. Complications of Prone Positioning During Extracorporeal Membrane Oxygenation for Respiratory Failure: A Systematic Review. Respir Care. 2016;61:249–54. https://doi.org/10.4187/respcare.03882.
69. Cheatham ML, De Waele JJ, De Laet I, De Keulenaer B, Widder S, Kirkpatrick AW, et al. The impact of body position on intra-abdominal pressure measurement: a multicenter analysis. Crit Care Med. 2009;37:2187–90. https://doi.org/10.1097/CCM.0b013e3181a021fa.
70. Yi M, Leng Y, Bai Y, Yao G, Zhu X. The evaluation of the effect of body positioning on intra-abdominal pressure measurement and the effect of intra-abdominal pressure at different body positioning on

organ function and prognosis in critically ill patients. J Crit Care. 2012;27:222.e1–6. https://doi.org/10.1016/j.jcrc.2011.08.010.

71. Barwing J, Pedroni C, Quintel M, Moerer O. Influence of body position, PEEP and intra-abdominal pressure on the catheter positioning for neurally adjusted ventilatory assist. Intensive Care Med. 2011;37:2041–5. https://doi.org/10.1007/s00134-011-2373-3.

72. Khir AW, Price S, Hale C, Young DA, Parker KH, Pepper JR. Intra-aortic balloon pumping: does posture matter? Artif Organs. 2005;29:36–40. https://doi.org/10.1111/j.1525-1594.2004.29013.x.

73. Chang AT, Boots RJ, Hodges PW, Thomas PJ, Paratz JD. Standing with the assistance of a tilt table improves minute ventilation in chronic critically ill patients. Arch Phys Med Rehabil. 2004;85:1972–6.

74. Hongrattana G, Reungjui P, Jones CU. Acute hemodynamic responses to 30° head-down postural drainage in stable, ventilated trauma patients: a randomized crossover trial. Heart Lung. 2014;43:399–405. https://doi.org/10.1016/j.hrtlng.2014.01.011.

75. Lizy C, Swinnen W, Labeau S, Poelaert J, Vogelaers D, Vandewoude K, et al. Cuff pressure of endotracheal tubes after changes in body position in critically ill patients treated with mechanical ventilation. Am J Crit Care. 2014;23:e1–8. https://doi.org/10.4037/ajcc2014489.

76. Chao YF, Chen YY, Wang KW, Lee RP, Tsai H. Removal of oral secretion prior to position change can reduce the incidence of ventilator-associated pneumonia for adult ICU patients: a clinical controlled trial study. J Clin Nurs. 2009;18:22–8. https://doi.org/10.1111/j.1365-2702.2007.02193.x.

77. Cooke M, Chaboyer W, Schluter P, Foster M, Harris D, Teakle R. The effect of music on discomfort experienced by intensive care unit patients during turning: a randomized cross-over study. Int J Nurs Pract. 2010;16:125–31. https://doi.org/10.1111/j.1440-172X.2010.01819.x.

78. Ahrens T, Kollef M, Stewart J, Shannon W. Effect of kinetic therapy on pulmonary complications. Am J Crit Care. 2004;13:376–83.

79. Ambrosino N, Janah N, Vagheggini G. Physiotherapy in critically ill patients. Rev Port Pneumol. 2011;17(6):283–8. https://doi.org/10.1016/j.rppneu.2011.06.004.

80. Delaney A, Gray H, Laupland KB, Zuege DJ. Kinetic bed therapy to prevent nosocomial pneumonia in mechanically ventilated patients: a systematic review and meta-analysis. Crit Care. 2006;10:R70. https://doi.org/10.1186/cc4912.

81. Prasarn ML, Horodyski M, Behrend C, Del Rossi G, Dubose D, Rechtine GR. Is it safe to use a kinetic therapy bed for care of patients

with cervical spine injuries? Injury. 2015;46:388–91. https://doi. org/10.1016/j.injury.2014.10.049.

82. Hamlin SK, Hanneman SK, Padhye NS, Lodato RF. Hemodynamic changes with manual and automated lateral turning in patients receiving mechanical ventilation. Am J Crit Care. 2015;24:131–40. https:// doi.org/10.4037/ajcc2015782.

83. Swadener-Culpepper L. Continuous lateral rotation therapy. Crit Care Nurse. 2010;30:S5–7. https://doi.org/10.4037/ccn2010766.

84. Brindle CT, Malhotra R, O'rourke S, Currie L, Chadwik D, Falls P, et al. Turning and repositioning the critically ill patient with hemodynamic instability: a literature review and consensus recommendations. J Wound Ostomy Continence Nurs. 2013;40:254–67. https://doi. org/10.1097/WON.0b013e318290448f.

# Chapter 9
# General Considerations About Infection Prevention

**Irene Comisso and Stefano Bambi**

Infections in the critically ill patients are challenging and increasing length of stay in ICU, subsequent morbidity, and mortality. It is widely recognized that all patients in ICU are prone to develop infections, both because of the severity of illness and treatments' invasiveness. A prevalence study [1] found a 51% prevalence of infection in ICU patients, with lungs being the most frequent site of infection (64%), followed by the abdomen, bloodstream, and urinary tract. Several factors increase the risk of infection for ICU patients (including length of stay, mechanical ventilation, medical or emergency surgery admission), and infection by itself is related to increased mortality and ICU and hospital length of stay. The infection prevalence varies significantly between continents and appears to be higher when the percentage of gross domestic product devoted to healthcare systems is low.

As for other critical care problems, the need to assess an infection risk became mandatory. At the same time, several factors may contribute to an infection development and mask other underlying conditions. A first attempt to predict infection in critically ill patients was tuned fine in 2003 [2], with the infection probability score (IPS). This simple tool (Table 9.1)

© Springer International Publishing AG, part of Springer Nature 2018    237
I. Comisso et al., *Nursing in Critical Care Setting*,
https://doi.org/10.1007/978-3-319-50559-6_9

**Table 9.1** IPS scoring

| IPS points | 0 | 1 | 2 | 3 | 6 | 8 | 12 |
|---|---|---|---|---|---|---|---|
| BT, °C | ≤37.5 | | <37.5 | | | | |
| HR, beats/min | ≤80 | | | | | 81–140 | 140 |
| RR, breaths/min | ≤25 | <25 | | | | | |
| WBC, ×$10^3$/mm$^3$ | 5–12 | <12 | | <5 | | | |
| CRP, mg/dl | ≤6 | | | | <6 | | |
| SOFA score | ≤5 | | <5 | | | | |

considers six variables commonly used in ICU daily care (heart rate, respiratory rate, white blood cells count, blood temperature, C-reactive protein, and SOFA score), whose total score can range between 0 and 26. Although fever is often suggestive for an ongoing infection, pooling together all of these variables provides clinician and nurses an adjunctive information to decide which patients should receive further diagnostic procedures, in order to quickly identify an infection. The validation process of this score reached high reliability (area under the ROC curve 0.962, with a 95% confidence interval between 0.806 and 0.923; sensitivity 90.0%, specificity 88.8%; positive predictive value 72.2%, negative predictive value 95.9%) with a cutoff value of 13.

IPS showed a higher prediction performance toward BSI in hematology-oncology patients, compared to APACHE II and Karnofsky score [3]. Comparisons between IPS and SOFA or APACHE II and III score showed a better performance of APACHE III score in predicting need for mechanical ventilation [4]. Despite these considerations, this tool could represent an adjunctive evaluation opportunity to intercept patients at higher risk of infection and decide concerning the antimicrobial therapy discontinuation [5].

Just as early identification of patients with high risk of infection is crucial, proper diagnosis should be obtained. Recently, an international consensus revised sepsis and septic shock definitions [6], overcoming the initial concept of sepsis as the presence of an infection together with at least two SIRS criteria. The new proposed definition describes sepsis as "life threatening organ dysfunction caused by a disregulated host response to infection," where "organ dysfunction can be identified as an acute change in total SOFA score $\geq 2$ points consequent to the infection."

Major efforts in fighting infections should tend first of all toward prevention, thus reducing the global cost of infections and other complications (such as increasing antimicrobial resistance). Guidelines for infection prevention [7] pointed their attention not only on correct patients' and devices' management but also on healthcare workers' behaviors and education.

Horizontal precautions embrace hospital environment and hand hygiene and staff and patients' education. A clean environment and proper selection of disinfectant agents for environment and shared equipments are recommended. Hand hygiene is widely known as one of the most important factors in reducing infections and cross infections, and therefore several campaigns (WHO) to increase adherence to this simple practice were undertaken. Traditional handwashing (water and soap) is only recommended when body fluids visibly or potentially contaminate hands or when caring for patients with diarrhea or vomiting. Hand rubbing with alcohol-based solutions is probably more advantageous, since it is easier to be performed and more effective in terms of hands contamination reduction. Staff and patients' education concerns both preparation and management of devices used for care, who's invasiveness (endotracheal tubes or intravascular catheters) is sometimes high and therefore predisposing to microbial invasion. When inserting such devices, proper aseptic technique (including maximum barrier precautions, when indicated) should be adopted, so as when devices are accessed (for blood sampling or endotracheal suctioning).

Great progresses on infection prevention came from bundles' introduction. Bundles are defined as a small group of interventions, aiming to provide patients with similar problems the best available care. Bundles differ according to the considered problem, but they generally consider the need to keep in the device, handwashing, and interventions for the device maintenance. More detailed information about bundles are provided in specific Chaps. 10, 11, and 12.

# References

1. Vincent JL, Rello J, Marshall J, Silva E, Anzueto A, Martin CD, Moreno R, Lipman J, Gomersall C, Sakr Y, Reinhart K, EPIC II Group of Investigators. International study of the prevalence and outcomes of infection in intensive care units. JAMA. 2009; 302(21):2323–9.
2. Peres Bota D, Mélot C, Lopes Ferreira F, Vincent JL. Infection probability score (IPS): a method to help assess the probability of infection in critically ill patients. Crit Care Med. 2003;31(11):2579–84. https://doi.org/10.1097/01.CCM.0000094223.92746.56.
3. Apostolopoulou E, Raftopoulos V, Terzis K, Elefsiniotis I. Infection probability score, APACHE II and KARNOFSKY scoring systems as predictors of bloodstream infection onset in hematology-oncology patients. BMC Infect Dis. 2010;10:135. https://doi.org/10.1186/1471-2334-10-135.
4. Safavi M, Honarmand A. Comparison of infection probability score, APACHE II, and APACHE III scoring systems in predicting need for ventilator and ventilation duration in critically ill patients. Arch Iran Med. 2007;10(3):354–60. https://doi.org/07103/AIM.0014.
5. Martini A, Gottin L, Mélot C, Vincent JL. A prospective evaluation of the infection probability score (IPS) in the intensive care unit. J Infect. 2008;56(5):313–8. https://doi.org/10.1016/j.jinf.2008.02.015.
6. Singer M, Deutschman CS, Seymour CW, Shankar-Hari M, Annane D, Bauer M, Bellomo R, Bernard GR, Chiche JD, Coopersmith CM, Hotchkiss RS, Levy MM, Marshall JC, Martin GS, Opal SM, Rubenfeld GD, van der Poll T, Vincent JL, Angus DC. The third international consensus definitions for sepsis and septic shock (Sepsis-3). JAMA. 2016;315(8):801–10. https://doi.org/10.1001/jama.2016.0287.

7. Loveday HP, Wilson JA, Pratt RJ, Golsorkhi M, Tingle A, Bak A, Browne J, Prieto J, Wilcox M, UK Department of Health. epic3: national evidence-based guidelines for preventing healthcare-associated infections in NHS hospitals in England. J Hosp Infect. 2014;86(Suppl 1):S1–70. https://doi.org/10.1016/S0195-6701(13)60012-2.

# Part III
# Care Quality Measurement: From Performance Indicators to Nursing Sensitive Outcomes

# Chapter 10
# Prevention of Hospital-Acquired Pneumonia and Ventilator-Associated Pneumonia

Stefano Bambi

## 10.1 Introduction

Healthcare-associated infections (HAIs) belong to hospital-acquired conditions (HACs) and account for patients' mortality ranging from 5% to 35% [1]. Their prevalence in ICUs ranges from 9% to 37%, with a mortality rate up to 50% [2].

In 2005, the American Thoracic Society published guidelines for management of three kinds of pneumonia in hospitalized patients: hospital-acquired pneumonia (HAP), ventilator-associated pneumonia (VAP), and healthcare-associated pneumonia (HCAP) [3] (Table 10.1).

HAP is the most frequent hospital infection after UTI, while it is at the first place in ICU [4]. Actually, a HAP in ventilated patients is a VAP. Consequently, the frequency of HAP in ICU can be split into VAP (86%) and non-VAP (14%) [5]. In general, VAP has an incidence rate of 8–28% [4]. HAP and VAP increase hospital LOS and costs [5]. VAP mortality rates vary from 20% to 76% [6].

© Springer International Publishing AG, part of Springer Nature 2018     245
I. Comisso et al., *Nursing in Critical Care Setting*,
https://doi.org/10.1007/978-3-319-50559-6_10

**Table 10.1** Definitions of patients' respiratory infective complications acquired during hospitalization [3]

| Typology of pneumonia | Definition |
| --- | --- |
| Hospital-acquired pneumonia (HAP) | Pneumonia that occurs 48 h or more after admission, which was not incubating at the time of admission |
| Ventilator-associated pneumonia (VAP) | Pneumonia that arises more than 48–72 h after endotracheal intubation |
| Healthcare-associated pneumonia (HCAP) | Includes any patient who was hospitalized in an acute care hospital for 2 or more days within 90 days of the infection; resided in a nursing home or long-term care facility; received recent intravenous antibiotic therapy, chemotherapy, or wound care within the past 30 days of the current infection; or attended a hospital or hemodialysis clinic |

About 30%–50% of the deaths related to HAP seem to be directly due to pneumonia [7]. The mortality rates of early- and late-onset HAP or VAP are comparable [5].

This chapter will focus mainly on the definitions, pathogenesis, risk factors, and prevention of HAP and VAP in ICU adult patients, with particular attention to the critical care nurses' contribution. The discussion about the treatment of pneumonia goes beyond the aims of this review.

## 10.2 Hospital-Acquired Pneumonia

HAP is classified as early onset (≤96 h from admission time) and late onset (>96 h) [3, 5].

HAP development is due to the impairment in the balance between patients' immunologic defense and the microorganism inclination to penetrate and colonize the lower airways [3].

The pathogenesis of HAP is through the spreading of microorganisms in the patient's lower airways and the overcoming of his/her defenses. Otherwise, the lowering of immunologic state can ease the infection by pathogens [5].

Responsible microorganisms can be exogenous or endogenous. HAP can develop more frequently from endogenous infection given by pathogens colonizing the airways, or through micro-aspiration of oropharyngeal secretions [5]. Staff and medical devices are responsible for the exogenous infection, especially in ICU. Lastly, bacteremia can be spread from other infection sites, or intravascular or urinary catheters through the bloodstream [5].

HAP is suspected when at least two of the following signs are detected: body temperature > 38 °C or <36 °C, leukopenia or leukocytosis, purulent airway secretions, or reduction in $PaO_2$ [5].

The inadequacy of initial antibiotic treatment of HAP (22%–73%) is the most influential factor on patients' prognosis [7]. The establishment and implementation of appropriate antibiotic treatment protocols and algorithms are fundamental for patients' survival [7].

## 10.3   Healthcare-Associated Pneumonia

Healthcare-associated pneumonia definition was formulated by the American Thoracic Society [3] (Table 10.1) to include the pneumonia acquired in healthcare environments outside of the traditional hospital setting, which have specific risk factors [8]. The concept of HCAP stands between CAP and HAP concerning to the causative pathogens and mortality rates (about 20% [9]) and mainly affects aging patients in healthcare facilities [10]. One of the principal physiopathologic mechanisms of pneumonia recognized in this category of patients is aspiration [10].

HCAP encompasses several conditions, and researches about HCAP have been performed on highly variable populations [9]. Later, another category was included in the HCAP: immunosuppressed patients (corticosteroid treatment, HIV infection, transplant, recent radiation or chemotherapy, inherited or acquired immunodeficiency) [9].

HCAP was originally treated with the same medical approach as CAP. Later studies suggested that HCAP could differ from CAP in terms of pathogens and prognosis while being similar to HAP and VAP [8], needing initial treatment with broad-spectrum antimicrobial agents [9].

A recent meta-analysis showed that HCAP was associated with increased mortality, compared with CAP [11]. HCAP was not a good predictor of resistant pathogens [11]; therefore, the higher mortality seemed to be due to higher mean age and comorbid illnesses associated with HCAP [9, 11].

As HCAP concept does not cover patients staying in critical care units, further discussion of this issue is beyond the aim of this chapter.

## 10.4 Ventilator-Associated Pneumonia

VAP is pneumonia that developed in MV patients 48–72 h after the time of intubation [12, 13].

Their classification is based on the onset time. Early VAP develops ≤96 h from intubation and has better prognosis, and the etiologic agents are usually community microorganisms [12]. Late VAP can occur >96 h after intubation and is often caused by multidrug-resistant pathogens [12].

VAP incidence rates represent a quality of care indicator in critical care [12, 14].

The use of incidence density of VAP is recommended over the simple incidence rate to perform optimal surveillance programs and benchmarking.

## 10.4.1   Pathogenesis of VAP and Risk Factors

There are two kinds of risk factors for development of VAP. Host factors are related to the patients' response to intubation and ventilation, while intervention factors come from the treatment and care provided to the patient by healthcare staff (Table 10.2) [15].

**Table 10.2**  Risk factors for development of VAP [12, 15]

| Host factors | Intervention factors |
| --- | --- |
| Oropharyngeal colonization | Emergency intubation[b] |
| Gastric colonization | Re-intubation[a,b] |
| Thermal injury (burns) | Tracheostomy[a,b] |
| Post-traumatic | Bronchoscopy |
| Head injury[a] | Nasogastric tube/enteral nutrition[b] |
| Postsurgical | Duration of hospital stay/ICU stay[b] |
| Neurosurgery[a] | Multiple central venous line insertions[b] |
| Impaired consciousness | Sedatives[b] |
| Immunosuppression | Stress ulcer prophylaxis[b] |
| (Multi-) organ failure[a] | Prior antibiotics/no antibiotic |
| Sinusitis | prophylaxis |
| Severity of underlying illness | Immunosuppressive medications |
| Old age ($\geq 60$ years)[a] | (corticosteroids) |
| Sex – male[a] | Supine head position |
| Presence of comorbidities | Contamination of ventilator circuits |
| Preexisting pulmonary disease[a] | Frequent patient transfers |
| Coma[a,b] | Low endotracheal tube cuff pressure |
| Gastric overdistension | |

[a]Nonmodifiable risk factors
[b]Independent risk factors

The etiological agents determining VAP can vary among different patient populations, hospitals, and countries [6]. These microorganisms can be endogenous or exogenous (coming from other patients, medical devices, and healthcare environment or staff) [6]. Bacteria frequently involved in the genesis of early VAP are *Streptococcus pneumoniae* (and other streptococcus species), *Haemophilus influenzae*, methicillin-sensitive *Staphylococcus aureus*, antibiotic-sensitive enteric Gram-negative bacilli, *Escherichia coli*, *Klebsiella pneumoniae*, *Enterobacter* species, *Proteus* species, and *Serratia marcescens* [13]. Late-onset VAP is generally caused by multidrug-resistant bacteria, such as methicillin-resistant *S. aureus*, *Acinetobacter*, *Pseudomonas aeruginosa*, and extended-spectrum beta-lactamase-producing bacteria [13]. A percentage of VAP ranging from 30% to 70% is caused by multiple microorganisms [6].

*Pseudomonas*, *Acinetobacter*, and methicillin-resistant *S. aureus* pneumonia are associated with higher rates of VAP mortality [6].

Infective agents reach the lower respiratory tract, adhere to the airways mucosa, and determine infections [16]. The mechanisms of airway contamination by pathogens are [6, 16]:

- Aspiration of microbes loaded secretions around the cuff of endotracheal tube (or tracheostomy tube). These secretions come from the nasopharynx and oropharynx or by gastroesophageal reflux.
- Presence of infective processes from contiguous anatomical structure.
- Contaminated medical aerosol or ambient air.
- Contaminated medical devices (e.g., bronchoscopes, breathing circuits, humidifiers, and suction catheters).
- Contaminated hands.
- Contaminated uniforms or gowns (e.g., from contact with other patients, taps, trolleys, etc.).
- Microorganisms from other remote sites of infection, e.g., intravascular catheter-related BSI.

## 10.4.2  Diagnosis

Currently, there is no gold standard for VAP diagnosis. The present clinical methods do not have the optimal sensitivity and specificity to identify VAP [13]. Chest radiography added to patient clinical assessment is not able to completely define VAP but only to be suggestive of it [13]. Up to about one third of VAP can be disregarded by clinical diagnostic criteria [13].

The clinical suspicion of VAP is given by new or persistent radiographic infiltrates or consolidation and at least two of the following elements [6, 13]:

- Body temperature > 38 °C
- Leukocytosis (WBC count $\geq$ 12,000 cells/mm$^3$) or leukopenia (WBC count <4000 cells/mm$^3$)
- Presence of purulent secretions

Since only about one third of clinically diagnosed VAP cases were confirmed by microbiological analysis results, the Clinical Pulmonary Infection Score has been designed to overcome this problem [6]. CPIS evaluates six items, each one ranging from 0 to 2 points: body temperature, leukocyte count, quantity and purulence of tracheal secretions (subjective visual scale), oxygenation status ($PaO_2/FiO_2$), type of radiographic abnormality, and results of endotracheal aspirate culture [6, 13]. A score of $\geq$ 6 showed a worthy correlation with VAP occurrence [16]. Currently, the diagnostic validity of this score is still debated because of interobserver variability [13].

Airway secretion samples for Gram stain, culture, and sensitivity can be obtained through [13]:

- Endotracheal aspirate. It is the simplest method.
- Bronchoalveolar lavage, performed under bronchoscopic guidance.

- Mini-bronchoalveolar lavage, performed without broncho-scopic guidance, in "blind" fashion.
- Protected specimen brush, through a brush at the tip of the catheter.

The American Thoracic Society 2005 HAP/VAP guidelines specified the need for lower airway tract samples for (qualitative or quantitative) microbiological culture and analysis of secretions [3].

## 10.4.3 From Ventilator-Associated Pneumonia to the Concept of Ventilator-Associated Conditions

The lack of gold standard in VAP diagnosis and the consequent difficulties in the surveillance programs and benchmarking processes, brought USA healthcare organs to make some changes aiming to improve the quality of data collection and analysis.

The Centers for Disease Control and Prevention recently drafted some new surveillance definitions, introducing a tiered classification of ventilator-associated events (VAEs) for adult patients [17].

The VAE concept is represented by a progressive and sustained augmentation of MV settings, coming after a clinical stability period [14]. VAEs include ARDS, pulmonary edema, atelectasis, and VAP (Table 10.3) [14]. VAE algorithm aims to identify different MV complications, improve surveillance and benchmarking, and reduce the risk of gaming [13]. CDC believes that VAE algorithm could reveal a more truthful VAP rate, despite some institution reports of (almost) zero VAP rate, probably due to economic and healthcare penalty reasons [13]. CDC clearly specified that "the VAE definition algorithm is for

**Table 10.3** CDC definition tiers for ventilator-associated event in adults [14, 17]

| Tier | Definition |
| --- | --- |
| Ventilator-associated event (VAE) | "VAEs are identified by using a combination of objective criteria: deterioration in respiratory status after a period of stability or improvement on the ventilator, evidence of infection or inflammation, and laboratory evidence of respiratory infection" "Patients must be mechanically ventilated for more than two calendar days to be eligible for VAE" |
| Ventilator-associated condition (VAC) | "VAC is defined by greater than or equal to 2 days of stable or decreasing daily minimum positive end expiratory pressure (PEEP) or daily minimum fraction of inspired oxygen ($FiO_2$) followed by an increase in daily minimum PEEP greater than or equal to 3 $cmH_2O$ or daily minimum $FiO_2$ greater than or equal to 0.20 points sustained for greater than or equal to 2 calendar days" |
| Infection-related ventilator-associated complication (IVAC) | "IVAC is triggered by the presence of possible infection indicators concurrent with VAC onset, namely, an abnormal temperature (below 36 ° C or above 38 ° C) or white blood cell count (less than or equal to 4000 or greater than or equal to 12,000 cells/$mm^3$) and 1 or more new antibiotic starts that continue for greater than or equal to 4 days" |
| Possible VAP | "Possible VAP is defined as Gram stain evidence of purulent pulmonary secretions or a pathogenic pulmonary culture in a patient with IVAC" |
| Probable VAP | "Probable VAP is defined as Gram stain evidence of purulence plus quantitative or semiquantitative growth of a pathogenic organism beyond specified thresholds. Probable VAP can also be triggered by positive tests for respiratory viruses, *Legionella* species, pleural fluid cultures, and suggestive histopathology with or without an abnormal Gram stain result" |

use in surveillance; it is not a clinical definition algorithm and is not intended for use in the clinical management of patients" [17].

The Society for Healthcare Epidemiology of America with the Infectious Diseases Society of America (SHEA/IDSA) paper specifies that the definition of VAC and IVAC was designed for public reporting or benchmarking, but more evidences about preventability and comparability are needed before their implementation [14]. On the contrary, possible and probable VAP definition should be employed only for quality improvement in single units or institutions. In fact, there are many differences in the methods used by clinicians to collect samples from patients under MV [14].

Finally, some study results indicate that the VAE definitions do not optimally perform in identifying many VAP cases [18]. Moreover, VAEs can detect many events without real hospital complications and are at risk of report artifacts [18].

### 10.4.4   VAP Prevention Strategies: What Works and What Does Not

In 2014 the SHEA/IDSA, the American Hospital Association, the Association for Professionals in Infection Control and Epidemiology, and the Joint Commission published an update of the recommendations about the strategies to prevent VAP in acute care hospitals, previously issued in 2008 [14]. The intervention levels of evidence were assessed through the Grades of Recommendation, Assessment, Development, and Evaluation (GRADE) [19] and the Canadian Task Force on Preventive Health Care [20].

This document covers two main issues: VAP surveillance strategies and VAP prevention interventions [14].

Currently, VAP preventive interventions focus on three areas: reducing the time at risk, preventing endotracheal tube colonization and minimizing contaminated, modulation of colonization [21].

Taking in account the current problems related to the accuracy and reproducibility of VAP diagnoses, SHEA/IDSA drafted their recommendations on the basis of published evidence on "hard" outcome as days of MV, ICU or hospital LOS, and mortality. Moreover, the authors assessed the balancing among costs, harms, benefit, and feasibility of interventions, distinguishing the interventions in four categories [14]. Basic practices collect all the interventions improving the hard outcomes with low risk of harm. Special approaches are interventions that can improve the outcomes with some risk of detriment for patients or reducing the VAP rates without data about the main outcomes and should be considered when basic practices fail to reach the desired outcomes [14]. Interventions generally not recommended for prevention are those able to reduce the VAP rates but with no influence on the "hard" outcomes [14]. Lastly, interventions without positive impact on VAP rates and outcomes are neither recommended nor discouraged [14]. SHEA/IDSA recommendations are summarized in Table 10.4, with a special column to show which interventions are under the complete commitment of nurses.

Some VAP interventions, especially those directly pertinent to nurses, deserve additional considerations.

NIV is a consolidated treatment to prevent intubation, finding its application in all hospital settings and increasing the evidence of effectiveness in lots of clinical conditions [22]. Given that NIV is a tool to avoid intubation, it prevents the main pathogenic mechanisms of VAP.

Five of the SHEA/IDSA basic practices (daily sedation interruptions, daily assessment of extubation readiness, spontaneous breathing trial performed with no sedatives, early mobilization)

**Table 10.4** Quality of evidence for VAP preventing strategies according to Society for Healthcare Epidemiology of America and Infectious Diseases Society of America (Modified from Klompas et al. [14])

| Recommendation | Intervention | Quality of evidence (GRADE) | Nursing care preserve |
|---|---|---|---|
| Basic practices | NIV in selected populations | High | |
| | Manage patients without sedation, whenever possible | Moderate | |
| | Daily sedation interruptions | High | √ |
| | Daily assessment of extubation readiness | High | √ |
| | Spontaneous breathing trial performed with no sedatives | High | √ |
| | Early mobilization | Moderate | √ |
| | Endotracheal tubes with subglottic drainage systems in patients requiring more than 48 or 72 h of MV | Moderate | |
| | Change of ventilator breathing circuits only when visibly soiled or in case of malfunctioning | High | √ |
| | HOB elevation to 30°–45° | Low | √ |

(continued)

**Table 10.4** (continued)

| Recommendation | Intervention | Quality of evidence (GRADE) | Nursing care preserve |
|---|---|---|---|
| Special approaches | Selective oral or digestive decontamination | High | |
| | Regular oral hygiene with chlorhexidine oral rinse | Moderate | √ |
| | Ultrathin polyurethane endotracheal tube cuffs | Low | |
| | Automated control systems of endotracheal tube cuff pressure | Low | |
| | Saline instillation before tracheal suctioning | Low | √ |
| | Mechanical tooth brushing | Low | √ |
| Generally not recommended | Silver-coated endotracheal tubes | Moderate | |
| | Kinetic beds | Moderate | √ |
| | Prone positioning | Moderate | |
| | Stress ulcer prophylaxis | Moderate | |
| | Early tracheotomy | High | |
| | Monitoring residual gastric volumes | Moderate | √ |
| | Early parenteral nutrition | Moderate | |
| No recommendation | Closed system/in-line endotracheal suctioning | Moderate | √ |

clearly belong to the ABCDE bundle [23]. These interventions aim to reduce MV duration and intubation and decrease LOS. An in-depth discussion about the ABCDE bundle is issued in Chap. 17.

The employment of endotracheal tubes with subglottic drainage systems represents a cost-saving intervention with high efficacy for VAP prevention in patients requiring at least 48 (or 72) hours of intubation [14]. These special tubes can be managed through intermittent or continuous suctioning, or mixed modes. The suction pressures reported in literature widely range from $-20$ to $-110$ mmHg for intermittent mode and from $-20$ to $-30$ mmHg for continuous mode [24]. A recent meta-analysis showed that subglottic secretion drainage is effective in preventing VAP (RR = 0.56, 95% CI 0.45–0.69, $p < 0.00001$) and early VAP (RR = 0.23, 95% CI 0.13–0.43, $p < 0.00001$) [25]. Subgroup analyses suggested a better reduction in incidence of VAP through intermittent vs. continuous suction system (RR = 0.49, 95% CI 0.34–0.71, $p = 0.0001$ vs. RR = 0.61, 95% CI 0.46–0.79, $p = 0.0003$) [25].

Data about possible adverse effects of these systems are still lacking. Moreover, there are no studies about the effectiveness of tracheostomy tubes with subglottic suction ports.

The scheduled change of ventilator breathing circuits can only increase the healthcare costs, since it has no impact on the VAP rates [26]. Hence, the recommendations to change the breathing circuits are only when visibly soiled or in case of malfunctioning [14].

Head of bed elevation to $30°$–$45°$, even if devoid of evidence about positive impact on VAP rates or other major outcomes [27], is a simple and low-cost intervention to implement [14]. The underlying rationale is to prevent the micro-inhalation of gastric content. The real problem, instead, lies in the conflict between VAP guidelines recommending the HOB elevation to prevent VAP and PU guidelines recommending the maintenance of HOB under $30°$ to limit the gliding of patients and the generation of friction forces [28]. Experts recommend to give priority to the HOB elevation upper than 30°, unless it conflicts with nursing tasks, doctors' interventions, or patients' desires [27].

Selective digestive and oral decontamination mainly by topical application of nonabsorbable antibiotics is a medical intervention with high level of evidence related to lowering mortality rates [14, 21]. However, the principal hindrance to the wide implementations of these practices is the potential occurrence of bacterial resistance [14, 21].

Oral hygiene with chlorhexidine is well discussed in Chap. 7. Chlorhexidine has a long-lasting effect, and a recent meta-analysis showed its dose-effect characteristics [29]. The subgroup analysis showed that the 2% concentration solution was associated with a significant reduction of RR of VAP, compared to 0.2%–0.12% solutions [29]. Moreover, the cardiosurgical patients showed better VAP prevention effects from oral antisepsis with chlorhexidine [29].

Low-level evidence is available for ETT with ultrathin polyurethane cuffs. However, the rationale for their implementation is the reduction of secretion gliding around the cuff. In fact, ultrathin polyurethane cuffs seal against the tracheal mucosa better than other kinds of tubes [14].

Similarly, the use of automated control of endotracheal tube cuff pressure for VAP prevention is based on a scant number of studies [14]. The tube cuff pressure should be maintained between 25 and 30 $cmH_2O$ [30]. Pressures higher than 30 $cmH_2O$ for more than 15 minutes determine ischemic damages on the tracheal mucosa [31]. Pressure values lower than 20 $cmH_2O$ are associated to more than the double increase of VAP rates [31]. Although there is still no consensus about the optimal frequency of cuff pressure monitoring [31], it seems reasonable to perform it more than once during the work shift. Furthermore, patient's oral hygiene, repositioning, and HOB momentary dropping should be preceded by the control of cuff pressure to prevent the risk of micro-aspiration. It's mandatory to use a manometer to control the cuff pressure, while the minimal occlusive volume or minimal leak technique should be limited only in emergency settings.

Saline instillation before endotracheal suctioning is another large controversial issue. While the recommendation of this intervention by SHEA/IDSA finds its evidence in a single RCT on oncological patients admitted in ICU [14], American Association of Respiratory Care guidelines on suctioning of MV patients currently suggest that "…routine use of normal saline instillation prior to endotracheal suction should not be performed." This is another case of conflict between different guidelines, making difficult the choice of the better (or less harmful) practice for patients [32].

Toothbrushing is also an intervention lacking of evidence. A recent meta-analysis showed that toothbrushing was not associated with the reduction of VAP rates nor any improved major outcome [33]. Nevertheless, the mechanical action of toothbrushing remains unique in the prevention and removal of the oral biofilm (dental plaque) [34]. Therefore, in spite of the decreased effectiveness of toothbrushing actions in orotracheal-intubated patients, nurses should perform this technique to eliminate as much dental plaque as possible.

Silver-coated endotracheal tubes can contrast the development of biofilm in their inner surface [21]. A recent Cochrane systematic review showed limited evidence that this kind of device reduces the risk of VAP, particularly during the first 10 days of MV [35].

The use of kinetic beds (continuous lateral rotational therapy and oscillation therapy) can reduce the incidence of VAP but does not affect patients' mortality [36]. Nonetheless some authors suggest that costs and feasibility can hinder the implementation of kinetic beds [37].

Similarly, prone positioning of critically ill patient as preventive measure of VAP, even if positively affecting its incidence, should consider the risk-benefit balance, before its implementation [36].

Stress ulcer prophylaxis is suggested to prevent gastrointestinal bleeding but has no impact on VAP rates or other major outcomes as LOS and mortality [14].

A Cochrane systematic review comparing the effectiveness and safety of early tracheostomy (performed ≤10 days after patient intubation) with late tracheostomy (performed >10 days after patient intubation) showed no difference in pneumonia rates but a significant reduced mortality rate in the early tracheostomy group [38]. These results are from a moderate level of evidence [38].

Although no consensus exists about gastric residual volume tolerance, some authors suggest that EN should be stopped with a GRV >500 mL. Adequate assessment and treatment should be undertaken to resolve this problem [39]. In MV patients, it seems prudent to not overcome the threshold of 250 mL [40]. Furthermore, the timely assessment of GRV should be always guaranteed, in spite of the results of a RCT showing that the absence of GRV monitoring was not associated with a higher VAP incidence than the routinely assessment [40]. In this study, the episodes of vomiting were 39.6% in the no GRV monitoring group, whereas only 27% in the routinely GRV monitoring group (difference 12.6%, 90% CI 5.4%–19.9%) [40].

Concerning the parenteral nutrition in critically ill patients, higher risks of mortality and infections are associated to an early start (≤ 48 hours from admission in ICU), than after 8 days [41].

SHEA/IDSA does not suggest any recommendation about the use (or not) of in-line suctioning system in intubated patients, since there is no evidence of lower association to VAP development or other major patient outcomes, compared to open suction system [14, 42]. However, closed suctioning systems have some points of strength that should be considered. There are some cost-effective evidences showing that in-line suctioning systems can be changed only when visibly soiled or malfunctioning [43]. Moreover, their adoption is suggested by AARC in adult patients ventilated with high levels of $FIO_2$ or

PEEP [32]. Finally, closed suction systems offer a valuable barrier toward exposure to respiratory infective agents during the suctioning maneuvers in patient with serious illnesses as tuberculosis.

There are other kinds of VAP prevention interventions that SHEA/IDSA document did not take in account: PEEP, chest physiotherapy, probiotics, iseganan, and intermittent or continuous suction of oral secretions. The application of prophylactic PEEP in non-hypoxemic ventilated patients showed a RRR of 63% for VAP rates but no impact on mortality, ICU and hospital LOS, and duration of MV [21]. None of the four studies evaluated in a recent literature review affected any major outcome [21]. Only a clinical trial revealed a RRR of 79% for VAP rates [44]. Probiotics are living microbial agents of human origins conferring a health benefit on the host if administered in adequate amounts. Probiotic administration determined a RRR of 47% for VAP rates but no effects on ICU LOS and duration of MV [21]. The employment of iseganan, a large specter antimicrobial peptide for oral care, failed to demonstrate any positive result on VAP rates and major patient outcomes [21]. Suctioning oral secretion before repositioning of patients seems to reduce significantly the VAP rates (2.6% in the studied group vs. 11% in the control group) and duration of MV [45]. However, this pilot study was performed with a before-after design and with a relatively small sample size (227 patients in the studied group, 237 in the control group) [45]. A pilot randomized controlled trial was performed to assess the effectiveness of a low-cost device (saliva ejector) on the reduction of VAP incidence. The device was inserted in the patients' oral cavity, between the cheek and teeth [46]. Suctioning was set to 100 mmHg to guarantee continuous drainage of saliva. The authors found a large difference in VAP rates between the studied and control groups (23.1% vs. 83.3%, $p = 0.003$), but this study was affected by a very small sample size (25 patients) [46]. Even if no damage to patients was reported, the safety of this device on ICU patients requires more studies [46].

Even if humidification of inspired gas is not considered as a tool of VAP prevention, it has been studied to evaluate which method, between passive (heated and moisture exchangers, HME) and active (heated humidifiers, HH) systems, is safer in terms of VAP incidence. A systematic review performed by the Cochrane Collaboration reported little evidence on the overall difference between HMEs and HHs [47]. However, hydrophobic HMEs may reduce the risk of pneumonia [47]. Unfortunately, the employing of HMEs has several limitations, due to the large differences in humidification performances among the make and models in the market (minimum standard 30 mgH$_2$O/L) and the contraindications (e.g., body temperature < 32 °C, low tidal volume ventilation, thick or copious airway secretions, spontaneous minute volumes >10 L/min) [48].

## 10.4.5   Bundle of Care: From the Evidence to Good Sense

In 2004, during the "save a 100,000 lives campaign," the Institute of Healthcare Improvement (IHI) introduced the "ventilator bundle," aimed to maximizing the critically ill patients' safety and outcomes [49]. The IHI bundles of care evidence-based interventions were four: HOB elevation over 30°, daily sedation interruptions and readiness to wean assessment, peptic ulcer disease (PUD) prophylaxis, and deep vein thrombosis (DVT) prophylaxis [49]. The concept at the basis of bundle of care is to implement a little cluster of evidence-based interventions (3–5) to improve the patients' outcomes [50]. Gathered interventions reach greater effectiveness than individual ones in obtaining the desired outcomes [49].

Bundles of care are useful tools for ICU staff, easing deci-
sional processes, diminishing the risk of errors in medical rea-
soning, supporting an outcome-oriented care, and offering
simple and solid interventions in ambiguity zones of clinical
practice [51].

Even if the implementation of IHI ventilator bundle was
associated with a decrease in VAP rates, some of the bundle elements (sedation interruptions and readiness to wean assessment,
PUD prophylaxis, DVT prophylaxis) are not directly involved in
reaching this outcome [50]. Therefore, some authors suggested
the addition of two evidence-based practices to the bundle: oral
hygiene with chlorhexidine antiseptic and ETT with subglottic
secretion drainage [50, 52].

After the introduction of the IHI ventilator bundle, a large
number of observational studies were performed using different
combinations of interventions to prevent VAP (Table 10.5). The
number of interventions included in the different VAP bundles
ranged from 4 to 11. Almost all studies showed a significant
reduction in VAP rates [49], but only one research showed
reduction of mortality [53].

The authors of a recent systematic review about VAEs recommend some key actions to improve the design and implementation of bundles [49]:

- Gathering the bundle with evidence-based interventions
- Choosing the bundle interventions on the basis of local availability of resources
- Increasing the adherence of healthcare staff through team-
  based strategies
- Considering that compliance to the interventions is more
  critical than the number of interventions to include in the
  bundle
- Using adequate education programs for the implementation
  phase, process and outcome indicator measurements, and

**Table 10.5** Different kinds of VAP bundles implemented in the studies from 2005 to 2014 [49]

| Interventions | Outcomes | Number of studies |
|---|---|---|
| *IHI ventilator bundle, composed by* | VAP rates ↓ | 11 |
| HOB elevation over 30° | Mean ventilation | |
| Daily sedation interruptions and | days ↓ | |
| readiness to wean assessment | ICU LOS ↓ | |
| PUD prophylaxis | Mortality rate ↓ | |
| DVT prophylaxis | | |
| HOB elevation 30° | VAP rates ↓ | 1 |
| Oral care | ICU LOS ↓ | |
| Hand hygiene | | |
| Glove use | | |
| Change/empty condensation in tubing | | |
| IHI ventilator bundle | VAP rates ↓ | 1 |
| Oral care every 2 h | ICU LOS ↓ | |
| Turning every 2 h | | |
| IHI ventilator bundle | VAP rates ↓ | 2 |
| Oral care | ICU LOS ↓ | |
| Hand hygiene | | |
| HOB elevation 30° | VAP rates ↓ | 1 |
| Oral care with chlorhexidine | ICU LOS ↓ | |
| Hand hygiene | | |
| Glove use | | |
| Tracheal cuff pressure maintenance >20 cm $H_2O$ | | |
| Use of orogastric tubes | | |
| Avoidance of gastric overdistension | | |
| Elimination of nonessential tracheal suction | | |
| HOB elevation 30° | VAP rates ↓ | 1 |
| Oral care | | |
| Daily sedation vacation and readiness to wean assessment | | |

(continued)

**Table 10.5** (continued)

| Interventions | Outcomes | Number of studies |
|---|---|---|
| HOB elevation 30° | VAP rates ↓ | 1 |
| Oral care | | |
| Hand hygiene | | |
| Condensation in ventilator tubing checked | | |
| Daily assessment of readiness to wean | | |
| DVT prophylaxis | | |
| PUD prophylaxis | | |
| HOB elevation 30° | VAP rates ↓ | 1 |
| Oral care | | |
| Daily sedation vacation and readiness to wean assessment | | |
| NIV use and duration minimization | | |
| Use of orotracheal intubation | | |
| Maintenance of endotracheal cuff pressure > 20-cm $H_2O$ | | |
| Removal of the condensate from ventilator circuits | | |
| Change of the ventilator circuit only when visibly soiled or malfunctioning | | |
| Avoidance of gastric overdistension | | |
| Avoidance of histamine receptor 2, (H)-blocking agents and proton 2 pump inhibitors | | |
| Use of sterile water to rinse reusable respiratory equipment | | |
| Oral care | VAP rates ↓ | 1 |
| Hand hygiene | ICU LOS ↓ | |
| No ventilator circuit changes unless clinically indicated | Duration of MV ↓ | |
| Daily sedation vacation and readiness to wean assessment | | |
| Intra-cuff pressure control | | |

(continued)

**Table 10.5**  (continued)

| Interventions | Outcomes | Number of studies |
|---|---|---|
| IHI ventilator bundle | VAP rates ↓ | 1 |
| Oral care | | |
| Maintenance of endotracheal cuff pressure > 20-cm $H_2O$ | | |
| Removal of the condensate from ventilator circuits | | |
| Change of the ventilator circuit only when visibly soiled or malfunctioning | | |
| Avoidance of gastric overdistension | | |
| Avoidance of histamine receptor 2, (H)-blocking agents and proton 2 pump inhibitors | | |
| Use of sterile water to rinse reusable respiratory equipment | | |
| HOB elevation 30° | VAP rates ↓ | 1 |
| Oral care | | |
| PUD prophylaxis | | |
| DVT prophylaxis | | |

scheduled feedback briefing to show the improvements and the goals still to reach
• Planning realistic aims

A cost-effectiveness analysis about the implementation of a ventilator bundle versus standard care was performed in a Danish ICU [54]. The ventilator bundle was composed of elevation of the head, a sedation protocol, an extubation protocol, oral decontamination, and DVT prevention. Authors found that the ventilator bundle, compared with standard procedures, was associated with an additional cost per avoided VAP case of EUR 4451 (95% CI 910–11,333) or an additional cost per avoided death of EUR 31,792 (95% CI 9,032–80,949) [54]. Setting a cost-effectiveness threshold of EUR 20,000 per avoided death or VAP case, the cost-effectiveness of the bundle was calculated in more than 50% of simulations per avoided death and more than 80% per avoided VAP case [54].

Recently some authors draw their attention on the potential conflict coming from the absence of effectiveness evidence about a bundle intervention and the need to implement it, emerging from the common sense, as the case of 30° HOB elevation [51]. However, it seems reasonable to adopt practices not based on evidence, only after having excluded any kind of harm for patients, and well balanced between risk and benefit [51]. Nurses should be aware that in similar circumstances, performance indicators could not represent adequate measures of quality of care [51].

## 10.4.6    Implementation Strategies of VAP Prevention

Appropriate strategies to change doctors and nurses' behaviors, and to encourage the adoption of new ones, are central issues to obtain the desired patient outcomes.

Four main categories of quality improvement (passive or active) strategies can be implemented alone or mixed [1]:

- Professional interventions

    - Educational material diffusion
    - Educational outreach visits
    - Educational meetings
    - Local opinion leaders
    - Local consensus processes
    - Patient-mediated intervention
    - Audit and feedback and reminders

- Organizational interventions

    - Multidisciplinary teams

- Modification of professional roles
- Skill mix changes
- Financial interventions
- Regulatory interventions

Even if the effectiveness of bundles is still controversial, due to the lack of randomized studies, lower infection rates seem to be associated with hospitals implementing policies, monitoring compliance, and with high compliance to care bundles [1].

Guideline implementation strategies can be passive (e.g., diffusion of educational materials, posters, toolkits, visual aids) or active (interactive workshops, academic detailing, audit and feedback, and reminders) [1]. Passive strategies cannot sustain long-lasting behavioral change, while active ones result in higher effectiveness [55].

Active educational interventions such as tutorials seem to be effective to increase adherence to VAP bundle [56].

Strategies involving at least two active educational interventions, with repeated administrations, seem to be effective in VAP prevention [1]. Single-time-administered and short educational interventions (an hour or less) did not show positive effects [1].

Finally, educational interventions conducted by specialized professionals, as evidence-based oral hygiene performed by dentists/dental auxiliaries, showed good results in preventing VAP [1].

A recent systematic review found moderate strength of evidence related to the effectiveness in lowering infection rates provided by the implementation of reminder systems or audit and feedback alone added to organizational change and provider education [57].

Nonetheless, some authors underline that, in addition to educational programs, the behavioral change process should consider the search of current practice gap and barriers to change and a behavior change model [1]. Moreover, institution should implement a new intervention at a time, to clearly understand its effectiveness without biases provided by simultaneous interventions [1].

The SHEA/IDSA recommendations identify the "accountability" and a top-down approach as the key elements for a successful implementation of an HAI prevention program [14]. In addition, there are other basic factors to facilitate the implementation of these programs: "engagement" (multidisciplinary team, involvement of local champions, use of peer networks), "education" (education sessions, educational materials), "execution" (standardization of care processes, creation of redundancy), and "evaluation" (performance measuring, feedback to staff) [14].

Even if lots of international studies reported compliance rates to VAP bundle implementation above 70% [49], except for a multicenter observational research performed in Spain with percentages <30% [58], a recent experience of VAP bundle implementation in ICU showed low compliance to the bundle application both in the pre-education and in the post-education period (36.5% and 41.2%, respectively, $p > 0.05$) [58]. When the researchers asked about the causes, more than 90% of nurses answered the lack of rigid monitoring of VAP care bundle adherence. Authors recommended frequent recall and continuous supervision of ICU staffs [59].

Some common obstacles to the implementation of VAP preventing strategies and bundles can be lack of resources, elevated costs, low levels of knowledge or trust in the evidence-based recommendations, nursing convenience, and worries about damages to patients [51].

Lastly, more studies are needed to estimate the effectiveness of interventions aimed to reduce the utilization of indwelling devices and the timely reassessment to the early removal [1].

Take-Home Messages

- HAP in ICU can be split into VAP (86%) and non-VAP (14%).
- The Centers for Disease Control and Prevention recently drafted some new surveillance definitions, introducing a tiered classification of ventilator-associated events for adult patients. VAEs include ARDS, pulmonary edema, atelectasis, and VAP.
- VAE algorithm aims to identify different MV complications, improve surveillance and benchmarking, and reduce the risk of gaming.
- The number of interventions included in the different kinds of VAP bundles ranges from 4 to 11. Almost all published studies reported a significant reduction in VAP rates.
- There is a potential conflict coming from the absence of evidence of effectiveness about some bundle interventions and the need to implement them, as sustained by the common sense (e.g., 30° HOB elevation).
- Passive strategies for guideline implementation cannot sustain long-lasting behavioral change, while active strategies result in higher effectiveness.

# References

1. Flodgren G, Conterno LO, Mayhew A, Omar O, Pereira CR, Shepperd S. Interventions to improve professional adherence to guidelines for prevention of device-related infections. Cochrane Database Syst Rev. 2013;3:CD006559. https://doi.org/10.1002/14651858.CD006559.
2. Majumdar SS, Padiglione AA. Nosocomial infections in the intensive care unit. Anaesthesia & Intensive Care Medicine. 2012;13:204–8. https://doi.org/10.1016/j.mpaic.2012.02.009.

3. American Thoracic Society, Infectious Diseases Society of America. Guidelines for the management of adults with hospital-acquired, ventilator-associated, and healthcare-associated pneumonia. Am J Respir Crit Care Med. 2005;171:388–416. https://doi.org/10.1164/rccm.200405-644ST.

4. Franzetti F, Antonelli M, Bassetti M, Blasi F, Langer M, Scaglione F, et al. Consensus document on controversial issues for the treatment of hospital-associated pneumonia. Int J Infect Dis. 2010;14:S55–65. https://doi.org/10.1016/j.ijid.2010.05.008.

5. Rotstein C, Evans G, Born A, Grossman R, Light RB, Magder S, et al. Clinical practice guidelines for hospital-acquired pneumonia and ventilator-associated pneumonia in adults. Can J Infect Dis Med Microbiol. 2008;19:19–53.

6. Joseph NM, Sistla S, Dutta TK, Badhe AS, Parija SC. Ventilator-associated pneumonia: a review. Eur J Intern Med. 2010;21:360–8. https://doi.org/10.1016/j.ejim.2010.07.006.

7. Torres A, Ferrer M, Badia JR. Treatment guidelines and outcomes of hospital-acquired and ventilator-associated pneumonia. Clin Infect Dis. 2010;51:S48–53. https://doi.org/10.1086/653049.

8. Kollef MH, Morrow LE, Baughman RP, Craven DE, McGowan JE Jr, Micek ST, et al. Health care-associated pneumonia (HCAP): a critical appraisal to improve identification, management, and outcomes-proceedings of the HCAP summit. Clin Infect Dis. 2008;46:S296–334. https://doi.org/10.1086/526355.

9. Ewig S, Welte T, Torres A. Is healthcare-associated pneumonia a distinct entity needing specific therapy? Curr Opin Infect Dis. 2012;25:166–75. https://doi.org/10.1097/QCO.0b013e32835023fb.

10. Komiya K, Ishii H, Kadota J. Healthcare-associated pneumonia and aspiration pneumonia. Aging Dis. 2015;6:27–37. 10.14336/AD.2014.0127.

11. Chalmers JD, Rother C, Salih W, Ewig S. Healthcare-associated pneumonia does not accurately identify potentially resistant pathogens: a systematic review and meta-analysis. Clin Infect Dis. 2014;58:330–9. https://doi.org/10.1093/cid/cit734.

12. Albertos R, Caralt B, Rello J. Ventilator-associated pneumonia management in critical illness. Curr Opin Gastroenterol. 2011;27:160–6. https://doi.org/10.1097/MOG.0b013e32834373b1.

13. Kalanuria AA, Zai W, Mirski M. Ventilator-associated pneumonia in the ICU. Crit Care. 2014;18:208. https://doi.org/10.1186/cc13775.

14. Klompas M, Branson R, Eichenwald EC, Greene LR, Howell MD, Lee G, et al. Strategies to prevent ventilator-associated pneumonia in acute

care hospitals: 2014 update. Infect Control Hosp Epidemiol. 2014;35:915–36. https://doi.org/10.1086/677144.

15. Charles MP, Kali A, Easow JM, Joseph NM, Ravishankar M, Srinivasan S, et al. Ventilator-associated pneumonia. Australas Med J. 2014;7:334–44. https://doi.org/10.4066/AMJ.2014.2105.

16. Efrati S, Deutsch I, Antonelli M, Hockey PM, Rozenblum R, Gurman GM. Ventilator-associated pneumonia: current status and future recommendations. J Clin Monit Comput. 2010;24:161–8. https://doi.org/10.1007/s10877-010-9228-2.

17. Center for Disease Control and Prevention. Ventilator-Associated Event (VAE). For use in adult locations only. January 2016. http://www.cdc.gov/nhsn/PDFs/pscManual/10-VAE_FINAL.pdf. Accessed 02 Jan 2016.

18. Guillamet CV, Kollef MH. Ventilator associated pneumonia in the ICU: where has it gone? Curr Opin Pulm Med. 2015;21:226–31. https://doi.org/10.1097/MCP.0000000000000151.

19. Guyatt GH, Oxman AD, Vist GE, Kunz R, Falck-Ytter Y, Alonso-Coello P, et al. GRADE: an emerging consensus on rating quality of evidence and strength of recommendations. BMJ. 2008;336:924–6. https://doi.org/10.1136/bmj.39489.470347.AD.

20. Canadian Task Force on Preventive Health Care. Grades of Recommendation, Assessment, Development, and Evaluation (GRADE). http://canadiantaskforce.ca/methods/grade/. Accessed 19 Dec 2015.

21. Bouadma L, Wolff M, Lucet JC. Ventilator-associated pneumonia and its prevention. Curr Opin Infect Dis. 2012;25:395–404. https://doi.org/10.1097/QCO.0b013e328355a835.

22. Cabrini L, Landoni G, Oriani A, Plumari VP, Nobile L, Greco M, et al. Noninvasive ventilation and survival in acute care settings: a comprehensive systematic review and metaanalysis of randomized controlled trials. Crit Care Med. 2015;43:880–8. https://doi.org/10.1097/CCM.0000000000000819.

23. Balas MC, Vasilevskis EE, Burke WJ, Boehm L, Pun BT, Olsen KM, et al. Critical care nurses' role in implementing the "ABCDE bundle" into practice. Crit Care Nurse. 2012;32:35–38, 40-7. https://doi.org/10.4037/ccn2012229.

24. Depew CL, McCarthy MS. Subglottic secretion drainage: a literature review. AACN Adv Crit Care. 2007;18:366–79. https://doi.org/10.1097/01.AACN.0000298629.15159.04.

25. Wang F, Bo L, Tang L, Lou J, Wu Y, Chen F, et al. Subglottic secretion drainage for preventing ventilator-associated pneumonia: an updated meta-analysis of randomized controlled trials. J Trauma

Acute Care Surg. 2012;72:1276–85. https://doi.org/10.1097/
TA.0b013e318247cd33.

26. Han J, Liu Y. Effect of ventilator circuit changes on ventilator-associated pneumonia: a systematic review and meta-analysis. Respir Care. 2010;55:467–74.

27. Niël-Weise BS, Gastmeier P, Kola A, Vonberg RP, Wille JC, van den Broek PJ, et al. An evidence-based recommendation on bed head elevation for mechanically ventilated patients. Crit Care. 2011;15:R111. https://doi.org/10.1186/cc10135.

28. Metheny NA, Frantz RA. Head-of-bed elevation in critically ill patients: a review. Crit Care Nurse. 2013;33:53–66. https://doi.org/10.4037/ccn2013456.

29. Labeau SO, Van de Vyver K, Brusselaers N, Vogelaers D, Blot SI. Prevention of ventilator-associated pneumonia with oral antiseptics: a systematic review and meta-analysis. Lancet Infect Dis. 2011;11:845–54. https://doi.org/10.1016/S1473-3099(11)70127-X.

30. Dullenkopf A, Gerber A, Weiss M. Fluid leakage past tracheal tube cuffs: evaluation of the new microcuff endotracheal tube. Intensive Care Med. 2003;29:1849–53. https://doi.org/10.1007/s00134-003-1933-6.

31. Rose L, Redl L. Survey of cuff management practices in intensive care units in Australia and New Zealand. Am J Crit Care. 2008;17:428–35.

32. American Association for Respiratory Care. AARC clinical practice guidelines. Endotracheal suctioning of mechanically ventilated patients with artificial airways 2010. Respir Care. 2010;55:758–64.

33. Gu WJ, Gong YZ, Pan L, Ni YX, Liu JC. Impact of oral care with versus without toothbrushing on the prevention of ventilator-associated pneumonia: a systematic review and meta-analysis of randomized controlled trials. Crit Care. 2012;16:R190. https://doi.org/10.1186/cc11675.

34. Hickman J, Millett DT, Sander L, Brown E, Love J. Powered vs manual tooth brushing in fixed appliance patients: a short term randomized clinical trial. Angle Orthod. 2002;72:135–40. https://doi.org/10.1043/0003-3219(2002)072<0135:PVMTBI>2.0.CO;2.

35. Tokmaji G, Vermeulen H, Müller MC, Kwakman PH, Schultz MJ, Zaat SA. Silver-coated endotracheal tubes for prevention of ventilator-associated pneumonia in critically ill patients. Cochrane Database Syst Rev. 2015;12(8):CD009201. https://doi.org/10.1002/14651858.CD009201.pub2.

36. Hess DR. Patient positioning and ventilator-associated pneumonia. Respir Care. 2005;50:892–8; discussion 898-9

37. Dodek P, Keenan S, Cook D, Heyland D, Jacka M, Hand L, et al. Evidence-based clinical practice guideline for the prevention of ventilator-associated pneumonia. Ann Intern Med. 2004;141:305–13.
38. Andriolo BN, Andriolo RB, Saconato H, Atallah ÁN, Valente O. Early versus late tracheostomy for critically ill patients. Cochrane Database Syst Rev. 2015;1:CD007271. https://doi.org/10.1002/14651858. CD007271.
39. Bankhead R, Boullata J, Brantley S, Corkins M, Guenter P, Krenitsky J, et al. Enteral nutrition practice recommendations. JPEN J Parenter Enteral Nutr. 2009;33:122–67. https://doi.org/10.1177/0148607108330314.
40. Reignier J, Mercier E, Le Gouge A, Boulain T, Desachy A, Bellec F, et al. Effect of not monitoring residual gastric volume on risk of ventilator-associated pneumonia in adults receiving mechanical ventilation and early enteral feeding: a randomized controlled trial. JAMA. 2013;309:249–56. https://doi.org/10.1001/jama.2012.196377.
41. Casaer MP, Mesotten D, Hermans G, Wouters PJ, Schetz M, Meyfroidt G, et al. Early versus late parenteral nutrition in critically ill adults. N Engl J Med. 2011;365:506–17. https://doi.org/10.1056/ NEJMoa1102662.
42. Subirana M, Solà I, Benito S. Closed tracheal suction systems versus open tracheal suction systems for mechanically ventilated adult patients. Cochrane Database Syst Rev. 2007;4:CD004581. https://doi. org/10.1002/14651858.CD004581.pub2.
43. Kollef MH, Prentice D, Shapiro SD, Fraser VJ, Silver P, Trovillion E, et al. Mechanical ventilation with or without daily changes of in-line suction catheters. Am J Respir Crit Care Med. 1997;156:466–72. https://doi.org/10.1164/ajrccm.156.2.9612083.
44. Ntoumenopoulos G, Presneill JJ, McElholum M, Cade JF. Chest physiotherapy for the prevention of ventilator-associated pneumonia. Intensive Care Med. 2002;28:850–6. https://doi.org/10.1007/ s00134-002-1342-2.
45. Tsai HH, Lin FC, Chang SC. Intermittent suction of oral secretions before each positional change may reduce ventilator-associated pneumonia: a pilot study. Am J Med Sci. 2008;336:397–401. https://doi. org/10.1097/MAJ.0b013e31816b8761.
46. Chow MC, Kwok SM, Luk HW, Law JW, Leung BP. Effect of continuous oral suctioning on the development of ventilator-associated pneumonia: a pilot randomized controlled trial. Int J Nurs Stud. 2012;49:1333–41. https://doi.org/10.1016/j.ijnurstu.2012.06.003.
47. Kelly M, Gillies D, Todd DA, Lockwood C. Heated humidification versus heat and moisture exchangers for ventilated adults and children.

Cochrane Database Syst Rev. 2010;4:CD004711. https://doi.org/10.1002/14651858.CD004711.pub2.

48. Restrepo RD, Walsh BK, American Association for Respiratory Care. Humidification during invasive and noninvasive mechanical ventilation: 2012. Respir Care. 2012;57:782–8. https://doi.org/10.4187/respcare.01766.

49. Chahoud J, Semaan A, Almoosa KF. Ventilator-associated events prevention, learning lessons from the past: a systematic review. Heart Lung. 2015;44:251–9. https://doi.org/10.1016/j.hrtlng.2015.01.010.

50. Wip C, Napolitano L. Bundles to prevent ventilator-associated pneumonia: how valuable are they? Curr Opin Infect Dis. 2009;22:159–66. https://doi.org/10.1097/QCO.0b013e3283295e7b.

51. Camporota L, Brett S. Care bundles: implementing evidence or common sense? Crit Care. 2011;15:159. https://doi.org/10.1186/cc10232.

52. Scottish Intensive Care Society Audit Group. VAP Prevention Bundle. Guidance for implementation. NHS National Services Scotland. 2012. http://www.sicsag.scot.nhs.uk/hai/VAP-Prevention-Bundle-web.pdf. Accessed 18 Dec 2015.

53. Hampton DC, Griffith D, Howard A. Evidence-based clinical improvement for mechanically ventilated patients. Rehabil Nurs. 2005;30:160–5.

54. Møller AH, Hansen L, Jensen MS, Ehlers LH. A cost effectiveness analysis of reducing ventilator associated pneumonia at a Danish ICU with ventilator bundle. J Med Econ. 2012;15:285–92. https://doi.org/10.3111/13696998.2011.647175.

55. Grimshaw JM, Thomas RE, MacLennan G, Fraser C, Ramsay CR, Vale L, et al. Effectiveness and efficiency of guideline dissemination and implementation strategies. Health Technol Assess. 2004;8:1–72.

56. Ranji SR, Shetty K, Posley KA, Lewis R, Sundaram V, Galvin C, et al. Closing the Quality Gap: A Critical Analysis of Quality Improvement Strategies (Vol. 6: Prevention of Healthcare–Associated Infections). Rockville (MD): Agency for Healthcare Research and Quality (US); 2007 Jan. (Technical Reviews, No. 9.6.) http://www.ncbi.nlm.nih.gov/books/NBK43982/ Accessed 14 Dec 2015.

57. Mauger B, Marbella A, Pines E, Chopra R, Black ER, Aronson N. Implementing quality improvement strategies to reduce healthcare-associated infections: a systematic review. Am J Infect Control. 2014;42:S274–83. https://doi.org/10.1016/j.ajic.2014.05.031.

58. Rello J, Afonso E, Lisboa T, Ricart M, Balsera B, Rovira A, et al. A care bundle approach for prevention of ventilator-associated pneumonia. Clin Microbiol Infect. 2013;19:363–9. https://doi.org/10.1111/j.1469-0691.2012.03808.x.

59. Hamishehkar H, Vahidinezhad M, Mashayekhi SO, Asgharian P, Hassankhani H, Mahmoodpoor A. Education alone is not enough in ventilator associated pneumonia care bundle compliance. J Res Pharm Pract. 2014;3:51–5. https://doi.org/10.4103/2279-042X.137070.

# Chapter 11
# Hospital-Acquired Catheter-Related Bloodstream Infection Prevention

**Irene Comisso and Alberto Lucchini**

## 11.1 Introduction

Intravascular catheters are widely used in ICU patients, both for monitoring (central venous pressure, arterial and pulmonary pressure) and treatment purposes (fluids, blood components, parenteral nutrition and drug administration, hemodialysis, and renal replacement therapy). According to a European survey, up to 70% of patients admitted to ICU undergoes arterial and central venous catheterization [1]. Although these devices are considered fundamental for ICU care, their use and indwelling remain affected by complications, one over all is infection. Regardless of hospital ward, central line-associated bloodstream infections (CLABSIs) account for an excess in variable costs of 33,000 US$ and a fourfold increased risk of death [2].

Throughout the years, infection incidence and prevalence strongly decreased, especially due to guidelines editing and dissemination [3, 4], although it still remains a challenge in some particular patient categories (onco-ematologic, hemodialyzed, burned, pediatric, critically ill).

© Springer International Publishing AG, part of Springer Nature 2018    279
I. Comisso et al., *Nursing in Critical Care Setting*,
https://doi.org/10.1007/978-3-319-50559-6_11

## 11.2   Definition and Diagnosis

A bloodstream infection (BSI) defines the recovery of microbial pathogens due to infection, and it is therefore different from a sample contamination [5].

Catheter-related bloodstream infection's (CRBSI) definition changed over the years, but it is generally assumed that a bacteremia deriving with an intravascular catheter (venous, arterial, umbilical, or pulmonary) defines a CRBSI. A clinical suspicion for CRBSI can occur in patients with infection signs and symptoms (fever, shivering), without other infection localizations. CRBSI is diagnosed by quantitative culture of catheter tip [5] or when the same phenotypic microorganism is isolated from an intravascular catheters and a peripheral blood culture sample (considering differences in growth) [4]. On the opposite, local skin infection arises with signs of inflammation (erythema, swelling), together with purulent secretions at the insertion site. Culturing the catheter exit-site might reflect the extraluminal colonization of the catheter, but its routinely use is not recommended [6].

CRBSI is suspected in a patient with an intravascular catheter presenting systemic inflammation signs and symptoms (such as fever, chills, hypotension) and without other possible infection localizations. Central line-associated bloodstream infection (CLABSI) describes a CRBSI subgroup and is defined as "a primary BSI in a patient with a central line within the 48 hours period before the development of the BSI and is not bloodstream related to an infection at another site" [7] (National Healthcare Safety Network). CLABSI also includes infections appearing within 48 h of CVC removal [5].

CRBSI and CLABSI are diagnosed keeping the catheter in place or culturing the catheter suspected for infection after its removal [6, 8]. Paired blood cultures (BC) (collected simultaneously from peripheral vein and from the intravascular catheter) should be obtained whenever a clinical suspicion for CLABSI is present. CRBSI diagnosis is confirmed when [8, 9]:

- The same microorganism is isolated (meaning both species and antibiogram).
- Microbial growth arises at least 2 h earlier in blood obtained from the CVC.
- The colony-forming units (CFU) are at least threefold higher in blood obtained from the CVC.

As any diagnostic test, BC are prone to false-negative and false-positive results. Mean contamination rates (i.e., the ratio between number of contaminated blood cultures and total blood cultures [10]) are around 3% [11]. Nurses are usually responsible for BC drawing. Ahead from general considerations, such as indications for obtaining BC, collection timing and number of sets collected, and antibiotic neutralization [10, 12], specific healthcare workers' behaviors have been associated with BC contamination and its reduction (Table 11.1). At the same time, as for many other situations requiring high adherence to a well-defined behavior, education strategies, feedback provision, dedicated phlebotomy teams, and compliance monitoring have been addressed as contributing to BC contamination reduction [10].

To date, it is well established that both endoluminal and extraluminal routes can have an impact on CRBSI occurrence but at different times: extraluminal route seems to have a heavier role during catheter insertion and soon after it, while endoluminal routes are more strongly involved in late catheter dwelling [9, 19].

When a CLABSI is suspected, the differential time to positivity between centrally and peripherally collected samples can help in diagnosing, with sensitivity and specificity higher than 90% when a 120-minute cutoff is used [20].

When CRBSI is suspected, a "watchful waiting approach" [21] can be safely adopted, reducing unnecessary catheter

**Table 11.1** Blood culture contamination sources and reduction strategies

| Intervention | Discussion |
| --- | --- |
| Skin antisepsis | Irrespective of chosen disinfectant agent (aqueous povidone iodine, iodine tincture, or 2% chlorhexidine gluconate with 70% isopropyl alcohol), proper skin antisepsis conducted by a trained phlebotomist team can significantly reduce BC contamination (overall rate 0.76%) [13] |
| | Alcohol provides an immediate antiseptic activity and can be therefore safely used (both alone or combined with other agents) to obtain BCs [14] |
| Sterile gloving | When collecting BC, both sterile and clean gloving have been described. Routine sterile gloving allows palpation of the venipuncture site even after skin disinfection, and when routinely used, it demonstrated a lower contamination rate compared to its optional use [15] |
| Masks | Currently, no evidence suggests to wear masks when collecting BC [10] |
| Rubber sept disinfection | Guidelines recommend to disinfect the rubber sept of BC bottles with 70% isopropyl alcohol [16], since it may significantly reduce BC contamination [17] |
| Number of sets, proper blood volume, and blood distribution | Current recommendation is to collect 2–3 sets per episode (i.e., 1 bottle for aerobic and 1 bottle for anaerobic pathogens) to increase the number of pathogen recovery rate [16]. The amount of growing pathogens is directly proportional to the blood volume collected. CLSI guideline recommends 20–30 ml from at least two separate venipunctures. When a small volume of blood is available, aerobic bottles should be inoculated first [16], since anaerobic bacteremia is rare (5%) and seems to be have been decreasing [16] during time [18] |

removal and avoiding subsequent complications related to new vascular catheterization. A prospective observational study revealed no statistically significant difference in mortality rates according to decision of, or timing of CVC removal, and irrespective of a suspected or confirmed CRBSI [22].

## 11.3 Epidemiology, Risk Factors, Etiology, and Pathogenesis

Several surveillance reports investigated CRBSI incidence, showing different rates through years, countries, and hospitals within the same country. Different incidences can be related to patients' case mix and severity of illness. Nevertheless, one must consider the role of different microbiologic testing procedures and healthcare workers adherence to samples collection and storage (pre-analytic phase) in determining different incidences.

In four European countries' ICUs, CRBSI incidence rate ranged between 1.23 and 4.4 per 1000 catheter days [23]. The NNIS (national nosocomial infection surveillance system) described varying incidence according to ICU's type, the highest (30.1/1000 catheter days) being recorded for burn units [24]. Arterial catheter-associated bacteremia was found to be 3.4/1000 catheter days [25]. For arterial catheters, the incidence in radial insertion site was more than double of femoral site (3.8/1000 catheter days vs. 1.65/1000 catheter days) [25, 26]. Pulmonary artery catheters seem to have a high colonization rate (15.5/1000 catheter day), although bacteremia was not diagnosed during an observational study [27].

Coagulase-negative staphylococci were found to be the most common pathogen in catheter-related BSI (arterial, venous, and pulmonary artery catheter) [25, 26, 28], followed by enterococci, Gram-negative bacilli, and yeasts [5].

Several factors, including catheter type, frequency and number of manipulations, and patient's characteristics, may lead to increased risk for catheter infection [29]. Evidence suggests that peripheral venous, arterial, midline, and PICC (peripherally inserted central venous catheters), as well as tunneled and totally implantable catheters, are less prone to BSI than central venous catheters and pulmonary artery catheters. According to a literature review, major controllable risk factors for CVC-related BSI include the inserter inexperience, jugular or femoral vein insertion site, catheter replacement over guidewire, limited use of sterile barriers, heavy colonization of the insertion site, hub contamination, and prolonged dwelling (>7 days) [29]. For pulmonary artery catheters, prolonged (>3 days) catheterization seems to have a high impact on catheter colonization and infection [27, 28].

Contamination routes play different roles in increasing the infection risk during catheter dwelling. In a prospective cohort study exploring the pathogenesis of CVC-related BSI, 45% of them were extraluminally acquired, 26% were intraluminal, and 29% had unclear origin [26]. For arterial catheter-related BSI, 63% were acquired extraluminally, 27% were intraluminal, and 9% had indeterminate origin [25]. Definitions used in both studies are summarized in Table 11.2.

When considering duration of catheter dwelling, endoluminal contamination (by healthcare worker's hands or skin flora) seems to be the most common for long-term (>10 days) catheters, while skin contamination appears as most frequent for

**Table 11.2** Contamination routes definition [25, 26]

| | |
|---|---|
| Extraluminally acquired BSI | Only isolates from the skin or catheter segment coincide with blood cultures |
| Intraluminally acquired BSI | Only isolates from catheter hub or infusate coincide with blood cultures |
| Indeterminate route of CRBSI | Both or neither routes of infection can be involved in BSI pathogenesis |

short-term catheters [19, 26]. Rarely, catheter contamination may occur from hematogenous migration from other sites or contamination of fluids (including PN and blood components) or drug incorrect preparation, storage, or management during administration [5].

Considering routes of colonization, it's easy to understand how most frequently contaminating organisms come from patient's or healthcare worker's skin (bacteria, mainly Gram-negative, or yeasts, mainly *Candida* spp.).

After accessing the device through its intraluminal or extraluminal surface, pathogens causing CRBSI adhere to it by forming a biofilm, in which microorganisms are irreversibly attached to the catheter's surface and produce extracellular polymeric substances [30]. Biofilm formation is also facilitated by catheter's inner surface imperfections or infusate residuals [31]. Biofilm allows bacterial growth and dissemination [26], and extracellular polymeric substances may have an important role in antimicrobial resistance [30].

## 11.4  Common Preventive Strategies

Intravascular catheter management is recognized as a nurse's responsibility. Despite this general consideration, diffusing a safe cathetrs' management culture within the entire healthcare workers involved in patients' care proved to be one of the most important approaches to significantly reduce catheter-related complications [32, 33]. The Keystone Intensive Care Unit Project [34] was developed at Johns Hopkins University School of Medicine, to implement a group of five evidence-based interventions (hand washing, full barrier precaution during central line insertion, skin disinfection with 2% chlorhexidine, femoral site avoiding, and removing of unnecessary catheters) to reduce CRBSI. One hundred three ICUs in Michigan provided data over an 18-month study period, including over 375.000 catheter days. During the study period, the incident-rate ratios significantly and continuously decreased, from 0.62 at 0–3 months to 0.34 ($p < 0.001$) at 16–18 months after intervention implementation. Basing on these successful results, a similar project (Bacteremia Zero project) was conducted in Spanish ICUs, leading to an approximate 50% CRBSI risk reduction (95% CI 0.39–0.63) and a statistically significant decrease (median 3.07 vs. 1.12 episodes per 1000 catheter days, $p < 0.001$) after 16–18 months from implementation [35].

Recommendations for catheter-related infection prevention are listed in detail in international guidelines [3, 4] and compared in Table 11.3.

## 11.4.1 General Precautions (Choice of Insertion Site and Device, Maximal Barrier Precautions, Skin Disinfection)

Recommendations from international guidelines also provide indications concerning general behaviors to be adopted before the catheter is inserted.

Catheter positioning should prefer upper-body sites, since they are more visible and accessible and generally considered cleaner than the lower-body ones. For non-tunneled central venous catheterization in adult patients, it is recommended to avoid femoral positioning and prefer subclavian vein (unless the patient needs a hemodialysis device or when medically contraindicated). Subclavian insertions have been associated with a lower risk for colonization when compared with jugular and femoral accesses, the latter being more prone (especially in obese patients) to bacterial colonization with subsequent increase of infection risk. Nonetheless, infection risk represents only one of several factors guiding the choice for an intravascular

**Table 11.3** Common preventive strategies for CRBSI prevention: comparison of main interventions reported in CDC 2011 and epic3 guidelines

| Intervention | Guideline (year) | |
| --- | --- | --- |
| | CDC (2011) [4] | EPIC (2012) [3] |
| Selection of catheter type and insertion site | Use a catheter with the minimum number of ports or lumens essential for the management of the patient | Select a catheter with the minimum number of ports for the management of the patient |
| | Avoid femoral access for CVC, and prefer subclavian site to reduce the infection risk | Use the upper extremities for non-tunneled catheters. In selecting the appropriate insertion site, weight both risks for infection and other complications, together with patients comfort |
| | | Currently, the issue concerning the use of a dedicated lumen for parenteral nutrition administration remains unresolved |
| Cutaneous antisepsis | >0.5% chlorhexidine with alcohol should be used to prepare skin prior CVC or peripheral arterial catheter insertion. Tincture of iodine, an iodophor, or 70% alcohol can be used when chlorhexidine is contraindicated | Skin should be decontaminated with 2% chlorhexidine gluconate in 70% isopropyl alcohol, and allow to air dry. Povidone iodine can be an option for patients with sensitivity to chlorhexidine |

(continued)

**Table 11.3** (continued)

| Intervention | Guideline (year) | |
| --- | --- | --- |
| | CDC (2011) [4] | EPIC (2012) [3] |
| Catheter dressing | Sterile gauze (for diaphoretic patients, or bleeding or oozing sites) or sterile, transparent, semipermeable dressing. Dressing should be replaced when it becomes damp, loosened, or visibly soiled. Gauze dressings should be replaced every 2 days, transparent ones every 7 days | Use a sterile, semipermeable, transparent polyurethane dressing and change them every 7 days or sooner (if no longer intact or moisture collects under the dressing) Sterile gauze dressing should be used for profuse perspiration or if the insertion site is leaking or bleeding. Gauze dressing should be changed when insertion site inspection is necessary, or when it becomes damp, loosened, or soiled 2% chlorhexidine gluconate in 70% isopropyl alcohol should be applied to clean the insertion site |

**Table 11.3** (continued)

| Intervention | Guideline (year) | |
| --- | --- | --- |
| | CDC (2011) [4] | EPIC (2012) [3] |
| Lines replacement | Continuously used administration sets should be no more frequently than 96 h but at least every 7 days. No recommendations can be made for intermittently used. Administration sets used for propofol should be changed every 6–12 h, according to the manufacturer's recommendations. Sets used for blood, blood products, or fat emulsions should be changed within 24 h of initiating the infusion | Administration sets in continuous use do not need replacements more frequently than 96 h, unless they are disconnected or the device is replaced. Sets for blood or blood components should be changed when the transfusion is complete or every 12 h. Administration sets for lipid-containing parenteral nutrition should be changed every 24 h |
| Hub management and needleless devices | Needleless connectors should be changed no more frequently than 72 h and as frequently as the administration sets. Ports should be accessed with sterile devices only, after decontamination with a proper disinfectant agent (chlorhexidine, povidone iodine, 70% alcohol) | 2% chlorhexidine gluconate in 70% isopropyl alcohol should be used to decontaminate the access port or catheter hub, with a minimum contact time of 15 s |

access site insertion. Healthcare workers should also consider patient's comfort and the risk for other complications (such as bleeding, thrombosis, occlusion) [36, 37]. When choosing a device, guidelines recommend to select central lines with the lowest lumen number, in order to reduce possible access ports for bacteria. In selected situations, antibiotic or silver-coated catheters might be chosen to reduce the infection risk. In any case, polytetrafluoroethylene (Teflon) and polyurethane catheters have shown a significantly lower infectious risk than polyurethane and polyvinyl chloride catheters.

Maximum barrier precautions (MBP) (sterile gown and gloves, cap, and full body drape) should be adopted when a central venous (including PICC and PAC) or a femoral artery catheter is placed, or guidewire exchange is performed. Insertion of a peripheral line does not require sterile gloves, unless a "no-touch" technique is adopted, while for peripheral artery insertion, cap, mask, and a small fenestrated drape should be used (although studies suggesting these conclusions are older than 5 years). Moreover, it has to be considered that arterial catheter colonization incidence did not significantly decrease with MBP and was similar to the CVC one [4].

Adequate skin preparation is required to reduce skin colonization (the density of skin flora), since it is considered the most important factor for CRBSI. When inserting a CVC or an arterial catheter, or anytime catheter dressings are renewed, the skin should be disinfected with chlorhexidine alcohol-based solution; other alcoholic or iodine disinfectant can be used when a peripheral catheter is positioned. A recent RCT demonstrated a higher power in reducing catheter colonization when using chlorhexidine compared to povidone and did not confirmed the need for skin scrubbing prior to skin disinfection [38]. A recent systematic review highlighted the important action of alcohol (both alone or combined with chlorhexidine or povidone), in reducing skin colonization. Particularly, alcohol has an immediate effect, while chlorhexidine and povidone provide persistent activity, with chlorhexidine showing a more prolonged activity, compared to povidone [14].

## 11.4.2  Catheter Dressing

Catheter dressing is important for several reasons: it provides a barrier between the insertion site and external environment; it helps securing the device to patient's skin; it provides an opportunity to evaluate insertion site's conditions. Insertion site's conditions should be reported within clinical documentation whenever they are inspected, in order to rapidly detect changes that might suggest an ongoing infection.

Both transparent polyurethane and gauze dressing can be used, without significant changes in infection rates [39], although a recent systematic review had showed a significant increase in CRBSI with transparent dressing application [40]. In addition to patient's preferences, the main criteria to guide a dressing's choice are related to insertion site evaluation: particularly, when there is bleeding, moisture, and purulent (or leaking) discharge, an absorbent dressing is recommended (gauze), while all other conditions suggest to use a transparent dressing, allowing a most frequent insertion site evaluation.

Transparent dressings should be renewed at least every 7 days (or whenever clinical judgment suggests it as necessary), while gauze dressings can stay no longer than 2 days and should be turned to transparent ones as soon as possible. A systematic review pooled the results of five studies and found no clear evidence to suggest longer (5–15 days) vs. shorter (2–5 days) dressing interval regimens [41]. In a prospective, single-center randomized controlled trial, catheter dressings were changed prior to 7 days when dressings' edges peeled off, thus inducing a lower securement and sealing of the catheter [42].

Guidelines [4] suggest to avoid topical use of antibiotic ointments, but choosing local application of chlorhexidine-impregnated sponge can be an option when other strategies fail in reducing CLABSI rates. Moreover, recent guideline updates [43] suggest the application of chlorhexidine-impregnated gel or sponge dressings to reduce skin and catheter colonization and CRBSI incidence. Despite this, a recent systematic review with meta-analysis found no statistically significant difference in CRBSI risk reduction comparing standard polyurethane and chlorhexidine gluconate-impregnated dressings [39].

## 11.4.3 Lines Replacement

Lines are connected to a central catheter hub for different purposes (administration of fluids, blood components, drugs, and total parenteral nutrition). Safety precautions are adopted to avoid common complications, such as interactions between molecules, catheter kinking, and occlusion. Periodic line replacement is required to avoid internal colonization, which might occur mainly when accessing and manipulating hubs. During the last two decades, several studies investigated the optimal frequency for line replacement, providing changes over time. Guidelines suggest to replace administration sets (used continuously) not earlier than 96 h but at least every 7 days for fluids and drugs [4, 44]. A recent retrospective observational study found no statistically significant difference in CRBSI occurrence between central venous and arterial catheters, and a significantly decreased incidence for pulmonary artery catheters with a 7-day interval replacement, thus suggesting that an increased interval is safe and may lead to cost reduction [45].

Adjunctive considerations concern blood and blood products, and fat emulsions, for which the administration set substitution should be provided 24 h after the infusion starts. Propofol sets should be changed every 6–12 h, in accordance to manufacturer indications [3, 4].

Total parenteral nutrition (TPN) represents the only alternative to administer nutrients when oral assumption or enteral nutrition (EN) is contraindicated. Current nutritional guidelines [46] suggest to avoid TPN in the first 7 ICU days, in the absence of preexisting malnutrition. BSI can reach high rates (up to 39%) [47] in patients receiving parenteral nutrition (PN). PN has been recognized as an independent factor for BSI. Particularly, multichamber bags showed a significantly lower risk for BSI when compared to compounding PN (both outsourced and pharmacy-prepared). Furthermore, increasing PN-days was associated with increased BSI risk [48]. Lipids are an optimal support for bacterial growth [49]. Interestingly, their role in increasing the risk for BSI has been recently reconsidered in a retrospective observational study, where similar BSI incidence in patients receiving premixed PN with or without lipids, after adjusting for the poorer health status of patients receiving PN with lipids [50], was found. Improved catheter care has also been recognized as a factor that may have reduced CRBSI associated with the use of PN [51].

## 11.4.4   Hubs Management

Catheter hubs are recognized as a source of contamination and therefore of possible infection development. As a general precaution, the number of catheter accesses should be reduced as much as possible, and a closed system (through a diaphragm) should be preferred to open ones (through a stopcock). Whenever accessing a catheter, hand hygiene with water and soap or with an alcoholic solution is recommended. Hub disinfection and scrubbing (with gauze and alcoholic solution) or alcohol-impregnated pads) reduces bacterial density and is therefore recommended by international guidelines [4], with a minimum recommended contact time of at least 5 s [52–54]. Nonetheless, recent systematic review highlighted the paucity of well-conducted randomized controlled trials.

### 11.4.4.1    Use of Needleless Devices

Stopcocks are widely used to increase hub number available for fluid and drug administration, in addition to blood samples collection. Needleless systems allow access to a catheter or an infusion line, without the use of needles, thus avoiding the needlestick injury risk for healthcare workers. Needleless connectors have different characteristics; particularly, simple connectors don't have internal moving parts, while complex connectors allow fluid flow by the presence of mechanical components (valves). In turn, fluid displacement within the connector is described as positive, negative, or neutral. Positive displacement connectors are provided with a fluid reservoir that avoids blood reflux when the administration set is disconnected. Negative displacement connectors allow blood to reflux and to be pulled back when they (or the administration sets) are connected or disconnected. Neutral displacements connectors prevent blood from moving into the catheter lumen upon connection or disconnection [55]. Precautions suggested for hub management can also be applied to needleless connectors. Needleless devices should be changed together with infusion lines. Several studies investigated the effectiveness of these devices in reducing hub, line, and catheter contamination, with conflicting results. Particularly, mechanical valve connectors are associated with a higher infection risk compared to split-septum devices. Adequate disinfection time and scrubbing appear as the most relevant factors in contamination reduction, although a definitive consensus about the best scrubbing time (described as ranging between 5 and 60 s) has not been reached [56]. Isopropyl alcohol has a dehydration action on bacterial cells and therefore acts immediately after its application, while alcoholic chlorhexidine has a more sustained effect and performs better than povidone iodine or sodium hypochlorite [57]. The combination of both agents showed superior effect when compared to a single-agent action. Furthermore, user expertise and knowledges about connector management relate with contamination and infection outbreak, underlining the need for adequate staff education. Recently, antiseptic-barrier caps have been introduced in the market. These plastic caps are placed over the needleless connectors after use, remain in place until next access, and contain a 70% isopropyl alcohol-impregnated sponge. Their purpose is both mechanical, protecting hubs from environmental contamination, and antimicrobial, providing a considerable reduction of microorganisms' density on connector's surface. Disinfection caps have been studied on hematology-oncology patients, demonstrating a significant reduction in CLABSI rates among high-risk oncology patients [58]. Interestingly, a significant reduction in BC contamination rates was also observed.

## 11.5    Selected Preventive Strategies

Some adjunctive intervention can be acted to maximize the infection prevention. Compared to standard interventions, an accurate evaluation of risks and benefits (with cost-effectiveness perspective) and patient selection are required.

### 11.5.1    Lock Therapy

In selected patients (premature neonates; hemodialysis, neutropenic patients), the injection of antimicrobial solutions (single or associated molecules) through the catheter lumen and their further lock and dwelling have been used to reduce internal colonization. The rate of CRBSI significantly decreased in hemodialysis and pediatric oncology patients, whose catheters were locked with antibiotics. Lock therapy seems to have a greater preventive effect than catheter flushing alone, and for certain molecules (such as trisodium citrate), collateral effects due to rapid injection of a great amount of solution are avoided. At the same time, lock therapy impedes a lumen access for the entire lock duration, thus requiring accessory devices positioning, or, when possible, delaying drug administration.

## 11.5.2 Antimicrobial and Antiseptic-Impregnated Catheters

Using impregnated or coated catheters should be designated to selected situations, mainly when education, the use of maximal barrier precautions, and skin antisepsis with chlorhexidine prior to catheter insertion do not result in a concrete CLABSI rate reduction. Disinfectants used to coat catheters (silver/sulfadiazine or platinum/silver, the latter only available in US market) are applied both on the external and internal surface and allow a prolonged release of such molecules. These devices showed a consistent reduction in CLABSI rates compared to standard catheters. Similarly, antimicrobial-coated catheters (minocycline/rifampin) proved a consistent effectiveness in reducing infection rates. A recently published systematic review [59] confirmed a significant reduction of CRBSI and catheter colonization rates using impregnated CVCs, particularly in ICU patients. In ICU patients, minocycline/rifampin CVCs have shown a significant CLABSI rate reduction compared to chlorhexidine/sulfadiazine CVCS [60]. Although their costs are significantly higher than the ones of a standard catheter, the real dwelling cost results reduced, due to infections rates decrease. Nonetheless, the decision to apply this kind of device should be weighed with considerations about general CLABSI rates, supposed dwelling time, and possible patient reactions to antimicrobials and disinfectants agents.

## 11.6 The Role of Bundles and Protocols

A bundle consists in a small group (3–5) of evidence-based recommendations, aiming to provide patients with similar problems or risks the best available care. According to the IHI (Institute for Healthcare Improvement), CVC bundles consist in five indications (hand hygiene, maximal barrier precautions, chlorhexidine skin antisepsis, optimal catheter site selection, daily review of line necessity), which might be integrated with other scientific recommendations [61]. Bundle adoption significantly reduced CLABSI rate in an emergency department [62], but experiences in ICU patients may differ between countries and patients (adults vs. pediatrics) [63]. Some [64, 65] also introduced bundle inherent catheter insertion, with promising results in CLABSI reduction.

Take-Home Messages
- Intravascular catheter-associated infections are threatening for ICU patients and account for increases in patient LOS, morbidity and mortality, and healthcare costs.
- Prevention still remains the best way to control catheter-related infections.
- Although evidence-based recommendations are widely disseminated and adopted, decisions about catheter management should always be personalized on patient conditions and weighted on staff and environmental resources.
- Provision of continuous education helps healthcare workers to update knowledges. Epidemiological surveillance keeps the attention on incidence and emerging resistance.

## References

1. Vincent JL, Sakr Y, Sprung CL, Ranieri VM, Reinhart K, Gerlach H, Moreno R, Carlet J, Le Gall JR, Payen D, Sepsis Occurrence in Acutely Ill Patients Investigators. Sepsis in European intensive care units: results of the SOAP study. Crit Care Med. 2006;34(2):344–53.

2. Stevens V, Geiger K, Concannon C, Nelson RE, Brown J, Dumyati G. Inpatient costs, mortality and 30-day re-admission in patients with central-line-associated bloodstream infections. Clin Microbiol Infect. 2014;20(5):O318–24. https://doi.org/10.1111/1469-0691.12407.

3. Loveday HP, Wilson JA, Pratt RJ, Golsorkhi M, Tingle A, Bak A, Browne J, Prieto J, Wilcox M, UK Department of Health. Epic3: national evidence-based guidelines for preventing healthcare-associated infections in NHS hospitals in England. J Hosp Infect. 2014;86(Suppl 1):S1–70. https://doi.org/10.1016/S0195-6701(13)60012-2.

4. O'Grady NP, Alexander M, Burns LA, Dellinger EP, Garland J, Heard SO, Lipsett PA, Masur H, Mermel LA, Pearson ML, Raad II, Randolph AG, Rupp ME, Saint S, Healthcare Infection Control Practices Advisory Committee. Guidelines for the prevention of intravascular catheter-related infections. Am J Infect Control. 2011;39(4 Suppl 1):S1–34. https://doi.org/10.1016/j.ajic.2011.01.003.

5. Shah H, Bosch W, Thompson KM, Hellinger WC. Intravascular catheter-related bloodstream infection. Neurohospitalist. 2013;3(3):144–51. https://doi.org/10.1177/1941874413476043.

6. Timsit JF. Diagnosis and prevention of catheter-related infections. Curr Opin Crit Care. 2007;13(5):563–71. https://doi.org/10.1097/MCC.0b013e3282efa03f.

7. Centers for Disease Control and Prevention. NHSN Patient Safety Component Manual. https://www.cdc.gov/nhsn/pdfs/validation/2016/pcsmanual_2016.pdf. Accessed 28 Apr 2016.

8. Timsit JF, Dubois Y, Minet C, Bonadona A, Lugosi M, Ara-Somohano C, Hamidfar-Roy R, Schwebel C. New challenges in the diagnosis, management, and prevention of central venous catheter-related infections. Semin Respir Crit Care Med. 2011;32(2):139–50. https://doi.org/10.1055/s-0031-1275526.

9. Mermel LA, Allon M, Bouza E, Craven DE, Flynn P, O'Grady NP, Raad II, Rijnders BJ, Sherertz RJ, Warren DK. Clinical practice guidelines for the diagnosis and management of intravascular catheter-related infection: 2009 update by the Infectious Diseases Society of America. Clin Infect Dis. 2009;49(1):1–45. https://doi.org/10.1086/599376.

10. Bekeris LG, Tworek JA, Walsh MK, Valenstein PN. Trends in blood culture contamination: a College of American Pathologists Q-tracks study of 356 institutions. Arch Pathol Lab Med. 2005;129(10):1222–5. https://doi.org/10.1043/1543-2165(2005)129[1222:TIBCCA]2.0.CO;2.

11. Garcia RA, Spitzer ED, Beaudry J, Beck C, Diblasi R, Gilleeny-Blabac M, Haugaard C, Heuschneider S, Kranz BP, McLean K, Morales KL, Owens S, Paciella ME, Torregrosa E. Multidisciplinary team review of

best practices for collection and handling of blood cultures to determine effective interventions for increasing the yield of true-positive bacteremias, reducing contamination, and eliminating false-positive central line-associated bloodstream infections. Am J Infect Control. 2015;43(11):1222–37. https://doi.org/10.1016/j.ajic.2015.06.030.

12. Self WH, Mickanin J, Grijalva CG, Grant FH, Henderson MC, Corley G, Blaschke Ii DG, McNaughton CD, Barrett TW, Talbot TR, Paul BR. Reducing blood culture contamination in community hospital emergency departments: a multicenter evaluation of a quality improvement intervention. Acad Emerg Med. 2014;21(3):274–82. https://doi.org/10.1111/acem.12337.

13. Washer LL, Chenoweth C, Kim HW, Rogers MA, Malani AN, Riddell J 4th, Kuhn L, Noeyack B Jr, Neusius H, Newton DW, Saint S, Flanders SA. **Blood culture** contamination: a randomized trial evaluating the comparative effectiveness of 3 **skin** antiseptic interventions. Infect Control Hosp Epidemiol. 2013;34(1):15–21. https://doi.org/10.1086/668777.

14. Maiwald M, Chan ES. The forgotten role of alcohol: a systematic review and meta-analysis of the clinical efficacy and perceived role of chlorhexidine in skin antisepsis. PLoS One. 2012;7(9):e44277. https://doi.org/10.1371/journal.pone.0044277.

15. Kim NH, Kim M, Lee S, Yun NR, Kim KH, Park SW, Kim HB, Kim NJ, Kim EC, Park WB, Oh MD. Effect of routine **sterile** gloving on contamination rates in **blood culture**: a cluster randomized trial. Ann Intern Med. 2011;154(3):145–51. https://doi.org/10.7326/0003-4819-154-3-201102010-00003.

16. Clinical and laboratory Standards Institute (CLSI). Principles and procedures for blood cultures: approved guideline. CLSI document M47-a. Wayne (PA): Clinical and Laboratory Standards Institute; 2007.

17. Schifman RB, Strand CL, Meier FA, Howanitz PJ. Blood culture contamination: a College of American Pathologists Q-probes study involving 640 institutions and 497134 specimens from adult patients. Arch Pathol Lab Med. 1998;122(3):216–21.

18. De Keukeleire S, Wybo I, Naessens A, Echahidi F, Van der Beken M, Vandoorslaer K, Vermeulen S, Piérard D. Anaerobic bacteraemia: a 10-year retrospective epidemiological survey. Anaerobe. 2016;39:54–9. https://doi.org/10.1016/j.anaerobe.2016.02.009.

19. Mermel LA. What is the predominant source of intravascular catheter infections? Clin Infect Dis. 2011;52:211–2. https://doi.org/10.1093/cid/ciq108.

20. Bouza E, Alvarado N, Alcala L, et al. A randomized and prospective study of 3 procedures for the diagnosis of catheter-related bloodstream

     infection without catheter withdrawal. Clin Infect Dis. 2007;44:820–6.
     https://doi.org/10.1086/511865.
21. Rijnders BJ, Peetermans WE, Verwaest C, Wilmer A, Van Wijngaerden E.
     Watchful waiting versus immediate catheter removal in ICU patients with
     suspected catheter-related infection: a randomized trial. Intensive Care Med.
     2004;30(6):1073–80. https://doi.org/10.1007/s00134-004-2212-x.
22. Lorente L, Martín MM, Vidal P, Rebollo S, Ostabal MI, Solé-Violán J,
     Working Group on Catheter Related Infection Suspicion Management
     of GTEIS/SEMICYUC. Should central venous catheter be systemati-
     cally removed in patients with suspected catheter related infection? Crit
     Care. 2014;18(5):564. https://doi.org/10.1186/s13054-014-0564-3.
23. Tacconelli E, Smith G, Hieke K, Lafuma A, Bastide P. Epidemiology,
     medical outcomes and costs of catheter-related bloodstream infections
     in intensive care units of four European countries: literature- and
     registry-based estimates. J Hosp Infect. 2009;72(2):97–103. https://doi.
     org/10.1016/j.jhin.2008.12.012.
24. NNIS System. National Nosocomial Infections Surveillance (NNIS)
     system report, data summary from January 1990-may 1999, issued
     June 1999. A report from the NNIS system. Am J Infect Control.
     1999;27(6):520–32.
25. Safdar N, O'Horo JC, Maki DG. Arterial catheter-related bloodstream
     infection: incidence, pathogenesis, risk factors and prevention. J Hosp
     Infect. 2013;85(3):189–95. https://doi.org/10.1016/j.jhin.2013.06.018.
26. Safdar N, Maki DG. The pathogenesis of catheter-related bloodstream
     infection with noncuffed short-term central venous catheters. Intensive
     Care Med. 2004;30(1):62–7. https://doi.org/10.1007/s00134-003-2045-z.
27. Blot F, Chachaty E, Raynard B, Antoun S, Bourgain JL, Nitenberg G.
     Mechanisms and risk factors for infection of pulmonary artery cathe-
     ters and introducer sheaths in cancer patients admitted to an intensive
     care unit. J Hosp Infect. 2001;48(4):289–97. https://doi.org/10.1053/
     jhin.2001.1014.
28. Mermel LA, McCormick RD, Springman SR, Maki DG. The pathogen-
     esis and epidemiology of catheter-related infection with pulmonary
     artery swan-Ganz catheters: a prospective study utilizing molecular
     subtyping. Am J Med. 1991;91(3B):197S–205S.
29. Safdar N, Kluger DM, Maki DG. A review of risk factors for catheter-
     related bloodstream infection caused by percutaneously inserted, non-
     cuffed central venous catheters: implications for preventive strategies.
     Medicine (Baltimore). 2002;81(6):466–79.
30. Lindsay D, von Holy A. Bacterial biofilms within the clinical setting:
     what  healthcare  professionals  should  know.  J  Hosp  Infect.
     2006;64(4):313–25. https://doi.org/10.1016/j.jhin.2006.06.028.

31. Marrie TJ, Costerton JW. Scanning and transmission electron micros-copy of in situ bacterial colonization of intravenous and intraarterial catheters. J Clin Microbiol. 1984;19:687–93.

32. Hansen S, Schwab F, Schneider S, Sohr D, Gastmeier P, Geffers C. Time-series analysis to observe the impact of a centrally orga-nized educational intervention on the prevention of central-line-associated bloodstream infections in 32 German intensive care units. J Hosp Infect. 2014;87(4):220–6. https://doi.org/10.1016/j.jhin.2014.04.010.

33. Pronovost P. Interventions to decrease catheter-related bloodstream infections in the ICU: the keystone intensive care unit project. Am J Infect Control. 2008;36(10):S171.e1–5. https://doi.org/10.1016/j.ajic.2008.10.008.

34. Pronovost P, Needham D, Berenholtz S, Sinopoli D, Chu H, Cosgrove S, Sexton B, Hyzy R, Welsh R, Roth G, Bander J, Kepros J, Goeschel C. An intervention to decrease catheter-related bloodstream infections in the ICU. N Engl J Med. 2006;355(26):2725–32. https://doi.org/10.1056/NEJMoa061115.

35. Palomar M, Álvarez-Lerma F, Riera A, Díaz MT, Torres F, Agra Y, Larizgoitia I, Goeschel CA, Pronovost PJ, Bacteremia Zero Working Group. Impact of a national multimodal intervention to prevent catheter-related bloodstream infection in the ICU: the Spanish experi-ence. Crit Care Med. 2013;41(10):2364–72. https://doi.org/10.1097/CCM.0b013e3182923622.

36. Parienti JJ, Mongardon N, Mégarbane B, Mira JP, Kalfon P, Gros A, Marqué S, Thuong M, Pottier V, Ramakers M, Savary B, Seguin A, Valette X, Terzi N, Sauneuf B, Cattoir V, Mermel LA, du Cheyron D, 3SITES Study Group. Intravascular complications of central venous catheterization by insertion site. N Engl J Med. 2015;373(13):1220–9. https://doi.org/10.1056/NEJMoa1500964.

37. Parienti JJ, du Cheyron D, Timsit JF, Traoré O, Kalfon P, Mimoz O, Mermel LA. Meta-analysis of subclavian **insertion** and nontunneled **central venous** catheter-associated infection risk reduction in critically ill adults. Crit Care Med. 2012;40(5):1627–34. https://doi.org/10.1097/CCM.

38. Mimoz O, Lucet JC, Kerforne T, Pascal J, Souweine B, Goudet V, Mercat A, Bouadma L, Lasocki S, Alfandari S, Friggeri A, Wallet F, Allou N, Ruckly S, Balayn D, Lepape A, Timsit JF, CLEAN trial inves-tigators. Skin antisepsis with chlorhexidine-alcohol versus povidone iodine-alcohol, with and without skin scrubbing, for prevention of intravascular-catheter-related infection (CLEAN): an open-label, mul-ticentre, randomised, controlled, two-by-two factorial trial. Lancet.

2015;386(10008):2069–77.          https://doi.org/10.1016/
S0140-6736(15)00244-5.0b013e31823e99cb.

39. Ullman AJ, Cooke ML, Mitchell M, Lin F, New K, Long DA, Mihala
    G, Rickard CM. **Dressings** and securement devices for central venous
    catheters (CVC). Cochrane Database Syst Rev. 2015;9:CD010367.
    https://doi.org/10.1002/14651858.CD010367.pub2.

40. Webster J, Gillies D, O'Riordan E, Sherriff KL, Rickard CM. Gauze
    and tape and transparent polyurethane dressings for central venous
    catheters. Cochrane Database Syst Rev. 2011;9:003827. https://doi.
    org/10.1002/14651858.CD003827.pub2.

41. Gavin NC, Webster J, Chan RJ, Rickard CM. Frequency of dressing
    changes for central venous access devices on catheter-related infec-
    tions. Cochrane Database Syst Rev. 2016;2:CD009213. https://doi.
    org/10.1002/14651858.CD009213.pub2.

42. Günther SC, Schwebel C, Hamidfar-Roy R, Bonadona A, Lugosi M,
    Ara-Somohano C, Minet C, Potton L, Cartier JC, Vésin A, Chautemps
    M, Styfalova L, Ruckly S, Timsit JF. Complications of intravascular
    catheters in ICU: definitions, incidence and severity. A randomized
    controlled trial comparing usual transparent dressings versus new-
    generation dressings (the ADVANCED study). Intensive Care Med.
    2016;42(11):1753–65. https://doi.org/10.1007/s00134-016-4582-2.

43. Loveday HP, Wilson JA, Prieto J, Wilcox MH. epic3: revised recom-
    mendation for intravenous catheter and catheter site care. J Hosp Infect.
    2016;92(4):346–8. https://doi.org/10.1016/j.jhin.2015.11.011.

44. Ullman AJ, Cooke ML, Gillies D, Marsh NM, Daud A, McGrail
    MR, O'Riordan E, Rickard CM. Optimal timing for intravascular
    administration set replacement. Cochrane Database Syst Rev.
    2013;9:CD003588. https://doi.org/10.1002/14651858.CD003588.
    pub3.

45. Lucchini A, Angelini S, Losurdo L, Giuffrida A, Vanini S, Elli S,
    Cannizzo L, Gariboldi R, Bambi S, Fumagalli R. The impact of closed
    system and 7 days intravascular administration set replacement on
    catheter related infections in a general intensive care unit: a before-after
    study. Assist Inferm Ric. 2015;34(3):125–33. https://doi.
    org/10.1702/2038.22138.

46. McClave SA, Taylor BE, Martindale RG, Warren MM, Johnson DR,
    Braunschweig C, McCarthy MS, Davanos E, Rice TW, Cresci GA,
    Gervasio JM, Sacks GS, Roberts PR, Compher C, Society of Critical
    Care Medicine, American Society for Parenteral and Enteral Nutrition.
    Guidelines for the provision and assessment of nutrition support ther-
    apy in the adult critically ill patient: Society of Critical Care Medicine
    (SCCM) and American Society for Parenteral and Enteral Nutrition

(a.S.P.E.N.). JPEN J Parenter Enteral Nutr. 2016;40(2):159–211. https://doi.org/10.1177/0148607115621863.

47. Opilla M. Epidemiology of bloodstream infection associated with parenteral nutrition. Am J Infect Control. 2008;36:S173.e5–8.

48. Turpin RS, Canada T, Rosenthal V, Nitzki-George D, Liu FX, Mercaldi CJ, Pontes-Arruda A, IMPROVE Study Group. Bloodstream infections associated with parenteral nutrition preparation methods in the United States: a retrospective, large database analysis. JPEN J Parenter Enteral Nutr. 2012;36(2):169–76. https://doi.org/10.1177/0148607111414714.

49. Melly MA, Meng HC, Schaffner W. Microbial growth in lipid emulsions used in parenteral nutrition. Arch Surg. 1975;110(12):1479–81.

50. Pontes-Arruda A, Liu FX, Turpin RS, Mercaldi CJ, Hise M, Zaloga G. Bloodstream infections in patients receiving manufactured parenteral nutrition with vs without lipids: is the use of lipids really deleterious? JPEN J Parenter Enteral Nutr. 2012;36(4):421–30. https://doi.org/10.1177/0148607111420061.

51. McCleary EJ, Tajchman S. Parenteral nutrition and infection risk in the intensive care unit: a practical guide for the bedside clinician. Nutr Clin Pract. 2016;31(4):476–89. https://doi.org/10.1177/0884533616653808.

52. Lockman JL, Heitmiller ES, Ascenzi JA, Berkowitz I. Scrub the hub! Catheter needleless port decontamination. Anesthesiology. 2011;114:958. https://doi.org/10.1097/ALN.0b013e3182054bd1.

53. Simmons S, Bryson C, Porter S. "Scrub the hub": cleaning duration and reduction in bacterial load on central venous catheters. Crit Care Nurs Q. 2011;34:31–5. https://doi.org/10.1097/CNQ.0b013e3182048073.

54. Rupp ME, Yu S, Huerta T, et al. Adequate disinfection of a split-septum needleless intravascular connector with a 5-second alcohol scrub. Infect Control Hosp Epidemiol. 2012;33:661–5. https://doi.org/10.1086/666337.

55. Hadaway L. Needleless connectors for IV catheters. Am J Nurs. 2012;112(11):32–44.; quiz 45. https://doi.org/10.1097/01.NAJ.0000422253.72836.c1.

56. Moureau NL, Flynn J. Disinfection of needleless connector hubs: clinical evidence systematic review. Nurs Res Pract. 2015;2015:796762. https://doi.org/10.1155/2015/796762.

57. Macias JH, Arreguin V, Munoz JM, Alvarez JA, Mosqueda JL, Macias AE. Chlorhexidine is a better antiseptic than povidone iodine and sodium hypochlorite because of its substantive effect. Am J Infect Control. 2013;41(7):634–7. https://doi.org/10.1016/j.ajic.2012.10.002.

58. Kamboj M, Blair R, Bell N, Son C, Huang YT, Dowling M, Lipitz-Snyderman A, Eagan J, Sepkowitz K. Use of disinfection cap to reduce central-line-associated bloodstream infection and blood culture con-

tamination among hematology-oncology patients. Infect Control Hosp Epidemiol. 2015;36(12):1401–8. https://doi.org/10.1017/ice.2015.219.

59. Lai NM, Chaiyakunapruk N, Lai NA, O'Riordan E, Pau WS, Saint S. Catheter impregnation, coating or bonding for reducing central venous catheter-related infections in adults. Cochrane Database Syst Rev. 2016;3:CD007878. https://doi.org/10.1002/14651858.CD007878. pub3.

60. Bonne S, Mazuski JE, Sona C, Schallom M, Boyle W, Buchman TG, Bochicchio GV, Coopersmith CM, Schuerer DJ. Effectiveness of mino-cycline and rifampin vs Chlorhexidine and silver sulfadiazine-impregnated central venous catheters in preventing central line-associated bloodstream infection in a high-volume academic intensive care unit: a before and after trial. J Am Coll Surg. 2015;221(3):739–47. https://doi. org/10.1016/j.jamcollsurg.2015.05.013.

61. Institute for Healthcare Improvement. How-to guide: preventing central-line associated bloodstream infection. http://www.ihi.org/resources/Pages/ Tools/HowtoGuidePreventCentralLineAssociatedBloodstreamInfection. aspx. Accessed 28 Apr 2016.

62. Theodoro D, Olsen MA, Warren DK, McMullen KM, Asaro P, Henderson A, Tozier M, Fraser V. Emergency department central line-associated bloodstream infections (CLABSI) incidence in the era of prevention practices. Acad Emerg Med. 2015;22(9):1048–55. https:// doi.org/10.1111/acem.12744.

63. Jeong IS, Park SM, Lee JM, Song JY, Lee SJ. Effect of central line bundle on central line-associated bloodstream infections in intensive care units. Am J Infect Control. 2013;41(8):710–6. https://doi. org/10.1016/j.ajic.2012.10.010.

64. Tang HJ, Lin HL, Lin YH, Leung PO, Chuang YC, Lai CC. The impact of central line insertion bundle on central line-associated bloodstream infection. BMC Infect Dis. 2014;14:356. https://doi.org/10.1016/j. jhin.2008.12.012.

65. Osorio J, Álvarez D, Pacheco R, Gómez CA, Lozano A. Implementation of an insertion bundle for preventing central line-associated bloodstream infections in an intensive care unit in Colombia. Rev Chil Infectol. 2013;30(5):465–73. https://doi.org/10.4067/S0716-10182013000500001.

# Chapter 12
# Catheter-Acquired Urinary Tract Infections

**Irene Comisso and Alberto Lucchini**

## 12.1 Introduction

Indwelling bladder catheters are widely used on intensive care unit (ICU) patients to monitor hourly urine output, thus allowing prompt identification and treatment of potentially life-threatening situations. As for other invasive procedures, bladder catheterization is prone to several complications, such as infections. In the United States, catheter-acquired urinary tract infections (CAUTIs) are considered a "never event," which means they are preventable and require creation and implementation of prevention programs [1]. In-hospital patients are frequently catheterized (15–25%), but catheterization is often unappropriated, and a survey [2] demonstrated that a high percentage of catheterized patients so as duration and discontinuation of the catheterization are not monitored. Urinary catheterization is frequent both in hospital and community settings (including patient's home), and a 30-day cutoff is used to differentiate between short- and long-term (or chronic) catheterization [3]. Guidelines suggest to adopt different approaches for insertion and management of urinary catheter (UC) according to the

© Springer International Publishing AG, part of Springer Nature 2018    305
I. Comisso et al., *Nursing in Critical Care Setting*,
https://doi.org/10.1007/978-3-319-50559-6_12

context where the procedure is performed. This chapter will only consider interventions related to acute settings. Although CAUTIs have a strong impact on hospitalized patients' outcomes, studies concerning the prevention of this problem are generally affected by poor-quality evidences and methodological issues. Therefore several research questions remain unresolved.

## 12.2 Definition

In 2009, the National Healthcare Safety Network (that refers to CDC safety surveillance system) narrowed the CAUTI definition (Patient Safety Component Manual) [4], excluding asymptomatic bacteriuria. CAUTIs are currently defined as "infections involving the urinary tract (including kidney) that develop in a person with an indwelling UC, thus not including Urinary Tract Infections (UTIs) developing when an alternative urinary drainage system (intermittent catheterization or external catheters) is adopted." The Infectious Diseases Society of America guidelines defined CAUTI as "the presence of symptoms or signs compatible with UTI with no other identified source along with $>10^3$ colony-forming units/mL…" with the symptoms and signs including "…new onset or worsening of fever, rigors, altered mental status, malaise, or lethargy with no other identified cause; flank pain; costovertebral angle tenderness; acute hematuria; pelvic discomfort…" [3]. According to CDC reports, CAUTIs are the most common (30%) type of healthcare-associated infections and are related to an increase in morbidity (as leading cause of secondary bloodstream infection, increased length of stay, costs, and antimicrobial use) and mortality (estimated 13,000 attributable deaths annually) [5].

Several definitions have been used from researchers when analyzing CAUTIs' incidence. It is fundamental to consider that a large portion of catheterized patients develops asymptomatic bacteriuria (ASB), a condition not requiring antimicrobial treatment, which, on the opposite, may lead to selection of resistant germs. ASB might evolve in a symptomatic UTI (SUTI). The recent changes in CAUTI definition provided by CDC substantially decreased CAUTI rates [6], since positive urine cultures were deemed as CAUTIs only when the patient was symptomatic or a bacteremia was present.

## 12.3  Epidemiology and Risk Factors

As for other infections, the incidence of CAUTIs widely varies between countries and hospitals, even according to resources' availability. It is estimated that in the United States, CAUTIs account for 36% of all hospital-acquired infections (HAIs) [7], and surveillance programs showed UTI as the most frequent infections in critically ill patients [8]. Recent data [9] confirmed that CAUTIs represent 23% of HAIs in ICU. Nonetheless, surveillance and educational programs seem to reduce CAUTI incidence only in non-ICU patients, while in critical care settings, incidence revealed an increasing trend from 2009, even if CAUTI definition change, and catheter use did not decrease [10].

CAUTIs are considered the leading cause of secondary acquired bacteremia, with an associated mortality of approximately 10%. In a cohort study, 21% of bloodstream infections derived from urinary infection [11]. ICU patients show different CAUTI rates, depending on ICU specialty (more frequent in burn and neurosurgical ICU) [12].

General risk factors indicate catheterization duration as the main responsible for CAUTI, since daily risk of bacteriuria acquisition when an indwelling catheter is in situ is of 3–7% [3]. While it is widely recognized that women have a greater risk for

UTI, a recent case-control study highlighted a higher predisposition for men. In fact they are more likely to develop urinary tract-related bloodstream infections [13]. In ICU patients, female gender (hazard ratio—HR 2.67, 95% CI 1.03–6.91; $p$ 0.043) and duration of urinary catheterization (HR 1.07 (per day), 95% CI 1.01–1.13; $p$ 0.019) were identified as risk factors for CAUTI acquisition alone [14]. Other independent risk factors identified in patients with other nosocomial infections are the presence of immune suppression and previous antibiotic usage [14]. In specific ICU populations (neurosurgery, cardiac surgery), CAUTI risk was significantly increased by older age, blood sugar >200 mg/dl, anemia requiring transfusion [15], cardiogenic shock, urgent or emergent surgery, and intensive care unit length of stay [16].

## 12.4  Pathogenesis and Diagnosis

Microorganisms generating CAUTIs can be endogenous (from rectal, vaginal, or meatal colonization) or exogenous (from professionals' contaminated hands). CAUTI onset can be both intra- and extraluminal [17]. Intraluminal onset may derive from a contamination of the collection bag and subsequent ascension into the bladder due to reflux, or an outbreak in closed drainage system, allowing germs to proceed along the internal lumen of the catheter. In extraluminal onset, the catheter can be contaminated during its insertion because of lack of asepsis or by capillary action (migration along the outer wall of the catheter) [17]. Subsequently, biofilm formation occurs and develops both intraluminally and extraluminally during the catheter's indwelling [17].

A recent retrospective study identified yeasts as the most frequent pathogens isolated in CAUTI (50%). Other isolated pathogens were *E. coli* (18%), *Enterococcus* spp. (12%), and *Pseudomonas* spp. (6%) [18]. In chronic catheterizations,

*Proteus mirabilis* is often isolated (up to 40% of collected samples). Its biofilm is more copious and persistent than the one of other microorganisms. A crystalline biofilm is characteristic for urease-producing microorganisms (*Proteus mirabilis*, *Pseudomonas aeruginosa*, *Klebsiella pneumoniae*), leading to catheter's obstruction [19].

According to recently published definitions, CAUTI is diagnosed when [4]:

- An indwelling UC had been in place for at least 2 days on the date of the event (and was present on the date of the event or removed the day before it).
- Fever, suprapubic tenderness, and costovertebral pain or tenderness are present.
- Positive urine culture with no more than two species or organisms, one of which is a bacterium of $\geq 10^5$ colony-forming unit (CFU).

Collection of urine specimens in a catheterized patient should be obtained aseptically through the catheter port. In chronically catheterized patients, urine specimens should be obtained after a new catheter is placed [3]. Recently, a survey reported that a considerable proportion of the interviewed nurses collected urine cultures from the urine bag (17%), or observed others acting this practice (41.6%), thus leading to a higher risk of sample contamination or irrelevant germs isolation and highlighting the need for knowledge assessment and dissemination and periodic audits [20].

## 12.5   Prevention

Although CAUTI has a strong impact on ICU patients' morbidity and mortality, and subsequently on global care costs, CDC guidelines were only recently updated [21], almost 30 years after the previous document [22]. During this long period, several societies and healthcare institutions developed guidelines to prevent CAUTI [23–26], and a recent review highlighted a substantial agreement within provided indications [27]. A further update of epic guidelines has also been released [28].

Listed below are interventions to prevent CAUTI; refer to the CDC guideline [21].

CAUTI's prevention is based on appropriate selection of patients undergoing catheterization. Particularly, catheterization should be considered when urinary retention or obstruction occurs or in case of prolonged immobilization. In critically ill and high-risk surgical patients, accurate assessment of hourly urine output remains an indication for permanent bladder catheter insertion [27], as it represents a tool to assess kidney perfusion and to manage fluid balance. For this reason, suggested alternatives to indwelling catheterization (such as intermittent catheterization or external catheters) are not applicable in ICU patients. In critically ill patients, bladder catheterization also can allow continuous monitoring of inner temperature (using a thermistor) or measurement of intra-abdominal pressure (IAP), although such maneuvers do not represent an indication for catheterization reported from guidelines.

On the other hand, catheterization should not be considered an intervention to manage urinary incontinence nor retention. In this case, other management strategies, such as intermittent catheterization, should be adopted.

Insertion of a bladder catheter in acute care settings requires the adoption of aseptic technique (including maximum barrier precautions) and sterile equipment. Prior to catheter insertion, adequate meatal hygiene is suggested, although no strong evidence is available concerning the best product for this practice (normal saline or a disinfectant agent). Concerning catheter's choice, researches comparing different catheter types are lacking, and results remain controversial [29]. Optimal catheter's characteristics should match retention systems together with reduced, or ideally cancelled, irritation, inflammation, or physical damage to the epithelium [30]. When considering resistance to kinking and flow rates, silicone catheters showed better in vitro performance compared to latex ones [31] and should be therefore preferred. In adjunction, in a prospective observational study, pure silicone catheters led to significantly lower bacterial colonization ($p = 0.03$) and biofilm formation ($p = 0.02$) compared to silicone-coated latex ones [32].

After catheter's insertion, one of the most important behaviors concerns maintenance of a closed drainage system (to avoid bacterial access) and of unobstructed urine flow (to avoid bacterial proliferation). Catheter's bag should always be positioned below the level of the bladder, avoiding contact with the floor.

As for other invasive devices, handwashing and use of non-sterile gloves are suggested whenever the catheter or the collection system is manipulated. Hygiene practices in catheterized patients do not require application of antiseptic soaps nor lubricants, and a recent RCT [33] demonstrated no significant reduction in CAUTI rates with chlorhexidine baths. Catheters should be properly ensured to the patient's leg, to avoid movements and secondary urethral and bladder trauma, thus increasing the risk of CAUTI [34].

UCs can be antiseptic-coated or antimicrobial-impregnated. Some studies evaluated the effects of these catheters on CAUTI reduction, also considering secondary endpoints such as asymptomatic bacteriuria, cost reduction, and patients' discomfort, reporting different results. A recently, published systematic review [35] found no substantial benefit regarding infection incidence when these catheters are used, although a small reduction in CAUTI incidence can be observed when nitrofurazone catheters are inserted, although more patients reported pain when catheters were in situ and after they were removed. These considerations suggest that no recommendations can be done regarding special UCs' insertion, and further research will be necessary to clarify their effect in CAUTI incidence reduction.

Ahead from those abovementioned, no routine interventions (such as catheter or collection bag changing, bladder irrigation, systemic and bladder antimicrobial administration) are recommended to prevent CAUTIs.

Bundles' implementation relates with a significant reduction in CAUTI incidence. The UC bundle includes the following five interventions [36]:

- Perform hand hygiene before insertion and manipulation of UC.
- Keep collection bag lower than the bladder level.
- Maintain unobstructed urine flow.
- Empty collecting bag regularly and avoid allowing the draining spigot to touch the collection catheter.
- Monitor CAUTIs using standardized criteria to identify patients with CAUTIs and to collect UC days as denominators.

Three larger studies [36–38] demonstrated a significant reduction in CAUTI rates after bundles' implementation. Ahead from bundles, other described interventions included the use of silver hydrogel UC and daily reminders to physicians to remove unnecessary catheters [39].

Both guidelines and observational before-after studies recommend the implementation of simple and not expensive interventions; in ICU patients, these interventions are mainly centered on daily evaluation of catheter's need and reminders to remove those no longer necessary [39]. Care interventions only concern the meatal hygiene and correct maintenance of the collection bag and closed collection system [39].

Take-Home Messages

- CAUTIs are increasing in ICU populations, even if improvement programs have been implemented.
- CAUTIs are a challenging problem, relating to patients' morbidity and mortality, but often underestimated.

- Simple and inexpensive interventions can significantly reduce CAUTI incidence.
- Education programs and surveillance should be implemented among care settings.

# References

1. Vacca M, Angelos D. Elimination of catheter-associated urinary tract infections in an adult neurological intensive care unit. Crit Care Nurse. 2013;33:78–80. https://doi.org/10.4037/ccn2013998.
2. Saint S, Kowalski CP, Kaufman SR, Hofer TP, Kauffman CA, Olmsted RN, et al. Preventing hospital-acquired urinary tract infection in the United States: a national study. Clin Infect Dis. 2008;46:243–50. https://doi.org/10.1086/524662.
3. Hooton TM, Bradley SF, Cardenas DD, Colgan R, Geerlings SE, Rice JC, et al. Diagnosis, prevention, and treatment of catheter-associated urinary tract infection in adults: 2009 international clinical practice guidelines from the Infectious Diseases Society of America. Clin Infect Dis. 2010;50:625–63. https://doi.org/10.1086/650482.
4. NHSN Patient Safety Component Manual. http://www.cdc.gov/nhsn/pdfs/pscmanual/pcsmanual_current.pdf. Accessed 19 Jun 2016.
5. Klevens RM, Edwards JR, Richards CL Jr, Horan TC, Gaynes RP, Pollock DA, et al. Estimating health care-associated infections and deaths in U.S. hospitals, 2002. Public Health Rep. 2007;122:160–6. https://doi.org/10.1177/003335490712200205.
6. Press MJ, Metlay JP. Catheter-associated urinary tract infection: does changing the definition change quality? Infect Control Hosp Epidemiol. 2013;34:313–5. https://doi.org/10.1086/669525.
7. Rebmann T, Greene LR. Preventing catheter-associated urinary tract infections: An executive summary of the Association for Professionals in Infection Control and Epidemiology, Inc, Elimination Guide. Am J Infect Control. 2010;38:644–6. https://doi.org/10.1016/j.ajic.2010.08.003.
8. Richards MJ, Edwards JR, Culver DH, Gaynes RP. Nosocomial infections in combined medical-surgical intensive care units in the United States. Infect Control Hosp Epidemiol. 2000;21:510–5. https://doi.org/10.1086/501795.

9. Burton DC, Edwards JR, Srinivasan A, Fridkin SK, Gould CV. Trends in catheter-associated urinary tract infections in adult intensive care units-United States, 1990-2007. Infect Control Hosp Epidemiol. 2011;32:748–56. https://doi.org/10.1086/660872.

10. Saint S, Greene MT, Krein SL, Rogers MA, Ratz D, Fowler KE, et al. A program to prevent catheter-associated urinary tract infection in acute care. N Engl J Med. 2016;374:2111–9. https://doi.org/10.1056/NEJMoa1504906.

11. Fortin E, Rocher I, Frenette C, Temblay C, Quach C. Healthcare-associated bloodstream infections secondary to a urinary focus: the Quebec provincial surveillance results. Infect Control Hosp Epidemiol. 2012;33:456–62. https://doi.org/10.1086/665323.

12. Dudek M, Horan T, Peterson K, Bridsonet KA, Morrell G, Anttila A, et al. National Health Care Safety Network (NHSN) Report, Data Summary for 2011, Device-associated Module. www.cdc.gov/nhsn/PDFs/dataStat/NHSN-Report-2011-Data-Summary.pdf. Accessed 19 Jun 2016.

13. Greene MT, Chang R, Kuhn L, Rogers MA, Chenoweth CE, Shuman E, et al. Predictors of hospital-acquired urinary tract-related bloodstream infection. Infect Control Hosp Epidemiol. 2012;33:1001–7. https://doi.org/10.1086/667731.

14. Temiz E, Piskin N, Aydemir H, Oztoprak N, Akduman D, Celebi G, et al. Factors associated with catheter-associated urinary tract infections and the effects of other concomitant nosocomial infections in intensive care units. Scand J Infect Dis. 2012;44:344–9. https://doi.org/10.3109/00365548.2011.639031.

15. Hagerty T, Kertesz L, Schmidt JM, Agarwal S, Claassen J, Mayer SA, et al. Risk factors for catheter-associated urinary tract infections in critically ill patients with subarachnoid hemorrhage. J Neurosci Nurs. 2015;47:51–4. https://doi.org/10.1097/JNN.0000000000000111.

16. Gillen JR, Isbell JM, Michaels AD, Lau CL, Sawyer RG. Risk factors for urinary tract infections in cardiac surgical patients. Surg Infect. 2015;16:504–8. https://doi.org/10.1089/sur.2013.115.

17. Maki DG, Tambyah PA. Engineering out the risk for infection with urinary catheters. Emerg Infect Dis. 2001;7:342–7. https://doi.org/10.3201/eid0702.700342.

18. Tedja R, Wentink J, O'Horo JC, Thompson R, Sampathkumar P. Catheter-associated urinary tract infections in intensive care unit patients. Infect Control Hosp Epidemiol. 2015;36:1330–4. https://doi.org/10.1017/ice.2015.172.

19. Nicolle LE. Catheter associated urinary tract infections. Antimicrob Resist Infect Control. 2014;3:23. https://doi.org/10.1186/2047-2994-3-23.

20. Jones K, Sibai J, Battjes R, Fakih MG. How and when nurses collect urine cultures on catheterized patients: a survey of 5 hospitals. Am J Infect Control. 2016;44:173–6. https://doi.org/10.1016/j.ajic.2015.09.003.

21. Gould CV, Umscheid CA, Agarwal RK, Kuntz G, Pegues DA. Guideline for prevention of catheter-associated urinary tract infections 2009. https://www.cdc.gov/infectioncontrol/pdf/guidelines/cauti-guidelines.pdf. Accessed 19 Jun 2016.

22. Wong ES. Guideline for prevention of catheter-associated urinary tract infections. Am J Infect Control. 1983;11:28–36.

23. Pratt RJ, Pellowe C, Loveday HP, Robinson N, Smith GW, Barrett S, et al. The EPIC project: developing national evidence-based guidelines for preventing healthcare associated infections. Phase I: guidelines for preventing hospital-acquired infections. Department of Health (England). J Hosp Infect. 2001;47:S3–82. https://doi.org/10.1053/jhin.2000.0888.

24. Pratt RJ, Pellowe CM, Wilson JA, Loveday HP, Harper PJ, Jones SRLJ, et al. EPIC 2: national evidence-based guidelines for preventing healthcare-associated infections in NHS hospitals in England. J Hosp Infect. 2007;65:S1–64. https://doi.org/10.1016/S0195-6701(07)60002-4.

25. Tenke P, Kovacs B, Bjerklund Johansen TE, Matsumoto T, Tambyah PA, Naber KG. European and Asian guidelines on management and prevention of catheter-associated urinary tract infections. Int J Antimicrob Agents. 2008;31:S68–78. https://doi.org/10.1016/j.ijantimicag.2007.07.033.

26. Lo E, Nicolle L, Classen D, Arias KM, Podgorny K, Anderson DJ, et al. Strategies to prevent catheter-associated urinary tract infections in acute care hospitals. Infect Control Hosp Epidemiol. 2008;29:S41–50. https://doi.org/10.1086/675718.

27. Conway LJ, Larson EL. Guidelines to prevent catheter-associated urinary tract infection: 1980 to 2010. Heart Lung. 2012;41(3):271–83. https://doi.org/10.1016/j.hrtlng.2011.08.001.

28. Loveday HP, Wilson JA, Pratt RJ, Golsorkhi M, Tingle A, Bak A, et al. epic3: national evidence-based guidelines for preventing healthcare-associated infections in NHS hospitals in England. J Hosp Infect. 2014;86(Suppl 1):S1–70. https://doi.org/10.1016/S0195-6701(13)60012-2.

29. Jahn P, Beutner K, Langer G. Types of indwelling urinary catheters for long-term bladder drainage in adults. Cochrane Database Syst Rev. 2012;10:CD004997. https://doi.org/10.1002/14651858.CD004997.pub3.

30. Feneley RC, Kunin CM, Stickler DJ. An indwelling urinary catheter for the 21st century. BJU Int. 2012;109:1746–9. https://doi.org/10.1111/j.1464-410X.2011.10753.x.

31. Lawrence EL, Turner IG. Kink, flow and retention properties of urinary catheters part 1: conventional foley catheters. J Mater Sci Mater Med. 2006;17:147–52. https://doi.org/10.1007/s10856-006-6818-0.

32. Verma A, Bhani D, Tomar V, Bachhiwal R, Yadav S. Differences in bacterial colonization and biofilm formation property of uropathogens between the two most commonly used indwelling urinary catheters. J Clin Diagn Res. 2016;10:PC01–3. https://doi.org/10.7860/JCDR/2016/20486.7939.

33. Noto MJ, Domenico HJ, Byrne DW, Talbot T, Rice TW, Bernard GR, et al. Chlorhexidine bathing and health care-associated infections: a randomized clinical trial. JAMA. 2015;313:369–78. https://doi.org/10.1001/jama.2014.18400.

34. Holroyd S. Innovation in catheter securement devices: minimising risk of infection, trauma and pain. Br J Community Nurs. 2016;21:256–60.

35. Lam TB, Omar MI, Fisher E, Gillies K, MacLennan S. Types of indwelling urethral catheters for short-term catheterisation in hospitalised adults. Cochrane Database Syst Rev. 2014;9:CD004013. https://doi.org/10.1002/14651858.CD004013.pub4.

36. Rosenthal VD, Todi SK, Álvarez-Moreno C, Pawar M, Karlekar A, Zeggwagh AA, INICC Members, et al. Impact of a multidimensional infection control strategy on catheter-associated urinary tract infection rates in the adult intensive care units of 15 developing countries: findings of the international nosocomial infection control consortium (INICC). Infection. 2012;40:517–26. https://doi.org/10.1007/s15010-012-0278-x.

37. Kanj SS, Zahreddine N, Rosenthal VD, Alamuddin L, Kanafani Z, Molaeb B. Impact of a multidimensional infection control approach on catheter-associated urinary tract infection rates in an adult intensive care unit in Lebanon: international nosocomial infection control consortium (INICC) findings. Int J Infect Dis. 2013;17:e686–90. https://doi.org/10.1016/j.ijid.2013.01.020.

38. Leblebicioglu H, Ersoz G, Rosenthal VD, Yalcin AN, Akan OA, Sirmatel F, et al. Impact of a multidimensional infection control approach on catheter-associated urinary tract infection rates in adult intensive care units in 10 cities of Turkey: international nosocomial infection control consortium findings (INICC). Am J Infect Control. 2013;41:885–91. https://doi.org/10.1016/j.ajic.2013.01.028.

39. Galiczewski JM. Interventions for the prevention of catheter associated urinary tract infections in intensive care units: an integrative review. Intensive Crit Care Nurs. 2016;32:1–11. https://doi.org/10.1016/j.iccn.2015.08.007.

# Chapter 13
# Venous Thromboembolism Prevention and Prophylaxis

**Matteo Manici, Giacomo Alemanno,
and Margherita I. Nuzzaco**

## 13.1 Introduction

Venous thromboembolism (VTE) is one of the most common complications for an intensive care inpatient. Primary thromboprophylaxis reduces the morbidity and mortality associated with deep vein thrombosis (DVT) and pulmonary embolism (PE). For those patients not receiving an adequate VTE prophylaxis, the incidence of DVT is 10–28% [1], and the incidence of PE is 7–27% [2]. The risk increases depending on the age, the weight, and a previous history of thromboembolic disease. The incidence could increase up to 85% if including the asymptomatic ones [3].

Base principles of VTE were known since the half eighth century. Virchow discussed about a "triad" made of vessel endothelial alterations, hematic flow stasis, and hypercoagulability: those three components are often present in critically ill patients [4, 5].

Nowadays the knowledge has enormously increased, but the adherence in the application of the two main guidelines [6, 7] is not satisfactory yet. In particular, with regard to the American

The original version of this chapter was revised. An erratum to this chapter can be found at https://doi.org/10.1007/978-3-319-50559-6_20

College of Chest Physicians (ACCP) guidelines [7], on its ninth edition now, the adherence hasn't improved over time even though, according to these recommendations, the decrease in percentage of the patient receiving VTE prophylaxis is quite significant, and this is true especially if it concerns an ambulatory environment (in a hospital environment, results seem to be better) [3].

Patients receiving intensive cares could be divided into groups according to their disease process:

- Acute illness with organ failure
- Need for higher level of observation and intervention
- After complex or prolonged surgery in need of prompt detection/management of complications
- End-of-life patients, with ongoing organ donation process

Inflammatory response to the physical stress, decreased mobilization, and intravascular devices increase the VTE risk.

For example, vasodilatation occurring during surgical procedures reduces the veins' hematic flow, causing venous stasis. Venous dilatation could lead to endothelial stretching that causes a tunica intima distress, resulting in an activation of platelets, coagulation factors, and other thrombogenic products related to tissue damage. Those factors, combined with traumatic surgical procedures and postoperative immobility, increase the risk to develop a thrombus in the veins [8].

At the same time, an increased bleeding risk (either because of a coagulopathy or as a consequence of illness or because of surgical procedure) could be present [6].

It is therefore necessary to get a good balance between the thromboembolic risk and the higher risk of bleeding. It is up to the Medical staff then to frequently assess those risks and consider the best VTE prophylaxis for each patient.

## 13.2 VTE Prevention

On the grounds of the above, the thromboembolic risk prevention could be made with medications, through a mechanical way, or, more often, with a combination of those.

Table 13.1 summarizes some recommendations for VTE prophylaxis in critically ill patient, adapted from AACP guidelines [7]. The pharmacological and physical therapies represent a continuum of care led according to patient's characteristics, past and current medical history, surgical and traumatological condition, bleeding risk, and contraindications to both ways of proceeding.

### 13.2.1 Pharmacological Prophylaxis

Pharmacological VTE prophylaxis could be made with low-dose ultrafractionated heparin (UFH), low-molecular-weight heparin (LMWH), fondaparinux (selective inhibitor of factor Xa), and oral vitamin K antagonist, chosen according to patient's risk. The right medication choice is not going to be discussed as it is not part of the purpose of this book.

On the contrary, the right administration of the prescribed therapies is part of the nurse professional's purpose to whom this book is addressed. In particular, the nurse while administering medications is responsible in preventing errors, so he is responsible for checking prescriptions, dispensary/medicine supply, and therapy administration and for monitoring the patient afterward [10]. Monitoring has to be carried out with particular attention as it needs to detect signs and symptoms of VTE (pain, redness, swollen legs, alterations of the breath and saturation, or the skin color) and of bleeding (external, visible internal, or not

**Table 13.1** Recommendations referred to venous thromboembolic prophylaxis in critically ill patients

| | | Prophylaxis | Recommendation | Considerations |
|---|---|---|---|---|
| Medical | Patient with medical disease | LMWH or UFH | Grade[a] 2C or grade 1B | Considering critical patient as acute case with high risk of VTE disease |
| | Patient with medical disease and high bleeding risk or contraindication to pharmacological prophylaxis | GCS or IPCS | Grade 2C | Switch to pharmacological prophylaxis once bleeding risk is resolved |
| Surgical | Patient with general surgical disease | LMWH or UFH | Grade 1B | Consider associating GCS or IPCS in case of high risk of VTE disease. Grade 2B |
| | Patient with surgical disease and high bleeding risk or contraindication to pharmacological prophylaxis | GCS or IPCS | Grade 2C | Switch to pharmacological prophylaxis once bleeding risk is resolved |

| Traumatologic surgical | Patient with | LMWH or UFH or IPCS | Grade 1B or grade 1C | Consider associating |
|---|---|---|---|---|
| | traumatologic surgical disease | | | GCS or IPCS in case of high risk of VTE disease. Grade 2B |
| | Patient with traumatologic surgical disease and high bleeding risk and/or contraindication to pharmacological prophylaxis | IPCS | Grade 2C | Switch to pharmacological prophylaxis once bleeding risk is resolved |

Adapted from ACCP 2012 guidelines in García-Olivares [9], reproduced with permission, modified

[a]Quality of evidence and strength of recommendation: Strong recommendation, high-quality evidence (1A); strong recommendation, moderate-quality evidence (1B); strong recommendation, low- or very-low-quality evidence (1C); weak recommendation, high-quality evidence (2A); and weak recommendation, moderate-quality evidence (2B)

visible internal bleeding, anemia, and signs of hemorrhagic shock). According to the kind of treatment and to the renal function, it is also necessary to check the full blood count and the coagulation blood tests, adding the anti-factor Xa assay when in treatment with LMWH (it is advisable to sample the patient at peak activity, from 3 to 5 h after the subcutaneous administration) [11].

UFH is administered intravenously; vitamin K antagonist requires oral administration, but it will not be discussed in this book.

LMWH and fondaparinux are administered subcutaneously; indications about prevention of bruise, hematoma, and pain in the injection site include:

- Lower abdomen is the eligible site. If this is not available, choose between the proximal area of the arm where the deltoid muscle is situated and area above the gluteus or the thigh.
- Inspect the injection for presence of lumps or pain and hygienic conditions.
- Carry out an antiseptic cleaning of the injection area.
- Use 25–27 gauge needles.
- Keep the air bubble into the syringe (when the syringe is in vertical position ready to inject, the bubble has to be close to the plunger tip).
- Insert the needle into the skin with an angle of 90° with a procedure less traumatic as possible.
- Avoid lesser maneuver (aspirate before injection when needle is in the skin).
- Keep pinching the skin while injecting the medication.
- Administer the medication slowly (30 s at least), and wait until the air bubble pushes the medication out of the needle.
- Once the needle is out, put some pressure on the site of injection, without rubbing [12].

## 13.2.2   Mechanical Prevention

Leading researches over the last three decades have shown that graduated compression stockings (GCSs), used alone or in combination with other external compression devices or medications, significantly reduce the DVT risk in surgical patients [13].

Mechanical prophylaxis is made by graduated compression stockings or pneumatic compression devices, aiming to reduce venous stasis.

### 13.2.2.1   Graduated Compression Stockings

GCSs are not simply elastic socks. They have been designed based on research studies trying to find the perfect balance between graduated compression, which helps the hematic flow, and the thrombosis risk reduction [13].

When correctly applied, GCSs speed the hematic flow up, reduce the risk of venous wall dilatation, improve the venous valve functionality, and could reduce the blood aggregation, leading to VTE risk reduction [13].

Since 1975, the compression stockings profile has been established, denominated as "the Sigel profile," which is about 8 mmHg at the ankle, 14 mmHg at the mid-calf, and 8 mmHg at the upper thigh, subsequently validated by other authors [14, 15], as shown in Fig. 13.1.

A recent Cochrane review highlighted that GCSs are effective in reducing the DVT risk in hospital inpatient, with strong evidence regarding their use in general and orthopedic surgery. The evidence of their effectiveness in medical patients is based on a single trial [16]. However, CLOTS1 study [17] conducted on acute-stroke inpatients hasn't demonstrated the same effectiveness. Therefore, benefits of GCSs combined with pharmacological prophylaxis in surgical patients are not clear [18].

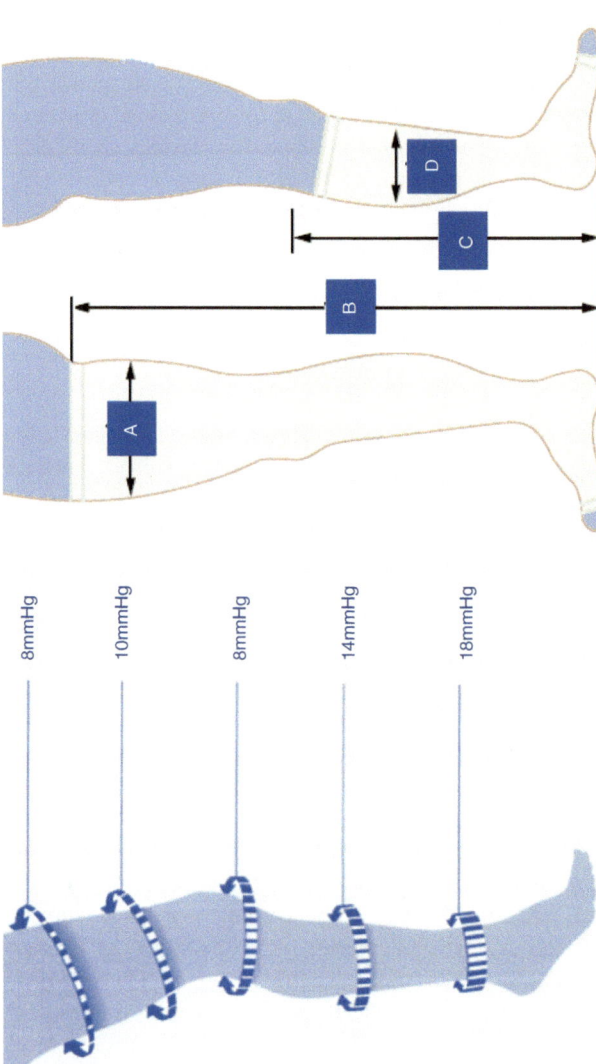

**Fig. 13.1** Left side: "Sigel profile." Right side: measurement of TL (A) thigh circumference and (B) length from the gluteal furrow to bottom of the heel, KL. (C) Length from bend of the knee to bottom of the heel and (D) calf circumference

GCSs are contraindicated in patients with peripheral vascular disease, arteriosclerosis, severe peripheral neuropathy, massive leg or pulmonary edema, edema secondary to congestive cardiac failure, local skin/soft tissue diseases such as recent skin graft or dermatitis, extreme deformity of the leg, gangrenous limb, Doppler pressure index <0.8, and gross limb cellulitis [19].

GCSs are produced in two lengths: thigh-length (TL) and knee-length (KL) stockings (Fig. 13.1).

The authors of a recent Cochrane review have considered the role of KL and TL in thromboprophylaxis in a postoperative patient group. No significant difference between the two groups has emerged. The heterogeneity and the small amount of primary studies suggest prudence regarding which one is the most effective in reducing DVT incidence [20].

The JBI [19] suggests that surgical patients should wear TL-GCSs from admission until they get back to their normal mobility, if those are not contraindicated. If the full length of the stockings is unsuitable because of thigh shape, the alternative is KL. Patients need to be encouraged to wear GCSs until they are back to their normal mobility.

Some authors indicate that nurses prefer KL and that they often use those, if not prescribed otherwise [13]. If TL are prescribed, but patients don't tolerate them, nurses put KL on or they lower TL down till the knee (even if this is not a correct procedure as the "Sigel profile" parameters are altered).

It is also important to guarantee that the stockings are correctly applied and worn and that the patient's skin and perfusion are monitored. To ensure a correct measurement and application of the stockings, manufacturer instructions should be followed. The measurement of the legs and of the sock size should be documented to keep a record and monitor the patient's leg size, to easily detect swelling. The most common complications are caused by sitting for a long period and by tourniquet effect made by multiple sock layers, which often produce an extended leg swelling. After application, the stockings need to be frequently checked to ensure that they are worn in the right way and that there are no wrinkles or folds along the length of the leg, especially in presence of leg swelling (the increase by 5 cm of the leg circumference could double the pressure applied by the stocking) [19].

The skin care is also important while wearing GCSs for a period of time. The stockings should be removed to assess skin condition and give appropriate hygienic care. There is no evidence about how often the legs need to be cleaned, but according to the experts, the skin should be inspected at least once a day. More frequent checks could be necessary in presence of particular skin conditions. Feet and legs need to be properly dried before putting the stockings on. Perfusion should be regularly checked, also through the GCSs inspection hole.

It's important that all the healthcare professionals that apply GCSs or teach the patients to do so are trained about how to put the stockings on and manage them, the reason why they are important, and the risks derived from a wrong use of those [19].

### 13.2.2.2 Intermittent Pneumatic Compression Systems

The use of intermittent pneumatic compression (IPC) systems had been described since 1934 from Reid and Hermann that proposed an archetype of the new alternating compression-decompression system, which they called "PAVEX" (passive vascular exercises), aiming to treat several kinds of lower limbs' arterial diseases [21].

The IPC is a therapeutic technique used in medical devices that consists of an inflatable sleeve wrapped around the calf (depending on the model, it could also be around the thigh and the foot) and an electrical pneumatic pump that inflates the sleeves with air, aiming to squeeze and push the blood in a centripetal way. The system's success presumes functioning venous valve. When the cuff inflates, the arteries are squeezed, and the blood flow is pushed forward; therefore, when the cuff deflates, it refills the veins, which in turn had been previously squeezed and emptied too [22]. Nowadays its main use is DVT prevention, but it can also be used in the treatment of venous ulcer, lymphedema, venous insufficiency, and other lower limb diseases.

There are several ways of applying IPC, using single or multiple chamber (also called as bladders) or using different kind of pumps, different compression cycles, or different inflation-deflation rates (Table 13.2). An example of IPC functioning could be the single posterior bladder designed for inflating uniformly at 40 mmHg (or at any pressure the operator sets it at)

**Table 13.2**  Types of IPC [21]

| Characteristics | Descriptions |
| --- | --- |
| Compression garments | • Circumferential bladder (encompasses the whole limb)<br>• Non-circumferential bladder (only compresses along part of the limb circumference) |
| Location of air bladder | • Thigh, calf, or foot compression<br>  – Or combination of these sites<br>  – Or the whole limb |
| Pump pressure cycles | • Uniform compression (a single pressure applied to all parts of the limb under compression simultaneously)<br>• Sequential compression (a single pressure applied to parts of the limb in sequence, with multiple bladders)<br>• Graded sequential compression (a gradient of pressure produced by inflating each bladder to different pressures) |
| Cycle length | • Duration of inflation time and deflation time<br>• Different cycling model such as automatic cycling devices (sequential compression device response compression system)<br>• Constant cycling devices |

in a cycle of 60 s (12 s for inflation, 48 s for deflation). The most common devices are often set up in a sequential way, starting from the ankle chambers inflated at 45–50 mmHg, following the calf one at 35 mmHg, and then the thigh one at 30 mmHg [21].

In any case, the IPC compressive strength is able to stimulate the systemic fibrinolytic ability and other circulation biochemical mechanisms able to reduce DVT (Fig. 13.2).

The thrombosis mechanical prophylaxis instruments are often used in the clinical practice. They are applied, monitored, and under the supervision of nurses and other healthcare providers [23]. It is strongly recommended to apply those devices in the right way and keep them continuously on (unless taken off for washing or for limbs assessment) [7, 24].

According to a study led by Elpern [23], for the 47% of cases, mistakes in IPC application are due to incorrect sleeve

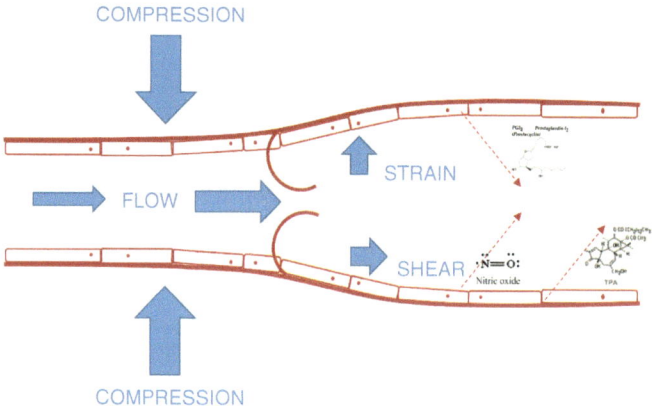

**Fig. 13.2** Mechanical effects of pneumatic compression on a vein or artery. The pneumatic compression increases intravascular flow, shear, and compressive strain on endothelial cells with the resulting release of many biochemical mediators

position, closing strap being worn and torn, and rotation along the leg axis. The author suggests that, with the aim of improving in applying IPC, it could be necessary to run some teaching sessions about how the mechanical thrombus prophylaxis works and about crucial moments during the application of this. Moreover, it could be useful to develop standard procedures that are evidence based and audit to evaluate the quality of the process [23].

## 13.3 Nursing Practice in VTE Prevention

The American Association of Critical-Care Nurses has published a "practice alert" regarding the VTE prevention [24], suggesting to assess the thromboembolic risk for all the patients on admission in ICU. It is necessary to mobilize the patient as soon as possible, reducing the number of immobile patients due to treatment reasons (because of pain, sedation, paralyzing agents, MV). It is also suggested to ensure the devices are correctly assembled and in good working condition all the time, except when removed during cleaning or skin inspection. Nurses should guarantee VTE prophylaxis policy availability, properly communicate with the patient, make sure that trainings and a regular assessment process exist about the correct use of mechanical prophylaxis devices, ensure to hand over those information to the ward the patient will go to after ICU discharge, guarantee the continuum of care, as well as monitor outcomes and compliance of the staff to the VTE policy.

In the English NICE guidelines of 2010 [6] there is a summary of the nursing cares, such as early mobilization, physiotherapy, and hydration, as shown in Table 13.3.

**Table 13.3** Nursing care for reducing the risk of venous thromboembolism (outlined by NICE guidelines) [6]

| Recommendation | Concept | Strong clinical evidence |
|---|---|---|
| Early mobilization and leg exercises | • Immobility and lack of exercise as risk factors for VTE (decreasing linear velocity of the blood, dilatation of the veins)<br>• Early mobilization prevents stasis and reduces subsequent risk of thrombi formation<br>• Leg exercises are a safe and effective method of increasing venous return to the heart, by particularly contracting the calf muscle pump, compressing the deep leg veins, and, with the aid of the venous valves, moving blood flow toward the heart | No RCTs |
| Leg elevation | • Leg elevation has a dual physiological effect: it reduces limb swelling and promotes venous return by its gravitational effect | No significant difference was found between leg elevation and no leg elevation (RR = 1.08, 95% CI 0.35 to 3.40, one study) |
| Hydration | • It is believed that dehydration predisposes to venous thromboembolism. There is a strong association between dehydration after acute ischemic stroke and VTE. Allowing a patient to become dehydrated during surgery may also be associated with VTE | Intravenous saline vs water by mouth associated with a significantly higher number of DVT events (RR = 4.50, 95% CI 1.06–19.11, one study) |

# References

1. Cook D, Crowther M, Meade M, Rabbat C, Griffith L, Schiff D, et al. Deep venous thrombosis in medical-surgical critically ill patients: prevalence, incidence, and risk factors. Crit Care Med. 2005;33(7):1565–71.
2. Geerts W, Selby R. Prevention of venous thromboembolism in the ICU. Chest J. 2003;124(6_suppl):357S–63S.
3. Farfan M, Bautista M, Bonilla G, Rojas J, Llinás A, Navas J. Worldwide adherence to ACCP guidelines for thromboprophylaxis after major orthopedic surgery: A systematic review of the literature and meta-analysis. Thromb Res. 2016;141:163–70. https://doi.org/10.1016/j.thromres.2016.03.029.
4. Virchow RLK. Die cellularpathologie: in ihrer begründung auf physiologische und pathologische gewebelehre. Unter den Linden No: Verlag von August Hirschwald; 1871. p. 68.
5. Welsby I, Ortel TL. Is it time for individualized thromboprophylaxis regimens in the ICU? Crit Care Med. 2015;43(2):500–1. https://doi.org/10.1097/CCM.0000000000000784.
6. The National Institute for Health and Care Excellence (NICE). Venous thromboembolism reducing the risk of venous thromboembolism (Deep Vein Thrombosis and Pulmonary Embolism) in patients admitted to hospital. London: National Clinical Guideline Centre - Acute and Chronic Conditions; 2010. https://doi.org/10.1136/hrt.2010.198275.
7. Guyatt GH, Eikelboom JW, Gould MK, Garcia DA, Crowther M, Murad MH, et al. Approach to outcome measurement in the prevention of thrombosis in surgical and medical patients: antithrombotic therapy and prevention of thrombosis: American College of Chest Physicians Evidence-Based Clinical Practice Guidelines. Chest J. 2012;141(2_suppl):e185S–94S. https://doi.org/10.1378/chest.11-2289.
8. The Joanna Briggs Institute. Graduated compression stockings: prevention of postoperative venous thromboembolism is crucial. Am J Nurs. 2006;106(2):72AA–DD.
9. García-Olivares P, Guerrero JE, Tomey MJ, Hernangómez AM, Stanescu DO. Prevention of venous thromboembolic disease in the critical patient: an assessment of clinical practice in the Community of Madrid. Med Intensiva. 2014;38(6):347–55. https://doi.org/10.1016/j.medin.2013.07.005.
10. Cousins d. Safety in doses: medication safety incidents in the NHS: the fourth report from the patient safety observatory. England: National Patient Safety Agency; 2007.
11. Boneu B, De Moerloose P. How and when to monitor a patient treated with low molecular weight heparin. Semin Thromb Hemost. 2001;27(5):519–22. https://doi.org/10.1055/s-2001-17961.

12. Ferri P, Davolio F, Panzera N, Corradini L, Scacchetti D. La somminist-razione sottocutanea di eparina: semplice procedura operativa, numerose variabilità. Evidence. 2012;4(1):e1000002.

13. Winslow EH, Brosz DL. Graduated compression stockings in hospitalized postoperative patients: correctness of usage and size. Am J Nurs. 2008;108(9):40–50; quiz 50-1. https://doi.org/10.1097/01. NAJ.0000334973.82359.11.

14. Sigel B, Edelstein AL, Savitch L, Hasty JH, Felix WR Jr. Type of compression for reducing venous stasis. A study of lower extremities during inactive recumbency. Arch Surg. 1975;110(2):171–5.

15. Horner J, Lowth LC, Nicolaides AN. A pressure profile for elastic stockings. Br Med J. 1980;280(6217):818–20.

16. Sachdeva A, Dalton M, Amaragiri SV, Lees T. Graduated compression stockings for prevention of deep vein thrombosis. Cochrane Database Syst Rev. 2014;12:CD001484. https://doi.org/10.1002/14651858. CD001484.pub3.

17. Dennis M, Sandercock PA, Reid J, Graham C, Murray G, Venables G, et al. Effectiveness of thigh-length graduated compression stockings to reduce the risk of deep vein thrombosis after stroke (CLOTS trial 1): a multicentre, randomised controlled trial. Lancet. 2009;373(9679):1958–65. https://doi.org/10.1016/S0140-6736(09)60941-7.

18. Mandavia R, Shalhoub J, Head K, Davies AH. The additional benefit of graduated compression stockings to pharmacologic thromboprophylaxis in the prevention of venous thromboembolism in surgical inpatients. J Vasc Surg. 2015;3(4):447–455. e1. https://doi.org/10.1016/j.jvsv.2014.10.002.

19. Joanna Briggs Institute. Graduated compression stockings for the prevention of post-operative venous thromboembolism. The JBI database of best practice information sheets and technical reports 2008;12(4):1–4.

20. Sajid MS, Desai M, Morris RW, Hamilton G. Knee length versus thigh length graduated compression stockings for prevention of deep vein thrombosis in postoperative surgical patients. Cochrane Database Syst Rev. 2012;5:CD007162. https://doi.org/10.1002/14651858.CD007162. pub2.

21. Chen AH, Frangos SG, Kilaru S, Sumpio BE. Intermittent pneumatic compression devices. Eur J Vasc Endovasc Surg. 2001;21(5):383–92. https://doi.org/10.1053/ejvs.2001.1348.

22. Zhao JM, He ML, Xiao ZM, Li TS, Wu H, Jiang H. Different types of intermittent pneumatic compression devices for preventing venous thromboembolism in patients after total hip replacement. Cochrane Database Syst Rev. 2014;12:CD009543. https://doi.org/10.1002/ 14651858.CD009543.pub3.

23. Elpern E, Killeen K, Patel G, Senecal PA. The application of intermittent pneumatic compression devices for thromboprophylaxis: an observational study found frequent errors in the application of these mechanical devices in ICUs. Am J Nurs. 2013;113(4):30–36; quiz 37. https://doi.org/10.1097/01.NAJ.0000428736.48428.10.
24. Martin B. Venous thromboembolism prevention. AACN practice alert. 2010.

# Chapter 14
# Hospital-Acquired Injuries: Device-Related Pressure Ulcers, Falls, and Restraints

Stefano Bambi

## 14.1 Introduction

Since quality indicators in healthcare systems are mainly oriented to the patients' safety area, lots of public and private institutes have promoted selected groups of outcome indicators. In the critical and intensive care settings, the outcome indicators should focus primarily on [1–4]:

- Reporting and analysis of standardized mortality ratio
- ICU readmission rate within 48 h from ICU discharge
- CVC-related bloodstream infection and VAP rate
- Rate of unplanned extubations
- Endotracheal re-intubation rate within 48 h from a planned extubation
- PU incidence (considered as institution-wide patient safety indicator)

Nevertheless, the above set of indicators, even if relevant for the ICU quality of care, are not completely centered on nursing. Rather, there is a special set of indicators called "nurse-sensitive outcomes," defined as "those outcomes that are relevant, based

© Springer International Publishing AG, part of Springer Nature 2018     335
I. Comisso et al., *Nursing in Critical Care Setting*,
https://doi.org/10.1007/978-3-319-50559-6_14

on nurses' scope and domain of practice, and for which there is empirical evidence linking nursing inputs and interventions to the outcome for patients" [5]. Among the most widespread nurse-sensitive outcome indicators, there are "pain," "patient falls," and "pressure ulcers" [5]. Some private institutions such as the National Quality Forum consider fundamental also the measure of "restraint prevalence" [6].

So, PUs (and the most peculiar device-related PUs), patient falls, and resorting to physical restraints (with related injuries) can be all collected under an idea that overcomes the generic "iatrogenic complications" concept, to embrace the more appropriate definition of "nursing-induced complications." Hence, we coined the term "hospital-acquired injuries (HAInj)" that currently does not exist in the literature. However, it can immediately recall a concept intimately linked to the adverse effects of nursing care.

This chapter will focus on these three important issues, tracing their conceivable cross trajectories and exploring their cause-effect relationships (Fig. 14.1).

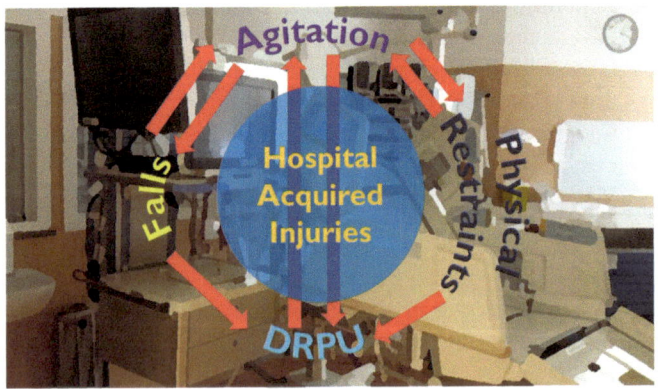

**Fig. 14.1** Hospital-acquired injuries vicious circle

## 14.2   Device-Related Pressure Ulcers

Device-related pressure ulcers (DRPUs) are a specific subset of hospital-acquired PUs, accounting for about 10% of the total PUs [7]. This issue is particularly challenging for critical care nurses, since ICU setting is characterized for a wide employment of diagnostic and therapeutic (invasive or noninvasive) equipment. DRPUs can involve patients' skin, mucous membranes, or both [8].

The prevalence of DRPUs reported in the literature is ranging from 0 to 85% [8], and some authors reported that 74% of DRPUs were discovered by healthcare staff when the ulcers were at the third or fourth stage or even unstageable [9].

Hospital devices causing PUs (summarized in Table 14.1) can be quite different [10, 18, 19]:

- Cervical collars, braces, splints, and other kinds of immobilizers (e.g., spinal boards)
- Nasal cannulas, oxygen tubing, and NIV interfaces (masks, helmets)
- Anti-embolic stockings or boots and sequential compression devices
- Endotracheal tubes, nasogastric tubes, and tube holders
- Pulse oximetry probes, artery catheters, and EKG wires
- Urinary catheters and fecal diversion systems
- Cooling mattress
- Restraints (wrist/ankles)
- Linen saver
- ECMO/ECLS tubes and catheters

However, 70% of these injuries affect anatomical areas located in the head, face, and neck [10].

Device features such as the materials used for its production, inadequate selection, anatomical sites of placement with scant fat tissue, modification of the physical condition of the skin under the device, and the securing method can concur in DRPU occurrence [20].

**Table 14.1** Device-related pressure ulcer typologies and prevention

| Device | Site and type of skin lesion | Prevention |
|---|---|---|
| Cervical collar [7, 10–12] | Occiputs, chin, clavicle, shoulder pressure ulcers | Optimize the efficiency of cervical spine clearance protocols |
| | | Remove hard collars as soon as possible, replacing it with softer ones |
| | | Padded collars seem to be effective in prevention of DRPU, if used appropriately, and routinely replacing the soiled and wet pads with clean and dry ones |
| | | Release braided or beaded hair before applying the collar |
| | | Try different kinds of cervical collars |
| | | Use correct collar and size |
| | | Use correct cervical collar placement techniques |
| | | Routine assessment of the skin under the collar (every 8–12 h), through its removal |
| | | Clean and dry the removable parts of the device |
| | | Reduce the prolonged pressure on the contact points of the skin |
| Elastic stocking [12] | Legs and feet skin pressure ulcers | Proper size of the device |
| | | Remove twice daily for an hour and contemporarily assess the skin under the stockings |

**Table 14.1** (continued)

| Device | Site and type of skin lesion | Prevention |
|---|---|---|
| Endotracheal tubes [7, 10, 12] | Neck, lips, mouth pressure ulcers | Routinely assess skin integrity and tension under the tube and the stabilizing device |
| | | Routine (at least every shift) change of orotracheal tube position (right, middle, left) |
| | | Some manufacturers recommend that endotracheal tube holders should not be used in patients with facial or lip edema and protruding teeth |
| Fecal diversion management system [7, 13, 14] | Perianal skin and mucosal breakdown, rectal damage (erosion) due to the presence of water-filled anchorage balloon, necrosis and hemorrhage of rectal mucosa | Routinely review the need of the fecal management system to remove it as early as possible (maximum 29 days) |
| | | Maintain the water-filled balloon according to the manufacturers' indication, avoiding overfilling |
| | | Caution should be used in patients with low platelet count or anticoagulation treatment |
| Nasal cannula/ oxygen mask [10] | Nares pressure ulcers | Routine inspection of the skin under the device |
| | Nasal bridge pressure ulcer | Routine cleaning of the nasal cannula |
| | Facial erythema | Decreasing mask strap tension |
| | | Use skin dressing behind the ears |
| Nasogastric tube [12] | Nares pressure ulcer | Routinely change the place of the NG tube standpoint on the nares |
| | | Splinting NG tube to suspend it from ala |

(continued)

**Table 14.1** (continued)

| Device | Site and type of skin lesion | Prevention |
|---|---|---|
| NIV mask [7, 15] | Facial erythema | Periodically readjust the mask straps |
| | | If possible, decrease pressure support levels |
| | | Allow some air leaks, adjusting the expiratory trigger setting to avoid the inspiratory hang-up phenomenon |
| | | Use skin dressing |
| | | Optimize mask active humidification to avoid condensation inside the interface |
| | | Routine cleaning of mask cushion |
| | | Interface rotation strategies |
| | Nasal bridge pressure ulcer | Use of correct interface size |
| | | Periodically readjust the mask straps |
| | | If possible, decrease pressure support levels |
| | | Allow some air leaks, adjusting the expiratory trigger setting to avoid the inspiratory hang-up phenomenon |
| | | Use foam skin dressing to reduce pressure and air leaks |
| | | Hydrocolloid dressing can be useful to reduce friction and shear forces, no direct pressure over the skin |
| | | Interface rotation strategies |
| NIV helmet [15, 16] | | Leaving the armpit out from the underarms and using a system with counterweights of 2 kg for each armpit (when set PEEP values do not exceed 10 $cmH_2O$) |
| | | Interface rotation strategies |

**Table 14.1** (continued)

| Device | Site and type of skin lesion | Prevention |
|--------|------------------------------|------------|
| Pulse oximeter [17] | Fingers, earlobe, forehead pressure ulcers | Frequent rotation of placement area |
| Tracheostomy straps/ties, flanges, and sutures [7, 10] | Stoma, around stoma skin, back neck skin, and skin under the flange pressure ulcers | Routine inspection of the skin interested by the device<br>Use of foam tracheostomy straps instead of ties or tape<br>Adequate management of suture in place<br>Use of foam dressing around the tracheostomy tube insertion, to prevent flange pressure and absorb the excess of exudate or secretion<br>Put a rolled towel under the ventilator tubing to prevent the flange pressure on the neck's skin |

Some other factors increase the risk of DRPU development, such as edema and moisture [10]. In fact, edema contributes to intensification of pressures and tension forces on the tissues under the device [10]. Instead, moisture caused by the permanence of body fluids around the device determines skin soaking [10]. Lastly, the frequent tightening of the devices to secure them, the materials used to fix them, and the force of friction coming from the movements can ease the DRPU onset [10, 18].

Some authors address reduced mobility, decreased sensory perception, and diminished perfusion as typical risk factors for the development of DRPUs in ICU settings [18]. Critically ill patients are often unable to communicate their discomfort, due to neurologic impairment, sedation, and neuromuscular blockage [21].

DRPUs usually evolve rapidly to full-thickness stage, for the areas of development are often lacking of adipose tissue, as on the neck, nasal bridge, occiput, and ears [10].

Finally, some DRPUs can be caused also by HCWs' imprudence and negligence acting as the unauthorized manumissions of medical devices (e.g., the case reports of gastric ulcer due to pressure necrosis related to a rigid and taut bumper applied to a percutaneous gastrostomy catheter) [22].

## 14.2.1   Noninvasive Ventilation Interface-Related Pressure Ulcers

NIV-related PUs can negatively affect the patients endurance toward this respiratory support.

A recently published systematic review on NIV complications summarized DRPUs' typologies and prevalence due to different NIV interfaces (oronasal, full face, and nasal masks or helmets) [15].

Facial skin erythema (incidence 20–34%) and nasal bridge ulcers (2–50%) are the most common NIV-related PUs, usually due to the compelling need to control the air leaks, increasing the tightening of the mask harnesses, the air volume in cushions, and the inspiratory pressures [15]. During NIV face PUs develop since the first hours, and nasal ulcers appear in almost the totality of patients with face mask within 48 h from the beginning of treatment [15].

Oronasal mask application longer than 26 consecutive hours was found as an independent risk factor for the development of skin breakdown in patients with ARF treated with NIV or CPAP [23].

Patients' risk factors for NIV interface-related PU development are BMI, diabetes, inotrope/vasoactive drugs, edema, vascular illnesses, nutritional status, chronic skin conditions, history of previous pressure lesions, steroid therapy treatment, and cytotoxic medications [24].

Helmets can early determine discomfort and pain under patients' armpits (mean NRS 4.8, after 5 min of helmet CPAP at

10 cmH$_2$O) [16]. Also, there's the risk of arm edema (incidence <5%) due to the armpit brace-induced venous and lymphatic stasis and DVT in the axillary vein [15].

With a NIV mask, the skin contact pressure is affected by contact area, respiratory pressure, and mask area during inspiration and expiration [25]; contact pressure is higher during expiration [25].

Both transparent and hydrocolloid dressings seem to be effective in preventing mask-related nasal bridge PUs if compared to a control group of patients treated without any dressing [26].

## 14.2.2   Cervical Collar-Related Pressure Ulcers

Some special DRPUs are those subsequent to the use of cervical spine collars in trauma patients. Their incidence varies from 6.8 to 38% [27]. Patients wearing cervical collars for more than 5 days have a risk to develop DRPUs from 38 to 55% [7].

An Australian ICU retrospective study on 299 major trauma patients showed that the most common site of Philadelphia collar-related PU was the occiput (59%). Other sites were the chin, clavicle, and shoulder [11]. The main predictor of ulcer development was the time to spinal clearance, since the probability of ulcer onset in patients meanly increased by 66% for every day with a collar on [11].

Other predictors for cervical collar-related PUs in major trauma patients were ICU admission, MV, and the need for cervical magnetic resonance imaging [28]. Even BMI is associated to the tissue interface pressure exerted by several typologies of cervical collars [28]. Interestingly the risk of collar-related PU development was 3.2 times in MV patients [11].

Even the choice of cervical collar type is likely to affect the chance of ulcer development [11].

A recent systematic review showed that only cervical collars can determine DRPUs, while other spinal immobilization devices, such as spinal boards and vacuum mattresses, are not associated with PU development, despite the increase of tissue interface pressure and the early onset of pain [28].

## 14.2.3   Device-Related Pressure Ulcer Prevention

The first way to prevent DRPUs is to suspect their presence or the risk of onset. Therefore, it's required to routinely assess the skin area in contact with the medical device and accurately register its conditions (aspect, stage, and extension of the lesions). An additional problem relates to the assessment of DRPU stage on mucous membranes, since the usual skin ulcer staging system cannot be used [8]. In fact, it's difficult to visually discriminate shallow from deep ulcer stages on the mucosa, and the presence of a coagulum can be confused with a full-thickness ulcer [8].

Beyond the risk assessment, other strategies should be implemented to fight the DRPUs: device selection (rigid vs soft materials), routine device repositioning, attentive device securing, shared and standardized protocols, device skin protective dressing, early withdrawal of the device as soon as it's no longer necessary, scheduled inspection of the skin area at risk of DRPUs and pain monitoring, patient education, and involvement of a multidisciplinary team [20].

The National Pressure Ulcer Advisory Panel (NPUAP) has dedicated a best practice document for DPRU in critical care. The synthesis of recommended interventions is reported below [29]:

- Choose the correct size of medical devices for every single patient.
- Shield the skin with dressings in high-risk areas.
- Assess the skin in contact with device routinely every day.

- Do not position devices over sites of pressure ulcers or preexisting lesions.
- Provide adequate education to the staff about the correct use of devices and the prevention and treatment of skin breakdown.
- Assess and identify edema under devices, recognizing the risk of skin breakdown.
- Control and confirm the position of the devices in a "free zone" that is not under a person who is bedridden or immobile.

Recently, recommendations from a panel of experts indicated the following needs [12]:

- Consider the use of dressings with effectiveness in pressure redistribution and moisture absorption from zones under or in contact with medical devices.
- Put dressings below medical device and temporarily remove or move (if it's possible) the device to assess the conditions of the underneath skin and provide a period of pressure relief.
- If the repositioning of devices does not reduce the pressure, avoid further pressure by applying dressing under tight devices.
- Report the onset and the clinical evolution of DRPUs.

Concerning DRPU reports, a recent explorative study showed that in 70.8% of National Health Service (NHS) inpatient facilities, PU monitoring systems do not differentiate PUs from DRPUs in nursing documentation [30].

Quality improvement programs seem to be associated to a decrement of the DRPU rates over time [18]. Focused checklists can be useful to address this issue. The checklist should address [31]:

- The routine assessment about the need to maintain the devices in place or replace it
- An accurate skin assessment and care every 8–12 h for all kinds of devices, except for NIV interfaces (every 2–4 h) and tracheal tubes (every 2 h)

- Systematic application of advanced wound dressing to protect the skin
- Limiting the moisture of skin through the use of protective products
- Use of pressure-relieving pads

Lastly, nurses' contribution to the redesigning of some medical devices could valuably aid to prevent DRPUs, since lots of device designs have not been reviewed for years by manufacturers [18].

## 14.3 Falls in Intensive Care Unit

The Institute for Clinical Systems Improvement (ICSI) defined a "fall" as "any unplanned descent to the floor" [32]. Falls can be assisted (with someone actively reducing its impact) and unassisted [33].

Usually, the fall of a patient from a hospital bed is a critical event potentially causing minor or major injuries (Table 14.2). Therefore, it represents one of the most common nursing-sensitive indicators, especially used for benchmarking aims [5]. This indicator should be calculated as incidence density (the total number of falls multiplied by 1000 and divided by the total number of patient days) [33].

**Table 14.2** Classification of falls with injuries [32]

| Point | Definition |
| --- | --- |
| 1 | No manifest injury |
| 2 | Minor: bruises or abrasions as consequences of the fall |
| 3 | Moderate: an injury causing tube or line displacement, fracture, or laceration requiring reparation |
| 4 | Major: injury requiring surgery or transfer to intensive care unit for monitoring a life-threatening injury |
| 5 | Death |

Falls are a principal cause of death in patients aged ≥65 years. Ten percent of deadly falls for the older patients happen in hospitals [34]. These kinds of adverse events are particularly feared by nurses, being directly responsible for patients' safety. The fall event is described by nurses as "upsetting" and "scary" [35]. Moreover, when a patient falls from the bed, it's easy to induce a guilt feeling in nurses, even if they have done all the possible interventions to prevent these adverse events. This occurrence can be even more dramatic, when a critical care patient falls from a bed in ICU.

Currently, patient fall in a hospital is the most common adverse event, ranging from 2.6 to 7.0 falls per 1000 patient days [36]. The injuries caused by these incidents vary from 23 to 42%. Fractures, traumatic brain injuries, and death account for percentages of 2–9% [36].

In a large observational study performed in the USA, falls were 3.32 per 1000 patient days across all nursing units. Falls were more frequent in rehabilitation wards, while ICUs accounted for the lowest rates. Seventy-two percent of patients had no injuries, 5% had moderate or major injury, and 23% had minor injury [37].

A recent descriptive study performed in Turkish ICUs showed that 13.6% of nurses experienced incidents with potential adverse effects for patients' safety, and the higher rate was represented by patient falls (48%) [38].

A quasi-experimental study has showed that nurse managers turnover does not play a role in patient fall occurrence. Medical and surgical wards are more affected by these adverse events than ICUs ($F_{1,11} = 15.9$, $p = 0.002$) [39].

A retrospective study performed in some ICU showed a falls incidence rate of 0.99/1000 patient bed days. Neuro/trauma critical care unit had instead an incidence of 1.97/1000 patient bed days [40]. The 43% of these episodes was related to falls from a chair, while falls from the bed accounted for the 33%. In the 83% of these events, there were no injuries as consequences [40].

Data from two ICUs in the USA reported that patient falls occurred mainly between 7 AM and 10:59 AM during early mobilization or routine hygiene practice. Sixty-eight percent of patients fell on the floor. Thirty-one percent of falls determined injuries [41]. The authors found that, if the staff had used the Hendrich II score, a threshold of 4 points would have predicted 95% of the occurred falls [41].

To date, no statistical association between nurse staffing and patient falls is known, despite few well-designed studies showing that lower rates of falls were associated to a better staffing condition [5]. Other significant associations were found between positive perceived interdisciplinary communication or higher levels of nursing education and lower patient falls, while an inverse relationship emerged between patient falls and levels of nursing experience [5].

A qualitative study revealed the stages of nurses coping with the falling event: denying responsibility, self-searching, facing reality, and accepting [35].

Nurses' point of view about the issue of patient falls is focused around the main concept of "knowing the patient as safe" [35]. This means to maintain their attention toward fall prevention through interventions in the spheres of assessment, monitoring, and communication [35].

Patient falls are an important outcome to be used in research about the optimization of nurse staffing in clinical settings with limited human resources [42]. The main features of nurse staffing are nurse staffing intensity, skill mix, and overtime use. The other two nursing staff characteristics are education level and experience [42].

### 14.3.1   Risk Factors for Patient Falls in ICU

The identification and assessment of patient fall risk factors are crucial to plan adequate prevention. In-hospital fall risk factors strictly depend on the clinical setting features (e.g., general ward, emergency department, ICU).

The risk of falls seems to be related to the amount of risk factors that are present at the moment of the incident [43].

Fall risk factors are classified as intrinsic (related to patient psychophysical condition) and extrinsic (related to hospital environment, supportive/assistive equipment, medications) [43].

The older patients are the most exposed category to these kinds of incidents. The general risk factors for patients falling are cognitive dysfunction (delirium, dementia), impaired mobility, medications (in particular, patients treated with four or more drugs have higher risks of falls), environmental obstacles, or physical hazards [32].

Currently, three main fall risk assessment tools are available for implementation in clinical settings.

The Hendrich II Fall Risk Model has a sensitivity of 70% and a specificity of 61.5% in acute care settings [43]. It explores seven categories (confusion/disorientation, depression, altered elimination, dizziness/vertigo, gender, antiepileptics/benzodiazepines, get up and go test/ability to rise in single movement), with 4 scale points from absent (0) to present (4). A threshold of 5 points indicates high risk of falls [43].

The Morse Fall Scale has a sensitivity of 88.3% and a specificity of 48.3% in acute care settings [43]. This scale includes six categories (history of falling, secondary diagnosis, ambulatory supports, intravenous saline lock, gait, mental status) [43]. The score of the Morse Fall Scale ranges from 0 to 125; the threshold for high risk of falling is 51 points [43].

The St. Thomas Risk Assessment Tool has a sensitivity of 55% and a specificity of 75.3% in acute care settings [43]. It evaluates the patient through five categories (history of falling, mental status, visual impairment, frequent toileting, transfer and mobility) [43]. This tool uses a binomial score (0 absent, 1 present) that can lead to a maximum point of 5. The threshold for high risk of falling is 2 [43].

A large number of risk factors (mainly drugs), not included in the above risk assessment tools (Table 14.3), were significantly related to falls. Therefore, they should deserve particular attention during patients' assessment. So, there is the need to improve the fall risk assessment tools through adequate research.

Within the critical care settings, intrinsic risk factors mainly concern the rapid beginning of patient deconditioning, early after admission [44]. Extrinsic factors are those related to the quantity and type of equipment attached to patients determining difficulties to increase patient mobilization [44].

In a study performed in a cardiac ICU, nurses addressed delirium as a contributing factor to this kind of adverse events (AE) [45]. In another research conducted on four critical care units, most frequent risk factors were confusion or agitation (60%) and the mobilization of patients against advice (38%) [40].

According to some authors, patient fall risk assessment in ICU should carefully consider: sedation or treatment with hypnotics; presence of confusion, delirium, or dementia; and previous falls [40].

**Table 14.3** Patient fall risk factors present in the literature and not included in the validated tools [32]

| Risk factors |
| --- |
| • Polypharmacy |
| • Lipid-regulating drugs |
| • Cardiac drugs |
| • Antiparkinson drugs |
| • Antidiabetic drugs |
| • Opioids/narcotic drugs |
| • Antidepressant drugs |
| • Diuretic drugs |
| • Antipsychotics |
| • Diagnosis of cancer |

## 14.3.2  Patient Fall Prevention in ICU

The general approach to patient fall prevention is adequate for all clinical settings and should consist of [45, 46]:

- Definition of fall
- Selection and implementation of a risk of fall assessment tool
- Communication of patient's fall risk between healthcare staff components (efficient handover)
- Implementation of universal strategies and interventions of fall prevention, including delirium prevention, assessment, and management
- Healthcare staff education about fall risk assessment, prevention, and reaction

Universal fall prevention interventions and general monitoring and surveillance recommendations are reported in Table 14.4. Appropriate preventive interventions in critical care setting are summarized in Table 14.5.

**Table 14.4**  Universal fall prevention interventions and general monitoring and surveillance recommendations [32]

| Fall preventive interventions | |
| --- | --- |
| Universal fall interventions | • Help patient with the environment familiarization |
| | • Patient "teach back" call light use |
| | • Maintain the call light within reach |
| | • *Maintain patient's personal effects within reach* |
| | • Strong handrails in patient bathrooms, rooms, and hallways |
| | • *Maintain the hospital bed in low position with brakes locked* |
| | • *Nonslip, well-fitting footwear for the patient* |
| | • *Night-light or supplemental lighting* |
| | • *Maintain floor surfaces clean and dry. Clean up all spills promptly* |
| | • *Maintain patient care areas uncluttered* |

(continued)

**Table 14.4** (continued)

| Fall preventive interventions | |
| --- | --- |
| Other fall precautions | • Do not leave alone the patient when in the bathroom<br>• *Intentional rounding behaviors at least hourly*<br>• *Transfer belts available at the bedside*<br>• Evaluate the need for home safety assessments, with physical and occupational consultation in the discharge planning<br>• *Evaluate the need for 1:1 monitoring*<br>• *Chair or bed alarm* |
| Behavioral interventions | • *In patients affected by dementia*<br>• *Regularity in procedures, routines and schedules, and staff allocation*<br>• *Identification of triggers for agitated behaviors*<br>• *Occupational and physical therapists to increase orientation, awareness, and function* and assess the need and the appropriate use of gait supports |
| Impaired mobility interventions | • *Patients should wear their shoes or nonskid footwear*<br>• *Physical therapy and occupational therapy consults*<br>• Educate the patient to rise slowly<br>• Early and regular ambulation of high-risk patients<br>• Periodic education of safety measures to the patient and family members<br>• Assist high-risk patients with transfers<br>• Use of patient's regular assistive devices<br>• Scheduled assistance with toileting<br>• Supportive chairs with armrests<br>• Hip protectors for patients at high risk for hip fracture<br>• *Adequate daytime and nighttime lighting*<br>• Elevated toilet seats<br>• Gait belt or transfer belt during mobility activities |
| Environmental interventions | • *Staff environmental round*<br>• Hip protectors<br>• *Removal of physical restraints*<br>• *Falls alarm devices*<br>• *Low height and alarmed bed* |

**Table 14.4** (continued)

| Fall preventive interventions | |
| --- | --- |
| Other environmental factors | • Adult assistive walking devices |
| | *• Convex mirrors to enable nursing staff visualization of all hallways from the nursing station* |
| | • Motion detectors at the bedside in patients' rooms |
| | *• Nonslip footwear* |
| | *• Upgrade of all bed-exit alarms* |
| **Observation and surveillance** | |
| Monitoring | *• Monitoring and reassessment on regular basis, also for patients that are not in high-risk groups: every shift and when patients' conditions change or after a fall* |
| Intentional timed rounding | *• Assessment of pain level* |
| | • Toileting assistance |
| | *• Repositioning and comfort* |
| | • Patient properties, call light, telephone, television remote, urinal, etc. within reach |
| | • Dressing checks |
| | *• Water refreshed and offered* |
| | *• Lighting and temperature of room* |
| | *• Checking room for environmental and hazardous elements* |
| | • Final question "Is there anything else I can do for you?" and scheduled time to return |

Legend: The interventions also suitable for critical care settings are in *italic font*

**Table 14.5** Fall preventive interventions for critical care settings [40]

| Preventive interventions |
| --- |
| • Maintain the patient in a safe position and guarantee adequate surveillance and observation |
| • Use of bed rails appropriately |
| • Mobilize the patients with the right equipment and number of staff adequate to the task |
| • Maintain footwear worn to the patients in chair |
| • Inform the patients about the risk of falling and educate them about self-mobilization to prevent falls |

There are positive experiences about the implementation of geriatric nurses as specialists with the aim to spread geriatric knowledge to ICU nurses, early identify the presence of geriatric syndrome in ICU patients, and detect those who are at higher risk of falls to trigger prevention protocols and AE audits [45].

The relationship between ICU patients' stay in high-visibility rooms (directly across from the nursing station) [47] and the fall from bed rates should deserve to be studied through well-designed observational research.

Some authors reported the effectiveness of comprehensive approach, including simulated case studies and real-time feedback, in dramatic reduction of ICU patient falls, reaching a real change in culture of safety practices [48].

Early mobilization consists in a stepwise-fashioned program of progressive mobility in patients still supported through MV [49]. According to a recent literature review, this important practice seems to be safe regarding the risk of patient falls, since no study reported any episode of patient fall in ICU (and no death nor cardiac arrest) [49].

A "post-fall" protocol, driving the right actions to implement immediately after the incidents, is a precious tool that all units should be provided with. These kinds of protocols should contain some basic elements such as immediate physical assessment, provider notification, treatment and diagnosis if necessary, enhanced safety measures, evaluation of nursing interventions at the time of the fall, proper documentation, and notification of the family [50].

## 14.4  Physical Restraints in Critical Care Settings

The need to protect patients from their self-harm behaviors in clinical settings implicates the use of chemical (pharmacological) and/or physical restraints (PR).

Some authors claim the lack of a clear and consistent definition for PR in the literature [51]. The Health Care Financing

Administration called PR as "any manual method or physical or mechanical device, material or equipment attached or adjacent to the residents' body that the individual cannot remove easily which restricts freedom of movement or normal access to one's body" [52].

A large prevalence study on ICU patient-initiated device removal ("treatment interference"), performed in the USA, showed that patients removed 1623 devices on 1097 occasions (22.1 episodes/1000 patient days) [53]. Forty-four percent of ICU patients were restrained at the time of device removal. Damages occurred in 250 (23%) events, while 10 determined a major harm [53].

The use of PR is the joining link between DRPUs and patient falls in the ICU settings. In fact, prevention of falls is considered by nurses as the principal reason for using restraints [54]. This is one of the most considerable issues for all nurses working in clinical settings, with important medicolegal implications. Moreover, beyond the risks for patients' safety in terms of injuries related to physical restraints, using such measures links an important ethical dilemma to nurses. Lastly, a large number of studies revealed a lack of evidence about the effectiveness of this practice, demanding the reduction and a more rational utilization of PR [51].

The most widespread techniques to institute PR in ICU are the boxing gloves, achieved through wrapping the hands with cotton bandages, with the aim of impeding patients to use their fingers, and tying the patient's arms to the bed frame, blocking their use but letting free the trunk, legs, and feet [55].

Other authors describe the tools used in PR as wrist, chest, and waist restraints, mitts, elbow splints, and sheets. In some studies, bedside rails are not considered as PR.

## 14.4.1  Epidemiological Features of Physical Restraints in ICU Settings

A survey performed on 38 critical care nurses from different countries in Europe in 2002 showed that 55.3% used PR in their units, often in the occurrence of patient agitation (73.7) [56]. PR use was at 100% for surveyed ICU nurses from Middle and Southern Europe, while it was at 44% for those from Scandinavia and 33% for those from the UK ($\chi^2$ =11.3; $p$ < 0.01) [56].

Some years later, the same authors designed a descriptive study about the use of restraints in 34 adult general ICUs from 9 European countries [57]. The point prevalence of PR in ICU patients was, at the moment of the study, 39%. PR were used mainly in MV patients ($\chi^2$ = 87.56, $p$ < 0.001), in sedated patients ($\chi^2$ = 34.66, $p$ < 0.001), and in units with lower nurse-to-patient ratio ($\chi^2$ = 17.17, $p$ = 0.001) [57]. In 89%, PR were made of commercial wrist restraints. The three most frequent reasons to initiate PR were, in diminishing order: prevention of self-extubation, patient pulling on tube and lines, and falls from bed prevention [57]. International data of PR prevalence and reasons of implementation in ICU settings are summarized in Table 14.6.

**Table 14.6** Use of physical restraints in ICU setting described in studies from different countries

| Authors (years) | Country | Prevalence of PR | Reason for PR |
|---|---|---|---|
| Benbenishty et al. [56] | Scandinavia | 44% | Patient's agitation All intubated patients |
| | UK | 33% | |
| | Middle Europe | 100% | |
| | Southern Europe | 100% | |
| Martin and Mathisen [58] | USA | 39% | NR |
| | Norway | 0% | |
| Minnick et al. [59] | USA | 9–351/1000 patient days | Prevent therapy disruption Confusion Fall prevention |
| Fogel et al. [60] | USA | 17–27% | NR |

**Table 14.6**   (continued)

| Authors (years) | Country | Prevalence of PR | Reason for PR |
|---|---|---|---|
| Benbenbishty et al. [57] | UK | 0% | Pulling on tubes/lines |
| | Switzerland | 43% | Preventing self-extubation |
| | Spain | 45% | Preventing from falling |
| | Italy | 100% | Danger to self |
| | France | 47% | Prevent falling from chair |
| | Portugal | 0% | Patient wandering off unit |
| | Finland | 12% | Reason unclear/other |
| | Greece | 21% | |
| | Israel | 28% | |
| Langley et al. [61] | South Africa | 48.3% | Agitation Treatment interference |
| De Jonghe et al. [62] | French | > 50% | Agitation |
| Kandeel and Attia [63] | Egypt | 6.2–46.2% | Patient's attempt to remove medical equipment Resisting treatment or care Patient's attempt to get out of bed Ensure patient safety Facilitate medical care Protect medical equipment Support the patient's position Compensate for deficiency in nursing staff |
| Krüger et al. [64] | Germany | 0–90% | NR |
| Pagliuco Barbosa et al. [65] | Brazil | From 9.4 to 40% | NR |
| van der Kooi et al. [66] | Dutch | 0–56% | Pulling on catheters/tubes Potential threat to airway Prevent patients' falling Unstable fracture Danger to self Danger to others or aggression Delirium |

Legend: *NR* Not Reported

As reported by a Dutch multicenter study, PR are applied mainly in the upper limb (98%) versus low rates of leg (5%) and torso (1%) restraints [66].

In USA there's a lack of education about PR in the current nursing curricula, despite the large employment of PR in critical care settings [67].

PR rates are usually low in most of European ICUs (26.4%) [57] but reach 92% in Dutch, even if only 31% of interviewed nurses stated that they used a PR protocol in every situation [66].

The sites of PR application in order of pattern frequency are usually bilateral wrist, bilateral wrist or four extremities alternately, unilateral wrist, four extremities, unilateral ankle, four extremities or chest restraint alternately, and bilateral wrist, four extremities, or chest restraint alternately [68].

## 14.4.2 Risk Factors for Use of Physical Restraints

The use of confusion assessment method for the intensive care unit (CAM-ICU) seems to be associated with a larger administration of PR and pharmacological restraints [69]. In fact, the incidence of delirium was higher in restrained patients, when compared with unrestrained ones (59 vs 33%, $p < 0.001$) [70].

Univariate analysis mode suggested that trauma or surgical ICU could be at risk of PR (hazard ratio (HR), 1.39; 95% CI, 1.02–1.90), so as patients with positive anamnesis for neurological pathologies (HR 1.71; 95% CI, 1.8–2.72) or psychiatric illnesses (HR 1.47; 95% CI, 1.11–2.00) [70].

## 14.4.3 Complications and Outcomes of Patients with Physical Restraints

The use of PR at admission time and during the 24 h before the onset was found to be significant predictors for patient agitation in ICU, scored as RASS $\geq$ +1 (respectively, OR = 3.77; 95% CI, 1.39–11.53; $p$ = 0.008; and OR =1.04; 95% CI, 1.01–1.08; $p < 0.001$) [71].

A study performed on 11 Egyptian ICUs revealed a complication rate related to PR from 19 to 25.3% [63]. Bruises were reported in 2%, redness in 16.5–22.4%, ulcers in 0.4–0.8%, and necrosis of the skin tissue in 0.1% [63]. The recorded behavioral consequences were crying/moaning (40.5–48.4%), increased agitation (14.3–18.3%), and calmness (33.3–44.9%) [63].

One study has demonstrated that the use of PR can be a risk factor for unplanned extubations, increasing it by 3.11 times [72], even if other authors showed that PR have a protective effect for AE, including unplanned self-extubations (OR = 0.28, CI 0.16–0.51) [73]. Other studies showed the association between PR and adverse events such as altered circulation, injuries to nerves, fractures, and death [74]. Some cases of DVT and PE associated to bed immobility due to the use of PR are reported in the literature, even in the absence of risk factors [75].

A multicenter follow-up study performed on five hospitals showed a higher incidence of post-traumatic stress disorder in surviving patients who were restrained during their ICU stay [76].

The Joint Commission identified six root causes for patients' injuries consequent to PR [77]:

- Insufficient patient assessment
- Equipment use
- Care planning
- Defective communication
- Insufficient orientation training
- Inappropriate use of staffing resources

In consideration of the abovementioned root causes for PR, four interventions were bundled together to improve performance and patients' outcome: products/equipment, rounds/consultation, dedicated resources, and education [77]. This kind of PR reduction program resulted in good compliance to process and some positive outcomes (restraint prevalence) in medical and surgical settings [77].

## 14.4.4 Ethical, Legal, and Educational Issues

Despite PR use being legitimized by the need to protect the patient from self-harming [78], critical care nurses daily struggle to find the right balance between the need to guarantee patient's safety and ethical and organizational mandates to limit the PR use [78]. Moreover, current dimensions of compassion, preserving patients' rights, and ethics have raised the heaviness of PR ethical dilemmas [79].

A descriptive study performed on 55 ICU nurses from 2 Turkish hospitals showed that 36.4% of nurses had some difficulties in taking decision about PR. The ethical dilemmas that they had to face were related to the principle of non-maleficence in 76.4%, beneficence and convenience in 45.5%, respect to the person in 18.2%, and autonomy in 9.1% [80].

The consequences of the use of PR, beyond physical and psychological injuries, are also related to the violation of individual rights: there is a total loss of autonomy and privacy, making thinner the boundaries with the risk of abuse in this exposed patient population [78].

In the UK there are three conditions in which restraining a patient could be considered lawful: protecting the patient from self-injury, actual risk of aggression for healthcare staff, and prevention of hazardous or menacing behaviors [81]. From a legal point of view, the overuse of PR as a defensive strategy is self-defeating, since PR can easily determine injuries in application sites [82].

Often the lack of discussion with patients and relatives violates the principle of informed consent [78]. Informed consent is mandatory for patient and/or surrogates, since PR are a practice at risk of patient injuries, and there's no high-level evidence on their effectiveness [78].

PR in critical care settings are frequently implemented under the principle of paternalism, which assumes that the benefits of PR, in terms of self-harm prevention, outweigh the patient's autonomy and liberty of action. This kind of behavior principle should be limited only to the real condition of danger for patients or when the patients become harmful to others. However, as soon as the hazard condition comes to an end, it's ethically mandatory to seek alternatives to PR [78].

Substantially, PR condition imposes harms to prevent larger ones. Nevertheless, in critical care patients, the analysis of risk-benefit can be hard, especially in case of dangers for third persons [55, 78].

PR influences the trust in the relationship between patients, relatives, and healthcare staff. In critical care settings, the recourse to PR can be sudden, so the discussion about the potential needs of PR should be anticipated at the moment of admission. Additionally, in case of emergent PR application, patients and surrogates should be widely informed to restore a climate of trust [78].

Nurses use several strategies to cope with the negative feelings associated to the use of PR: paying attention to expected benefit for patients rather than the restriction of patients' liberty; the nurses' perceptions of PR vary with the degree of limitations induced by the devices; searching the approval of other colleagues for the use of PR limits the feelings of individual responsibility [54].

## 14.4.5  Best Management of Physical Restraints, Alternative Interventions, and Prevention

The first approach to prevent the use of PR is to perform a comprehensive patient assessment, through five steps [83]:

1. Identification of behaviors at risk of restraints: treatment interference, agitation, risk of falls, and confusion/altered mental state

2. Identification of factors affecting patients' behaviors and intervention to improve their conditions or encounter their needs
3. Recording of patients' health history and eventual coping behaviors
4. Medication history to identify drugs affecting the risk of delirium, agitation, and falls

5. Patient's cognitive status and environment and social factors

Gaps in PR application training and documentation and lack of reassessment of patients' anatomical sites for restraints are reported in the literature [51]. Moreover, nurses express the need of some support in the decision-making process for PR [51].

A recent systematic review showed that nurses, if in doubt, often choose to apply restraints [54].

Critical care nurses perceive PR patients as significantly requiring more workload than restrained ones (4.2 vs 3.3 on a visual analog workload scale ranging from 0 to 10, $p < 0.0001$) [70].

Beyond an improvement of nurse-to-patient ratio, a real alternative to PR could be the direct observation and physical presence of a clinical nurse at high-risk patient's bedside [84].

Since restraint use should not compensate for lack of staffing or environmental resources [81], the presence of significant others at patient's bedside can be a valid choice in agitated ICU patients [78].

Open visiting policies can ease this kind of humanizer intervention. Family members should be accurately informed and involved in the decision to implement PR [79] but avoiding to delegate the patient surveillance responsibilities. Moreover, they can provide important information about intubated patient's behaviors and gestures, to ease the nursing care planning and avoid excessive restraint measures [79].

A recent study performed in a trauma ICU showed that educational programs about the implementation of non-pharmacological alternative strategies to the use of PR (Table 14.7) can significantly reduce their rate of utilization in

**Table 14.7**  Non-pharmacological alternative strategies to the use of PR [85–87]

| Alternative interventions |
| --- |

*Non-pharmacological interventions*
- Visual and hearing supports
- Repeated communication and frequent reorientation
- Personal and familiar stuffs from patient's home in the room
- Adequate nurse staffing
- Availability of television during the daytime and daily news
- Instrumental music
- Tubing and equipment out of patients' view
- Reassuring presence of relatives or significant others at patient's bedside
- Call an interpreter for foreigner patients, as necessary
- Adequate assessment and management of discomfort and pain (non-pharmacological sedation)
- Comfortable position and thermal status
- Eyeglasses and hearing aids, if the patient is awake
- Giving information before doing interventions to the patient
- Sleep quality assessment
- Adequate electrolyte status
- Preventing drug withdrawal syndromes
- Early removing invasive devices, as soon as they are no more useful for patient treatment and care
- Let the patient touch and feel the bed and the objects around him/herself, indicating him/her the position of lines and tubes
- Management of hypoxemia, ventilator setting adjustment
- Early oral feedings, as soon as possible
- Early physical exercise and mobilization
- Suspension of treatment inducing discomfort, as soon as possible

*Environmental approaches*
- Calm and reassuring environment
- Sleep quiet time
- Lights on during daytime and no lights during the nighttime
- Avoid excess of noise
- Reduced utilization of bedside rails if patients are trying to climb them
- Increasing the frequency of supervision
- One-to-one supervision
- Early and often walking patients

(continued)

**Table 14.7** (continued)

| Alternative interventions |
| --- |

*Alternative devices*
- Handheld tools to be twisted and shape-changed by patients; these tools can be moved and squeezed with varying degrees of resistance
- Lap devices (activity lap blankets, favorite photo frame, buckles, belts, zippered coin purse, key ring, and textured fabric)
- Soft baby dolls, stuffed animals with and without a built-in sound device

ICU patients (restraints per 1000 patient days were 314.1, SD $\pm$ 35.4, in pre-intervention, while in post-intervention they were 237.8, SD $\pm$ 56.4, $p = 0.008$), except for adult aged from 20 to 40, admitted with head injuries and/or multiple vehicle accidents [85].

Large efforts in research focusing toward the effectiveness of alternatives to PR are needed.

Some authors suggested a three-tier strategy to assess the need of restraints in ICU patients [88]:

- Level 1: Devices are present, but patient is alert and oriented, or unconscious, or paralyzed. No need of restraints.
- Level 2: Patient with nonlife treatment/devices—Do not apply restraints if patient is alert/oriented. Try another alternative to restraints in case of agitation or confusion or aggressive behaviors. Apply traditional PR if alternative methods fail.
- Level 3: Patient with life-support treatment/devices—Do not apply restraints if alertness/orientation, or unconsciousness, or paralysis is present. Apply restraints if the above conditions are not present.

PR should be implemented only after adequate patient assessment, correction of contributing factors, activation of other professional consultants, and pain and discomfort reduction [83]. Furthermore, restraints should be considered only after the failure of alternative interventions [81]. Lastly the presence of individual contraindications to PR implementation should be excluded [83].

Guidelines about the use of restraints in critical care settings drafted by the American College of Critical Care Medicine give some useful guide to manage PR [87].

Bedside monitoring of agitated patient should accurately check the following every 15 min [87]:

- Skin color, capillary refill time, and the presence of pulse in the restrained extremities
- Movement ability and sensation of the restrained extremities
- Adequate body alignment and repositioning
- Adequate documentation

Moreover, every 2 h, in agitated patients, these interventions should be provided [87]:

- Assessment of the need for drugs to manage pain, anxiety, agitation, and delirium
- Assessment of elimination needs
- Food and fluids in patients capable of oral nutrition or artificial administration of fluids and nutrients in those not able to take food orally
- Release of restrained extremities and assessment of range of motion

In every condition of PR, it is mandatory to make a record on the patient's chart and physician order and perform patient reassessment of PR reduction or suspension at least every 8 h [87].

Lastly, some authors hope for the establishment of meaningful collaborations between clinical nurses and restraint device manufacturers to design safer tools for patients [78].

Take-Home Messages
- A bidirectional vicious circle involves patient's agitation, physical restraints, device pressure ulcers, and falls from ICU beds.

- DRPU is a specific subset of the larger problem represented by hospital-acquired PUs, accounting for about 10% of the total PUs. A large amount of DRPUs is discovered by health-care staff when the ulcers are at the third or fourth stage or even unstageable.
- Falls are a principal cause of death in patients aged ≥65 years. Ten percent of deadly falls for the older patients happen in hospitals. The patient fall risk assessment in the ICU should carefully consider these elements: if the patient is sedated or treated with hypnotics; if there is presence of confusion, delirium, or dementia; and if the patients have previously fallen.
- There's lack of statistical association between nurse staffing and patient falls.
- Forty-four percent of ICU patients were restrained at the time of unplanned device removal.
- PR is an important issue for all the nurses working in clinical settings, with important medicolegal implications and ethical dilemmas. PR can induce adverse events such as agitation, increased risk of falls from bed, unplanned extubations, skin necrosis, altered circulation, injuries to nerves, fractures, and death.

# References

1. Rhodes A, Moreno RP, Azoulay E, Capuzzo M, Chiche JD, Eddleston J, et al. Prospectively defined indicators to improve the safety and quality of care for critically ill patients: a report from the Task Force on Safety and Quality of the European Society of Intensive Care Medicine (ESICM). Intensive Care Med. 2012;38:598–605. https://doi.org/10.1007/s00134-011-2462-3.
2. Critical Care Services Ontario. Critical care unit balanced scorecard toolkit. Critical Care Secretariat. 2012. https://www.criticalcareontario.ca/EN/Toolbox/Toolkits/Critical%20Care%20Unit%20Balanced%20Scorecard%20Toolkit%20%282012%29.pdf. Accessed 04 Mar 2016.

3. de Vos M, Graafmans W, Keesman E, Westert G, van der Voort PH. Quality measurement at intensive care units: which indicators should we use? J Crit Care. 2007;22:267–74.

4. Tsang C, Palmer W, Aylin P.. Patient safety indicators: a systematic review of the literature. Centre for Patient Safety and Service Quality. London: Imperial College London. 2008. https://www1.imperial.ac.uk/resources/147E3ECA-1FD2-4AF8-BA34-08AAF1FBCAB1/psireportv3.pdf. Accessed 03 Mar 2016.

5. Stalpers D, de Brouwer BJ, Kaljouw MJ, Schuurmans MJ. Associations between characteristics of the nurse work environment and five nurse-sensitive patient outcomes in hospitals: a systematic review of literature. Int J Nurs Stud. 2015;52:817–35. https://doi.org/10.1016/j.ijnurstu.2015.01.005.

6. Savitz LA, Jones CB, Bernard S. Quality indicators sensitive to nurse staffing in acute care settings. In: Henriksen K, Battles JB, Marks ES, et al., editors. Advances in patient safety: from research to implementation (volume 4: programs, tools, and products). Rockville: Agency for Healthcare Research and Quality (US); 2005. p. 375–85.

7. Cooper KL. Evidence-based prevention of pressure ulcers in the intensive care unit. Crit Care Nurse. 2013;33:57–66. https://doi.org/10.4037/ccn2013985.

8. Coyer FM, Stotts NA, Blackman VS. A prospective window into medical device-related pressure ulcers in intensive care. Int Wound J. 2014;11:656–64. https://doi.org/10.1111/iwj.12026.

9. ECRI Institute. Medical devices' role in causing pressure ulcers. Published 8/1/2014. https://www.ecri.org/components/PSOCore/Pages/PSONav0814.aspx?tab=2. Accessed 01 Mar 2016.

10. Apold J, Rydrych D. Preventing device-related pressure ulcers: using data to guide statewide change. J Nurs Care Qual. 2012;27:28–34. https://doi.org/10.1097/NCQ.0b013e31822b1fd9.

11. Ackland HM, Cooper DJ, Malham GM, Kossmann T. Factors predicting cervical collar-related decubitus ulceration in major trauma patients. Spine (Phila Pa 1976). 2007;32:423–8.

12. Black J, Alves P, Brindle CT, Dealey C, Santamaria N, Call E, Clark M. Use of wound dressings to enhance prevention of pressure ulcers caused by medical devices. Int Wound J. 2015;12:322–7. https://doi.org/10.1111/iwj.12111.

13. Sammon MA, Montague M, Frame F, Guzman D, Bena JF, Palascak A, et al. Randomized controlled study of the effects of 2 fecal management systems on incidence of anal erosion. J Wound Ostomy Continence Nurs. 2015;42:279–86. https://doi.org/10.1097/WON.0000000000000128.

14. Mulhall AM, Jindal SK. Massive gastrointestinal hemorrhage as a complication of the Flexi-Seal fecal management system. Am J Crit Care. 2013;22:537–43. https://doi.org/10.4037/ajcc2013499.

15. Carron M, Freo U, BaHammam AS, Dellweg D, Guarracino F, Cosentini R, et al. Complications of non-invasive ventilation techniques: a comprehensive qualitative review of randomized trials. Br J Anaesth. 2013;110:896–914. https://doi.org/10.1093/bja/aet070.

16. Lucchini A, Valsecchi D, Elli S, Doni V, Corsaro P, Tundo P, et al. The comfort of patients ventilated with the Helmet Bundle. Assist Inferm Ric. 2010;29:174–83.

17. Wounds UK. Device related pressure ulcers made easy. 2012; 8. http://www.wounds-uk.com/made-easy/device-related-pressure-ulcers-made-easy. Accessed 29 Feb 2016.

18. Black JM, Cuddigan JE, Walko MA, Didier LA, Lander MJ, Kelpe MR. Medical device related pressure ulcers in hospitalized patients. Int Wound J. 2010;7:358–65. https://doi.org/10.1111/j.1742-481X.2010.00699.x.

19. Ham WH, Schoonhoven L, Schuurmans MJ, Leenen LP. Pressure ulcers in trauma patients with suspected spine injury: a prospective cohort study with emphasis on device-related pressure ulcers. Int Wound J. 2016;14:104–11. https://doi.org/10.1111/iwj.12568.

20. Dyer A. Ten top tips: preventing device-related pressure ulcers. Wounds. Int J. 2015;6:9–13.

21. Makic MBF. Medical device-related pressure ulcers and intensive care patients. J Perianesth Nurs. 2015;30:336–7. https://doi.org/10.1016/j.jopan.2015.05.004.

22. Cappell MS, Inglis B, Levy A. Two case reports of gastric ulcer from pressure necrosis related to a rigid and taut percutaneous endoscopic gastrostomy bumper. Gastroenterol Nurs. 2009;32:259–63. https://doi.org/10.1097/SGA.0b013e3181b0a1af.

23. Yamaguti WP, Moderno EV, Yamashita SY, Gomes TG, Maida AL, Kondo CS, et al. Treatment-related risk factors for development of skin breakdown in subjects with acute respiratory failure undergoing noninvasive ventilation or CPAP. Respir Care. 2014;59:1530–6. https://doi.org/10.4187/respcare.02942.

24. Bambi S, Peris A, Esquinas AM. Pressure ulcers caused by masks during noninvasive ventilation. Am J Crit Care. 2016;25:6. https://doi.org/10.4037/ajcc2016906.

25. Dellweg D, Hochrainer D, Klauke M, Kerl J, Eiger G, Kohler D. Determinants of skin contact pressure formation during non-invasive ventilation. J Biomech. 2010;43:652–7. https://doi.org/10.1016/j.jbiomech.2009.10.029.

26. Weng MH. The effect of protective treatment in reducing pressure ulcers for non-invasive ventilation patients. Intensive Crit Care Nurs. 2008;24:295–9. https://doi.org/10.1016/j.iccn.2007.11.005.

27. Ham HW, Schoonhoven LL, Galer AA, Shortridge-Baggett LL. Cervical collar-related pressure ulcers in trauma patients in intensive care unit. J Trauma Nurs. 2014;21:94–102. https://doi.org/10.1097/JTN.0000000000000046.

28. Ham W, Schoonhoven L, Schuurmans MJ, Leenen LP. Pressure ulcers from spinal immobilization in trauma patients: a systematic review. J Trauma Acute Care Surg. 2014;76:1131–41. https://doi.org/10.1097/TA.0000000000000153.

29. National Pressure Ulcer Advisory Panel (NPUAP). Best practices for prevention of medical device-related pressure ulcers in critical care. 2013. http://www.npuap.org/wp-content/uploads/2013/04/BestPractices-CriticalCare1.pdf. Accessed 04 Mar 2016.

30. Coleman S, Smith IL, Nixon J, Wilson L, Brown S. Pressure ulcer and wounds reporting in NHS hospitals in England part 2: survey of monitoring systems. J Tissue Viability. 2016;25:16–25. https://doi.org/10.1016/j.jtv.2015.11.002.

31. Glasgow D, Millen IS, Nzewi OC, Varadarajaran B. Device-related atypical pressure ulcer after cardiac surgery. J Wound Care. 2014;23:383-4–6-7. 10.12968/jowc.2014.23.8.383.

32. Degelau J, Belz M, Bungum L, Flavin PL, Harper C, Leys K, et al. Institute for clinical systems improvement. Prevention of falls (acute care). Updated April 2012. https://www.icsi.org/_asset/dcn15z/Falls.pdf. Accessed 01 Mar 2016.

33. Cangany M, Back D, Hamilton-Kelly T, Altman M, Lacey S. Bedside nurses leading the way for falls prevention: an evidence-based approach. Crit Care Nurse. 2015;35:82–4. https://doi.org/10.4037/ccn2015414.

34. Pearson KB, Coburn AF. Evidence-based falls prevention in critical access hospitals. Policy Brief #24. 2011. http://www.flexmonitoring.org/wp-content/uploads/2013/07/PolicyBrief24_Falls-Prevention.pdf. Accessed 01 Mar 2006.

35. Rush KL, Robey-Williams C, Patton LM, Chamberlain D, Bendyk H, Sparks T. Patient falls: acute care nurses' experiences. J Clin Nurs. 2009;18:357–65. https://doi.org/10.1111/j.1365-2702.2007.02260.x.

36. Falen T, Alexander J, Curtis D, UnRuh L. Developing a hospital-specific electronic inpatient fall surveillance program: phase 1. Health Care Manag (Frederick). 2013;32:359–69. https://doi.org/10.1097/HCM.0b013e3182a9d6ec.

37. Lake ET, Shang J, Klaus S, Dunton NE. Patient falls: association with hospital magnet status and nursing unit staffing. Res Nurs Health. 2010;33:413–25. https://doi.org/10.1002/nur.20399.
38. Yilmaz Z, Goris S. Determination of the patient safety culture among nurses working at intensive care units. Pak J Med Sci. 2015;31:597–601. 10.12669/pjms.313.7059.
39. Warshawsky N, Rayens MK, Stefaniak K, Rahman R. The effect of nurse manager turnover on patient fall and pressure ulcer rates. J Nurs Manag. 2013;21:725–32. https://doi.org/10.1111/jonm.12101.
40. Richardson A, Carter R. Falls in critical care: a local review to identify incidence and risk. Nurs Crit Care. 2015. https://doi.org/10.1111/nicc.12151.
41. Taylor S, Sayre C, Nasenbeny K, Sisco K. A step toward decreasing falls and preventing injuries in critical care. Crit Care Nurse. 2008;28:e47.
42. Rochefort CM, Buckeridge DL, Abrahamowicz M. Improving patient safety by optimizing the use of nursing human resources. Implement Sci. 2015;10:89. https://doi.org/10.1186/s13012-015-0278-1.
43. Callis N. Falls prevention: identification of predictive fall risk factors. Appl Nurs Res. 2016;29:53–8. https://doi.org/10.1016/j.apnr.2015.05.007.
44. Flanders SA, Harrington L, Fowler RJ. Falls and patient mobility in critical care: keeping patients and staff safe. AACN Adv Crit Care. 2009;20:267–76. https://doi.org/10.1097/NCI.0b013e3181ac2628.
45. Mullin SG, Chrostowski W, Waszynski C. Promoting safety in the cardiac intensive care unit: the role of the geriatric resource nurse in early identification of patient risk for falls and delirium. Dimens Crit Care Nurs. 2011;30:150–9. https://doi.org/10.1097/DCC.0b013e31820d2230.
46. McCarter-Bayer A, Bayer F, Hall K. Preventing falls in acute care: an innovative approach. J Gerontol Nurs. 2005;31:25–33.
47. Pettit NR, Wood T, Lieber M, O'Mara MS. Intensive care unit design and mortality in trauma patients. J Surg Res. 2014;190:640–6. https://doi.org/10.1016/j.jss.2014.04.007.
48. Kozub E, Ravelo A, Gamboa M, Worthy K. Reducing patient falls in a surgical intensive care unit. Crit Care Nurse. 2015;35:e41–2.
49. Nydahl P, Ewers A, Brodda D. Complications related to early mobilization of mechanically ventilated patients on Intensive Care Units. Nurs Crit Care. 2014. https://doi.org/10.1111/nicc.12134.
50. Bonuel N, Manjos A, Lockett L, Gray-Becknell T. Best practice fall prevention strategies. CATCH! Crit Care Nurs Q. 2011;34:154–8. https://doi.org/10.1097/CNQ.0b013e3182129d3a.
51. Freeman S, Hallett C, McHugh G. Physical restraint: experiences, attitudes and opinions of adult intensive care unit nurses. Nurs Crit Care. 2016;21:78–87. https://doi.org/10.1111/nicc.12197.

52. Li X, Fawcett TN. Clinical decision making on the use of physical restraint in intensive care units. Int J Nurs Sci. 2014;1:446–50.
53. Mion LC, Minnick AF, Leipzig R, Catrambone CD, Johnson ME. Patient-initiated device removal in intensive care units: a national prevalence study. Crit Care Med. 2007;35:2714–20.
54. Möhler R, Meyer G. Attitudes of nurses towards the use of physical restraints in geriatric care: a systematic review of qualitative and quantitative studies. Int J Nurs Stud. 2014;51:274–88. https://doi.org/10.1016/j.ijnurstu.2013.10.004.
55. Nirmalan M, Dark PM, Nightingale P, Harris J. Editorial IV: physical and pharmacological restraint of critically ill patients: clinical facts and ethical considerations. Br J Anaesth. 2004;92:789–92.
56. Benbenishty J, DeKeyser Ganz F, Adam S. Differences in European critical care nursing practice: a pilot study. Intensive Crit Care Nurs. 2005;21:172–8.
57. Benbenbishty J, Adam S, Endacott R. Physical restraint use in intensive care units across Europe: the PRICE study. Intensive Crit Care Nurs. 2010;26:241. https://doi.org/10.1016/j.iccn.2010.08.003.
58. Martin B, Mathisen L. Use of physical restraints in adult critical care: a bicultural study. Am J Crit Care. 2005;14:133–42.
59. Minnick AF, Mion LC, Johnson ME, Catrambone C, Leipzig R. Prevalence and variation of physical restraint use in acute care settings in the US. J Nurs Scholarsh. 2007;39:30–7.
60. Fogel JF, Berkman CS, Merkel C, Cranston T, Leipzig RM. Efficient and accurate measurement of physical restraint use in acute care. Care Manag J. 2009;10:100–9.
61. Langley G, Schmollgruber S, Egan A. Restraints in intensive care units--a mixed method study. Intensive Crit Care Nurs. 2011;27:67–75. https://doi.org/10.1016/j.iccn.2010.12.001.
62. De Jonghe B, Constantin JM, Chanques G, Capdevila X, Lefrant JY, Outin H, et al. Physical restraint in mechanically ventilated ICU patients: a survey of French practice. Intensive Care Med. 2013;39:31–7. https://doi.org/10.1007/s00134-012-2715-9.
63. Kandeel NA, Attia AK. Physical restraints practice in adult intensive care units in Egypt. Nurs Health Sci. 2013;15:79–85. https://doi.org/10.1111/nhs.12000.
64. Krüger C, Mayer H, Haastert B, Meyer G. Use of physical restraints in acute hospitals in Germany: a multi-centre cross-sectional study. Int J Nurs Stud. 2013;50:1599–606. https://doi.org/10.1016/j.ijnurstu.2013.05.005.
65. Pagliuco Barbosa T, Artuzi Arantes de Oliveira G, Neves de Araujo Lopes M, Aparecida Poletti NA, Marinilza Beccaria LM. Care practices for patient safety in an intensive care unit. Acta Paul Enferm. 2014;27:243–8.

66. van der Kooi AW, Peelen LM, Raijmakers RJ, Vroegop RL, Bakker DF, Tekatli H, et al. Use of physical restraints in Dutch intensive care units: a prospective multicenter study. Am J Crit Care. 2015;24:488–95. https://doi.org/10.4037/ajcc2015348.

67. Stinson KJ. Nurses' attitudes, clinical experience, and practice issues with use of physical restraints in critical care units. Am J Crit Care. 2016;25:21–6. https://doi.org/10.4037/ajcc2016428.

68. Choi E, Song M. Physical restraint use in a Korean ICU. J Clin Nurs. 2003;12:651–9.

69. Micek ST, Anand NJ, Laible BR, Shannon WD, Kollef MH. Delirium as detected by the CAM-ICU predicts restraint use among mechanically ventilated medical patients. Crit Care Med. 2005;33:1260–5.

70. Rose L, Burry L, Mallick R, Luk E, Cook D, Fergusson D, et al. Prevalence, risk factors, and outcomes associated with physical restraint use in mechanically ventilated adults. J Crit Care. 2016;31:31–5. https://doi.org/10.1016/j.jcrc.2015.09.011.

71. Burk RS, Grap MJ, Munro CL, Schubert CM, Sessler CN. Predictors of agitation in critically ill adults. Am J Crit Care. 2014;23:414–23. https://doi.org/10.4037/ajcc2014714.

72. Chang LY, Wang KW, Chao YF. Influence of physical restraint on unplanned extubation of adult intensive care patients: a case-control study. Am J Crit Care. 2008;17:408–15.

73. Perren A, Corbella D, Iapichino E, Di Bernardo V, Leonardi A, Di Nicolantonio R, et al. Physical restraint in the ICU: does it prevent device removal? Minerva Anestesiol. 2015;81:1086–95.

74. Hofsø K, Coyer FM. Part 2. Chemical and physical restraints in the management of mechanically ventilated patients in the ICU: a patient perspective. Intensive Crit Care Nurs. 2007;23:316–22.

75. Laursen SB, Jensen TN, Bolwig T, Olsen NV. Deep venous thrombosis and pulmonary embolism following physical restraint. Acta Psychiatr Scand. 2005;111:324–7.

76. Jones C, Bäckman C, Capuzzo M, Flaatten H, Rylander C, Griffiths RD. Precipitants of post-traumatic stress disorder following intensive care: a hypothesis generating study of diversity in care. Intensive Care Med. 2007;33:978–85.

77. Antonelli MT. Restraint management: moving from outcome to process. J Nurs Care Qual. 2008;23:227–32. https://doi.org/10.1097/01.NCQ.0000324587.53719.2f.

78. Reigle J. The ethics of physical restraints in critical care. AACN Clin Issues. 1996;7:585–91.

79. Martin B. Restraint use in acute and critical care settings: changing practice. AACN Clin Issues. 2002;13:294–306.

80. Yönt GH, Korhan EA, Dizer B, Gümüş F, Koyuncu R. Examination of ethical dilemmas experienced by adult intensive care unit nurses in physical restraint practices. Holist Nurs Pract. 2014;28:85–90. https://doi.org/10.1097/HNP.0000000000000013.
81. Bray K, Hill K, Robson W, Leaver G, Walker N, O'Leary M, et al. British Association of Critical Care Nurses position statement on the use of restraint in adult critical care units. Nurs Crit Care. 2004;9:199–212.
82. Kapp MB. Physical restraint use in critical care: legal issues. AACN Clin Issues. 1996;7:579–84.
83. Park M, Tang JH. Changing the practice of physical restraint use in acute care. J Gerontol Nurs. 2007;33:9–16.
84. Happ MB. Further considerations regarding the effects of physical restraint in the intensive care unit. Crit Care Med. 2004;32:1977.
85. Johnson K, Curry V, Steubing A, Diana S, McCray A, McFarren A, et al. A non-pharmacologic approach to decrease restraint use. Intensive Crit Care Nurs. 2016;34:12–9. https://doi.org/10.1016/j.iccn.2015.08.004.
86. Hurlock-Chorostecki C, Kielb C. Knot-So-Fast: a learning plan to minimize patient restraint in critical care. Dynamics. 2006;17:12–8.
87. Maccioli GA, Dorman T, Brown BR, Mazuski JE, McLean BA, Kuszaj JM, et al. Clinical practice guidelines for the maintenance of patient physical safety in the intensive care unit: use of restraining therapies-American College of Critical Care Medicine Task Force 2001-2002. Crit Care Med. 2003;31:2665–76.
88. Vance DL. Effect of a treatment interference protocol on clinical decision making for restraint use in the intensive care unit: a pilot study. AACN Clin Issues. 2003;14:82–91.

# Chapter 15
# Enteral Nutrition and Bowel Management

Irene Comisso and Stefano Bambi

## 15.1 Introduction

Artificial nutrition is commonly used in ICU patients, since several factors, such as altered state of consciousness or inability to self/nourishment, impede normal nutrients assumption. In ICU patients, nutritional support can help keep the immunitary system more efficient and balance anabolism and catabolism [1]. Although the association between malnutrition and ICU mortality is not clearly demonstrated, a recently published systematic review [2] confirmed the association between malnutrition (diagnosed through validated tools) and ICU-LOS.

Artificial nutrition can be administered both parenterally and enterally. The first requires adequate venous accesses (particularly, total parenteral nutrition can only be administered via a CVC), while enteral nutrition is administered using a feeding (gastric or intestinal) tube.

Enteral nutrition (EN) is normally preferred, since it is more physiological and apparently less prone to infectious complications [3] and protective toward liver and gut function, even in patients treated with vasopressor medications [1]. Despite these

© Springer International Publishing AG, part of Springer Nature 2018      375
I. Comisso et al., *Nursing in Critical Care Setting*,
https://doi.org/10.1007/978-3-319-50559-6_15

considerations, it is important to underline that EN is associated to complications in 80% of patients receiving it.

## 15.2 Nutritional Assessment

Several observations have been traditionally used to determine nutritional status. Patient's assessment includes recording of daily nutrient intake, actual weight, recent weight changes, and body measurements. These include body mass index (BMI), triceps skin fold (TSF) thickness, mid-upper arm circumference (MUAC), and mid-arm muscle circumference (MAMC). Table 15.1 summarizes parameters' characteristics.

A retrospective study involving 1373 patients found a significant correlation between MUAC and BMI (Pearson correlation coefficient 0.78; 95% CI: 0.76–0.80), stating that MUAC can be easily used as a surrogate indicator for malnutrition (cutoff value ≤22.5 cm) and as a predictor of BMI [7]. In another prospective study [10] on 1363 ICU patients' BMI used as continuous variable, MUAC, MAMC, and the SGA "muscle wasting" and "subcutaneous fat loss" categories showed predictive ability and clinical utility toward hospital mortality. Conversely, BMI and TSF did not perform adequately [10], thus suggesting that their absolute value might not always indicate a malnutrition condition, often depending on individual's physical constitution.

Recently published guidelines [11] suggest to perform nutritional assessment in ICU patients whose voluntary intake might be insufficient. In these guidelines, proposed nutrition assessment tools include the Nutritional Risk Screening (NRS) 2002 or the *Nut*rition *Ri*sk in *C*ritically Ill (NUTRIC) score.

NRS 2002 [12] score was created analyzing retrospectively the indications used for nutritional support and related outcomes in 128 studies. The score grades two variables (severe undernutrition and severe disease) from 0 to 3 points, with a correction factor

**Table 15.1** Main body measurement characteristics

| | BMI [4] | TSF thickness [5] | MUAC | MAMC |
|---|---|---|---|---|
| Formula/measurement | Weight (kg/height (m)$^2$ | Measurement (using a caliper) of a skin fold at the midpoint between olecranon process of the ulna and acromion process of the scapula | Measurement (using a nonelastic tape) of nondominant arm, at midpoint between acromion and olecranon, in sitting or standing position [7] | MAMC = MUAC−($\pi$*TSF) [8] |
| Normal values | 18.5–24.99 kg/m$^2$; values lower than 16 kg/m$^2$ describe a severe anorexia condition; values higher than 30 kg/m$^2$ describe obese conditions | Male: 11–12.5 mm Female: 15–16.5 mm [5] | Male: 26–29 cm Female: 26–28.5 cm [5] | Male: 23–25 cm Female: 20–23 cm [5] |
| Limitations for use | Does not consider differences related to sex, age, and body proportions | Considerably influenced by vertical or horizontal displacement of the site of measurement and from the limb position (medial or lateral) chosen for the measurement [6] | Cutoff used for malnutrition may significantly vary between adult and elder patients No definitive consensus exists about the cutoff value for malnutrition [7] | No international values are available [9] |

(1 point) for patients aged ≥70. A total score ≥3 suggests to begin nutritional support. It is important to underline that some information used to determine patient's actual nutritional status (such as recent weight loss or habitual food intake) might be difficult to obtain in ICU patients. Moreover, BMI calculation could be imprecise when real weight and height are not available.

NUTRIC score was firstly validated in 2011 [13] on 597 ICU patients. The score aims to define patients that might benefit from nutrition therapy. NUTRIC score considers six variables: age, baseline APACHE II score, baseline SOFA score, number of comorbidities, days from hospital to ICU admission, and interleukin 6 (IL-6). Other variables (procalcitonin, C-reactive protein, % of oral intake in the previous week, weight loss, and BMI) were studied but not included in the final model because they do not significantly increase the discriminative ability of the score. Mortality and days on mechanical ventilation were significantly associated with increased NUTRIC score. A further modified score, omitting IL-6, was validated [14], confirming score's attitude in identifying ICU patients that might benefit from nutritional support optimization.

NUTRIC score has been used within a quality improvement project [15], together with the institution routine screening method and the subjective global assessment (SGA) to determine nutrition risk in ICU patients. Findings from this study confirm that patients with highest NUTRIC scores had the longest hospital and ICU-LOS, probably related to a more severe clinical condition.

A comprehensive nutritional assessment should also include patient's energy requirement. Indirect calorimetry (IC) is considered the gold standard for energy requirements measurement. Nonetheless, IC equipment is costly and not available in all hospitals. IC measures the respiratory quotient (i.e., the ratio between carbon dioxide excretion and oxygen consumption, both in mL/min). Normally, the respiratory quotient ranges between 0.7 and 1.

Oxygen consumption and carbon dioxide excretion are also used to determine the [16],

$$\text{Resting energy expenditure} \left(\text{REE}\right) \left(\text{kcal / d}\right)$$
$$= 1.44 \left(3.9\text{VO}_2 + 1.1\text{VCO}_2\right)$$

Several equations have been used to predict energy requirements in hospitalized patients [17], with different, but not adequate, accuracy levels. Current guidelines [11] suggest to target energy requirements on 25–30 kcal/kg/d.

Bowel sounds are daily assessed to determine GI dysfunction. Nonetheless, bowel sounds accuracy might significantly differ between doctors and nurses and mislead the correct interpretation of GI function [18]. A recent observational study found low accuracy for bowel sounds assessment in patients with bowel obstruction. Also, judgment's agreement between involved doctors was found to be low [19]. Absent or reduced bowel sounds alone should not impede EN start. Nonetheless, absent or reduced bowel sounds might indicate an underlying dysfunction, and therefore a more complex GI evaluation (including abdominal distention, vomiting, pain) should be performed.

## 15.3   EN Administration

Recently released guidelines recommend EN initiation within 24–48 h from ICU admission [11]. ICU patients usually receive continuous EN at slow rates during the 24 h, and flows are gradually increased during the days after EN starts until the desired hourly volume is reached. This approach is susceptible for many interruptions, related, for example, to medical or nursing procedures or drug administration through the feeding tube. Recent approaches [20] suggest to target EN delivery on desired daily volume, with hourly rates managed by nurses according to duration of planned and unplanned interruptions. Furthermore, literature findings show that EN can be started at target rates without complications. When high gastric volumes are not tolerated, a trophic feed, aiming to keep the GI tract functioning, can be adopted. In a recent meta-analysis, initial enteral full feeding compared to initial enteral intentional underfeeding does not seem to improve major outcomes such as mortality, hospital LOS and ICU-LOS, duration of mechanical ventilation, and incidence of infectious complications [21].

EN formulas contain both macro- (carbohydrates, proteins, lipids) and micronutrients and have different compositions according to calories, proteins, and micronutrients provided [22].

Main feeding tube characteristics refer to diameter, insertion site, and tip position and are listed in Table 15.2 [23–25].

Choice of feeding tubes should be oriented on patient's conditions and device's tolerance. Currently, no clear benefit can be addressed to post-pyloric feeding tubes. A recent systematic review and meta-analysis revealed lower incidence of pneumonia (moderate quality of evidence) and higher percentage of administered nutrients (low quality of evidence) when post-pyloric feeding was compared to gastric one; nevertheless, major outcomes such as ICU mortality or LOS do not seem to be affected by feeding site, so as complications affecting the GI tract and those related to tube insertion and management [26]. Confirmation of tube's position is a crucial point. Currently, chest radiograph is considered the gold standard to determine tip-tube position, especially in patients with altered consciousness and impaired reflexes [27]. Incorrect insertion of a NG feeding tube through the airways can lead to severe complications such as pneumothorax [28]. Other methods are suitable for this purpose, with stomach auscultation and determination of aspirated pH being most widely used [29]. Also, patient observation during and after

**Table 15.2**  Characteristics of feeding tubes

| Bore | Insertion | Tip position |
| --- | --- | --- |
| Large (≥14 Fr): preferred when gastric emptying is required; esophageal ulceration may occur | Nasal: common route for insertion; allows better oral care (intubated) and patient's conversation (non-intubated) Saliva reduction, mouth dryness, and thirst may occur | Stomach: common route for feeding in ICU; allows administration of hypertonic solutions |
| Small (5–12 Fr): more comfortable for the patient; more at risk for incrustation and obstruction; preferred in patients ad greater risk for aspiration | Oral: commonly used in premature neonates or small infants Transcutaneous: preferred when long-term artificial feeding is required | Jejunal/duodenal: preferred when higher risk for aspiration is present |

tube's positioning may provide information about incorrect positioning in the airways.

A cross-sectional study revealed poor correlation between chest radiograph NG tip-tube position confirmation and auscultatory method performed by a nurse (Prevalence and Bias Adjusted Kappa (PABAK) 0.188, $p = 0.111$) [30]. In this study, duodenal positioning was frequent (27.4%), and potentially harmful positioning (distal esophageal portion and lung) was not entirely negligible (1.3 and 1.3%, respectively). Furthermore, a low agreement between position assessment performed by doctors and nurses (Kappa = 0.215; $p = 0.118$), doctor and nursing researcher (Kappa = 0.142; $p = 0.114$), and nurses and nursing researcher (Kappa = 0.052; $p = 0.107$) confirmed poor interrater reliability of this method [30].

Measurement of gastric pH in 44 ICU patients revealed a mean value (± SD) of 4.2, with 59.1% of patients with values between 0 and 4 [31], although a statistically significant difference ($p < 0.05$) in gastric pH was observed whether patients were treated with antacid drugs (4.6 ± 1.7) or not (3.5 ± 1.8) [32]; pH ≤5.5 had a positive predictive value for correct gastric positioning of 98.9%, although two false-positive tests with esophageal positioning were identified. Although helpful, gastric pH measurement has limitations related to inability to obtain gastric aspirate, influence of feeding, drugs, and small bowel or esophageal positioning that may require chest radiograph confirmation [32, 33].

## 15.3.1 Prevention of Feeds Contamination

Incorrect feeds management can result in potentially harmful contamination. Currently, contamination from enteral formulas can be considered rare, since industrial preparations are usually administered. External sources of contamination can come from professionals' hands or water. The importance of correct handwashing and gloves utilization has been explored in Chap. 9. Water administration in enterally fed patients is common, both for dilution of formulas in order to reduce nutrients' concentration and therefore minimize the intolerance risk (diarrhea), administer drugs, and flush NG tube when nutrition is interrupted. For all of these purposes, bottled water should be preferred, and sterile water should be used with immunocompromised patients. Several studies documented infections from *Legionella pneumophila* and *Pseudomonas aeruginosa* from tap water. For this reason, reusable devices (such as tablet crushers) should be accurately dried after rinsing. When administering EN, feeding bags or bottles are connected to feeding sets. A recent retrospective observational study found a statistically significant reduction in diarrhea occurrence risk (HR = 0.27, 95% CI: 0.12–0.61, $p = 0.002$) when the set hang time was reduced from 72–96 h to 24 h [34]. Feeds contamination might also occur due to retrograde microorganism migration from patient's GI tract toward NG tubes.

## 15.4  EN Complications

Up to 80% of patients receiving EN develop complications [35]. The term nutritional intolerance describes situations in which an increased gastric residual volume (GRV), together with vomiting, is detected, thus reducing the total nutrients amount administered [36]. To date, a definitive nutritional intolerance definition is not available, as underlined in a recent systematic review [37] reporting 43 different definitions of nutritional intolerance. The authors classified nutritional intolerance in three different categories, i.e., high gastric residual volume, presence of gastrointestinal (GI) symptoms, and inadequate enteral nutrition administration.

In a retrospective analysis [38], 30.5% of patients developed feeding intolerance, with a median occurring time of 3 days (range 1–12) from EN start. Feeding intolerance was associated with lower caloric and protein intake and significantly related with decreased median ventilator-free days (11.2 vs. 2.5; $p < 0.0001$), ICU-LOS (11.3 vs. 14.4; $p < 0.0001$), and days to discharge alive from hospital (20.3 vs. 23.8; $p = 0.0002$). Although nonstatistically significant, 60-day mortality was higher in patients with feeding intolerance.

### 15.4.1  High Gastric Residual Volume

Gastric residual volume (GRV) measurements are recommended to determine EN tolerance [39, 40], predict inhalation risk [41], and monitor the functional status of digestive tract. Delayed gastric emptying is common in enterally fed patients, involving up to

50% of MV patients, and comes from altered GI motility, drugs, surgery [42], altered state of consciousness, reduced coughing reflex, and indwelling ETT [43].

Ninety-seven percent of nurses measure GRV [35], to quantify and qualify [44] gastric content and identify intolerance to EN [45].

GRV measurement is normally performed by aspirating the stomach with a 50 mL syringe or connecting a collection bag to NG tube for at least 10 min [35]. Several factors, including tube diameter [46] and position [47] and fluid viscosity [45], influence the amount of detected GRV. High GRV (defined as gastric aspirates ≥200 mL) does not seem to be affected by continuous or bolus EN administration (13.3 vs. 20%, respectively, $p = 1$) [48].

Normally, GRV is classified as mild (<150 mL/6 h), moderate (251/350 mL/6 h), and severe (>350 mL/6 h). To date, the maximum tolerable GRV amount has still not been defined, so as the usefulness of this measurement. In fact, no statistically significant association was found between different GRV amounts and number of episodes of inhalation or regurgitation [41], and an increased GRV tolerance up to 500 mL did not influence diarrhea, abdominal distention, regurgitation, nor pneumonia [49].

Optimal timing to check GRV has also not been identified [50]. In many ICUs, GRV measurements are performed three times a day, after interrupting EN for 1 h [51]. Also, more frequent (every 6 h) GRV assessment is suggested during the first EN day, while a daily measurement can be adopted from the third, when no complications are detected [49]. Since higher GRVs are detected during the first EN hours [52], a more strict control is suggested within this period [29].

GRV < 250 mL should not be discarded but reintroduced. In fact, discarding gastric content seems to be associated to a higher delayed gastric emptying and hypokalemia incidence. When GRV is higher than 250 mL, the exceeding volume is discarded.

As high GRV is the main EN intolerance feature (61.6%) of observed patients, treatment with prokinetic agents can be adopted to facilitate nutrition admixtures proceeding through the GI tract [38].

## 15.4.2   Gastrointestinal Symptoms

Vomiting is defined as "an objective event that results in the forceful evacuation of gastric contents from the stomach, up and out of the mouth" [53]. In ICU patients, vomiting has been described as "any regurgitation," irrespective of the amount [54]. Several factors, including surgery, medications, CNS, and gut disorders, have been addressed as possible causes for vomiting. In ICU patients, vomiting and regurgitation represent, respectively, 12.2% and 5.5% of EN-associated complications [40]. Higher prevalence (38.2%) has been observed in a more recent observational study [54], without statistically significant difference in vomiting occurrence between survivors and non-survivors (37.3% and 40.9%, respectively; $p = 0.13$). In this study, vomiting was found to significantly reduce the mortality risk (OR 0.44, 95% CI: 0.29–0.68; $p < 0.001$). Vomiting rates do not relate with EN type of administration (continuous vs. bolus, 6.7% vs. 6.7%, $p = 1$) [48].

Vomiting is addressed as causing 6.8% of EN interruptions [52].

Abdominal distention is not clearly defined among studies exploring GI complications. It is generally assumed that abdominal distention can be diagnosed radiologically or clinically, and although less frequent when compared to vomiting (10.6%), it has been associated with a significantly higher risk of death (OR 1.64, 95% CI: 1.07–2.53; $p = 0.025$) [54].

Although not widely reported from the literature, vomiting and abdominal distention can lead to increased patient discomfort. Thus, proper assessment and treatment of these symptoms are required.

### 15.4.3   Inadequate EN Administration

Inadequate EN delivery is frequent in ICU patients. Currently, a homogeneous definition for inadequate EN administration does not exist, and findings from a literature review underlined how prescription goals for enterally fed patients vary from 70 to 110% [55].

According to a literature review, inadequate EN administration refers to:

- Patient's factors: age, sex, nutritional status, disease severity, and mechanical ventilation
- Feeding methods: feeding formula and tube location
- Feeding process: time to initiation, feeding underprescription, and EN interruption [55]

Patient-related factors do not seem to significantly affect EN delivery. Particularly, disease severity nor nutritional status influences the achievement of optimal caloric intake [56].

No clear benefit has been evidenced by nutrient-dense formulas administration. Particularly, a prospective study revealed a highest caloric intake with hypertonic formulas, but not adequate protein provision [57]. Use of hypertonic formulas should therefore balance potential risks (diarrhea) and benefits (administration of smaller volumes). Similarly, post-pyloric tubes did not demonstrate significant improvements in caloric and protein goals achievements [58].

A recent retrospective observational trial [59] examined process-related barriers to optimal EN volume administration. In this study, a high number of interruptions (49% of observed days, 198 total interruptions) were intercepted. Interruptions are also related to accidental device removal (ETT or enteral access) [59, 60] or need for device positioning [60], bedside or radiology procedures [59, 60], problems with small-bore feeding tubes [61], weaning [61], or presence of GRV [59, 61]. GRV ≥500 mL was related to the largest EN loss (77%) and the longest interruption (18.5 h) [59]. EN interruptions seem to be a predisposing factor for under-feeding (OR, 2.89; 95% CI: 1.03–8.11) and prolonged ICU-LOS (IRR, 1.53; 95% CI: 1.41–1.67) [60]. Underfeeding is significantly predicted by delays in EN start after ICU admission, total amount of prescribed calories, and total interruption time [62]. Duration of interruptions varies between 1 and –24 h [63], thus compromising the final amount of calories and proteins received by the patient. In a prospective observational study, 62% of patients received lower caloric intake than required (according to Harris-Benedict equation requirement) [62].

When EN management is supported by a shared protocol, goals achievement in terms of use of more EN alone [20], earlier initiation [20, 64], and amount of prescribed and delivered EN [20, 65] significantly increases. Despite these considerations, a recent systematic review highlighted the need for more well-designed randomized studies, in order to ascertain the effects of protocol-driven EN on major outcomes (mortality, ICU-LOS, and hospital LOS) [66].

## 15.5 Drug Administration via Feeding Tubes

Oral and feeding tubes administration are often not interchangeable, and specific considerations concerning drug crushing and mixing, proper water-volume dilution, NG tube flushing, and compatibility with EN formulas should be highlighted.

### 15.5.1 Drug Crushing and Mixing

Oral medications can be available as solid or liquid form [33]. Solid forms include both products with immediate release (few minutes after reaching the stomach) both those with modified release (extended or delayed) [33]. Oral medications form may impact on the possibility to crush them. Tablets can be provided with an enteric-resistant coat or be designed to slowly release the active medication or allow resistance to gastric pH. Crushing such medications may lead to altered drug effect, in terms of bioavailability, therapeutic effect, and toxicity, and should therefore be avoided. Moreover, coat chipping can be difficult and provoke aggregation between small particles, thus increasing the NG tube obstruction risk [33].

A recent randomized crossover study on 36 healthy volunteers demonstrated higher ticagrelor (and its metabolite) plasma concentrations when the crushed drug was administered orally or via NG tubes compared to whole tablet administration [67]. Although no relevant AEs were observed, caution should be used when transferring these results to the critically ill population.

Oral medications are crushed using dedicated crushers. Oral medication mixing occurs because of simultaneous prescription. Crushing together two or more medications might generate chemical reaction, with subsequent changes in drugs' properties, and similar considerations can be applied for liquid forms [33].

## 15.5.2 *Proper Water-Volume Dilution*

Oral suspensions and solutions osmolality can be up to 25-fold greater than the one in the GI tract [68]. When administering such drugs using a transpyloric tube, it is important to adopt adequate drug's dilution's volume to avoid intolerance [68], meaning that 150–250 mL of water could be required to achieve adequate osmolality [69]. Suspensions dilution might also be necessary to reduce their viscosity and facilitate proceeding through NG tubes [69], although adequate dilution volume can be difficult to establish. Immediate-release tablets, so as the content of immediate-release gelatine capsule, should be fine-crushed and then diluted in sterile water [69].

### 15.5.3  Compatibility with EN Formulas and Feeding-Tube Flushing

Limited informations about compatibility and stability of oral medications and EN formulas admixtures are available. Both drug's and EN formulas' characteristics may interfere with medication's stability. For this reason, admixture of oral medications and EN formulas is discouraged [70], and administration of EN formulas should be temporarily withheld when giving oral medications through NG tube [33, 70].

In a recent in vitro study, the compatibility between an EN formula and 62 suspensions and solutions has been tested [68]. Drugs with pH <4 can interact with diet proteins, leading to precipitate formation in NG tubes [70]. Acid pH is typical for oral liquid drugs (excluding antacid ones and potassium iodide), thus suggesting adequate NG tube flushing after medication's administration in order to avoid tube's occlusions [68]. Appropriate feeding tube flushing (before and after drug's administration) with at least 15 mL of sterile water is recommended to avoid interactions between drugs, drugs and EN, and drugs and feeding tubes (as for diazepam) [70]. Feeding tube's flushing may also prevent drug clotting (clonazepam, carbamazepine, phenytoin) within the tube [70]. Also, when administering drugs through a feeding tube, evaluation of tube diameter and tip positioning should be considered. Small-bore tubes are more likely to clog, although more comfortable for the patients [25]. Tip position (gastric, duodenal, or jejunal) could interfere with drug absorption, especially for those with gastric effect or absorption (lowered effect and absorption) or those with extended hepatic first-pass effect (increased absorption and effect) [25].

EN administration should be restarted not earlier than 30 minutes after drug's administration [33], but in case of drugs with well-established EN interaction (fluoroquinolones, hydralazine, warfarin, carbamazepine, hydrochlorotiazide, theophylline, gabapentin), feeds should be withheld 1 and 2 h after administration (2 h for phenytoin) [25, 70].

### 15.5.4   Considerations About Nursing Practices

Noncompliant practices in oral medications administration through feeding tubes have been highlighted. Particularly, verification of tube position prior drug administration, proper medication preparation (including crushing only when appropriate and appropriate dilution), and tube's flushing were identified as susceptible for improvement, since nurses did not perform consistently with available evidences [71]. Moreover, lack of knowledge concerning pharmaceutical form and the importance of tip-tube position has been shown [72]. Nurses often refer to their experience (80%), while hospital policy, pharmacists, or more experienced nurses consult lightly influenced (40.9, 37.6, and 33.7, respectively) nursing practices [71]. Multidisciplinary interventions including pharmacy support and provision of detailed instructions for administration proved to be effective in reducing (although not statistically significant) the incidence of tube obstructions (HR 0.22, 95% CI: 0.047–1.05) and administration errors (23% before intervention; 82% after intervention) [73].

## 15.6   Bowel Management

Bowel care is no longer perceived as priority in ICU staff, and lack of knowledge has been highlighted during focus groups oriented to examine in depth staff's attitudes toward bowel care [74]. Implementation of a bowel management protocol in three Australian ICUs led to significant increase in knowledge concerning bowel management, frequency of bowel function assessment, and proper decision (suppository or enema administration) to take following a *per rectum* exam [75]. Conversely, effects on patients in terms of duration and episodes of constipation and episodes of diarrhea did not change significantly after a bowel management protocol [76].

## 15.6.1 Diarrhea

Diarrhea has been defined as three or more loose bowel motions, or four or more bowel motions of any consistency, or more than 300 mL of stool on at least two consecutive days [77]; recently, the ESICM group on abdominal problems referred to diarrhea as three or more loose or liquid stools with a stool weight greater than 200–250 g/day (or 250 mL/day) [78]. A recently proposed definition [79] adds consideration of feces based on the Bristol Stool Chart (categories 5–7). The Bristol Stool Chart was originally developed to categorize stool according to consistency and form in seven different items [80] and later validated on a general population [81]. To our knowledge, no validation on the critically ill population has been conducted, and proper assessment of stool amount and characteristics in bedridden patients could be affected by loss or absorption of feces from bed linen. Similarly, estimation of stool volume/weight could represent a limit in the application of these definitions.

An observational study on MV patients documented loose stool (Bristol types 5–7) in 36.9% of study days, with diarrhea occurrence of 12% [82]. Nonetheless, the authors conclude that liquid stools are a common finding within critically ill patients due to common administration of EN and laxatives and should therefore not be considered a feature of diarrheic condition [82]. More recent observational studies reported a 12.9–14% prevalence of diarrhea on admitted patients [83, 84] or a 5.2% per 100 patient-days incidence [84].

Pathogenesis of diarrhea can be osmotic, motoric, secretory/ inflammatory, or from altered absorption [22] (also deriving from reduction of intestinal surface). Two main underlying mechanisms can explain the pathogenesis of diarrhea, the action of osmotically active substances and the electrolyte imbalance, resulting in a larger amount of water in the intestinal lumen [85].

Previously described causes for diarrhea [77] have been revisited during the last 10 years. Well-recognized causes can nowadays be referred to:

- **Medications**: 20.0% of patients with diarrhea received laxatives prior to its occurrence, and 11.4% had enemas administered [83]. Diarrhea could also be referred to administration of liquid drugs containing sorbitol, saccharose, mannitol, lactose, and magnesium through a NG tube [70].
- **Enteral nutrition**: the role of EN in diarrhea onset is nowadays unclear; on one side, EN seems to have a protective effect on intestinal mucosa, but, on the other side, EN may have an osmotic effect; nonetheless, research findings suggest that EN per se does not increases the risk of diarrhea (RR 0.87%, 95% CI: 0.46–1.66), but EN delivery >60% of energy target does (RR 1.75, 95% CI: 1.02–3.01; $p = 0.042$). Administering continuous or bolus EN does not affect the incidence of diarrhea (13.3% vs. 33.3%, $p = 0.39$) [48].
- **Antibiotic and antifungal therapy** is associated with an incidence rate of 8.94/100 patient-days and 25.35/100 patient-days, respectively. Estimated RR for diarrhea significantly increases when antibiotics (RR 3.64, 95% CI: 1.26–10.51, $p = 0.017$) and antifungal drugs (RR 2.79, 95% CI: 1.16–6.70; $p = 0.022$) are administered [84]. Authors also reported that the administration of EN >60% of energy target together with antibiotics or antifungal drugs increases the incidence risk ratio for diarrhea by 4.8 or 5.0 times, respectively [84].

- **Intestinal infections**: the most commonly reported infectious agent for ICU is *C. difficile* (0.7 [84]–1% [83] of the ICU population); other agents can be intestinal viruses, *Salmonella* and *Campylobacter* [83].

Patients with diarrhea have longer ICU-LOS (9.5 vs. 1.7 days, $p < 0.001$) and higher mortality (22.5 vs. 8.7%, $p < 0.001$) [83]. The role of fiber administration to reduce diarrhea is still controversial. Fibers act both as bulking agents (insoluble fiber) and by increasing water absorption (soluble fiber) [22].

Recently published guidelines do not suggest routine use of fiber formulas, since no consistent evidence concerning diarrhea reduction with fiber use is currently available [11]. Hemodynamically stable patients might benefit from a 10–20 g/ fiber addition, as it helps maintain the intestinal flora [11]. Caution should be kept toward hemodynamically unstable patients, since increasing intestinal mass could impair bowel perfusion [22].

According to the findings of a recent systematic review and meta-analysis, administration of probiotics has no effect on diarrhea reduction (RR 0.97, 95% CI 0.82–1.15, $P = 0.74$) [86].

## 15.6.2 Bowel Constipation

Although frequent in ICU patients, bowel constipation (BC) is often ignored. Nonhomogeneous definition of BC is still available, and previously reported definitions refer both to need for laxatives or enemas and days between stool passage (3, 6, or 9 days, according to studies). Recently the Working Group on Abdominal Problems from the European Society of Intensive Care Medicine (ESICM) refers to the term "paralysis of the lower GI tract," meaning the absence of stool passage for three or more consecutive days without mechanical obstruction, regardless of bowel sounds [78]. Further observational studies distinguished between early (3–5 days) and late (≥6 days) onset for constipation [87].

Recently, the concept of impaired gastrointestinal transit (IGT) has been introduced in enterally fed (for at least 3 days) and mechanically ventilated (for at least 2 days) patients; IGT bounds the absence of bowel movements for ≥days and BC treatment, together with at least other clinical criteria (radiological confirmation, feeding intolerance, abdominal distention, or need for gastric decompression) [88].

Prevalence of constipation in ICU population varies widely according to the setting and the definition used, thus leading to a difficult measurement of real impact of this problem. Nonetheless, constipation affects a significant proportion of ICU patients. Two observational studies revealed a constipation incidence (defined as "failure of bowel to function for 3 or more days") of 69.9% in surgical ICU patients [89] and of 83% in medical-surgical ICU patients. A more recent observational study investigating constipation in ICU patients found a global 51.9% incidence [87]. The abovementioned studies do not refer to patient's previous bowel habits.

Individual factors such as age and sex are not considered as predisposing factors for late defecation [90]. Table 15.3 summarizes predisposing factors for bowel constipation.

Constipation incidence is significantly reduced by early EN [89] and spontaneous breathing [87]. Therefore, attention to feeding and weaning from MV could also result in better GI outcomes. Interestingly, in a pseudo-randomized controlled trial [48], the incidence of constipation was significantly higher when EN was administered continuously compared to bolus (66.7% vs. 20%, $p = 0.025$).

Disease severity (measured by SOFA or APACHE II scores) has been addressed as responsible for delayed defecation [93]. Irrespective of stool-passage intervals considered (3–5 days or ≥6 days), constipation is significantly associated with invasive MV, use of vasopressors, continuous sedation, neuromuscular

**Table 15.3** Predisposing factors for bowel constipation

| | |
|---|---|
| Drugs | Exogenous opioids adhere to enteric opioid receptors, leading to altered motility and bowel dysfunction [91] and increasing water absorption from the GI tract, with consequent harder and drier feces [92]; moreover, opiates strongly impact on patient's LOC, leading to a reduced sensation of need for defecation |
| | Dopamine and norepinephrine can lead to reduced intestinal motility [93] |
| | Dehydration associated with diuretics can result in harder feces [94] |
| Environment | ICU environment often does not provide adequate privacy, leading to patient's embarrassment |
| | Reduced motility is common in ICU patients |
| Perfusion and oxygenation | Hypotension (SBP < 90 mmHg) and hypoxemia ($PaO_2/FiO_2$ ratio < 150 mmHg) impact on intestinal perfusion and oxygenation and are independently associated with late ($\geq 6$ days) passage of stool [95] |
| Surgery | Abdominal surgery per se [94, 96] and other site surgeries [90] can alter the brain-gut-microbiota axis |
| Late enteral nutrition | Delay in EN start could alter intestinal peristalsis [90] |

blocking agents, enteral feeding, ICU-LOS, and mortality [87]. Although nonstatistically significant, MV duration increases in constipated patients [87]. Prolonged constipation ($\geq 6$ days) is significantly associated with increased MV duration, ICU-LOS [87, 93, 97], risk of VAP [87], and bacterial infections at any site [95]. Feces passing through the gut allow intestinal "cleaning" [98], thus contributing to reduced bacterial overgrowth and increased bacterial translocation.

The association between late constipation and mortality is controversial [87, 90, 97]. When considering severity of disease, no clear assumption can be considered about which one is the causative agent and which one is the consequence [98].

Delay in stool passage has also been independently associated (adjusted HR 1.14, 95% CI 1.06–1.12; $p < 0.01$) with the onset of delirium [99].

Since bowel constipation is potentially life-threatening and causes discomfort to patients, maintenance of a regular intestinal function is essential to prevent potential complications. Correction of causative agents is the first step to manage the problem. Awareness of the problem so as proper consideration of risk factors (including daily review for opiates need) is crucial to keep adequate attention [94].

Constipation can be treated by administering laxatives, suppositories, or enemas. Laxatives include [91, 100]:

- Bulking agents (methylcellulose, psyllium): increase stool bulk
- Stimulant agents (senna, bisacodyl): stimulate peristalsis and increase water and electrolyte secretion at intestinal mucosa
- Osmotic agents (lactulose or polyethylene glycol (PEG)): increase water content in stool
- Emollient agents: create a slippery covering on stool, thus decreasing the amount of water absorbed at intestinal level

Currently, few data on effectiveness of laxatives in the critically ill population are available.

In a RCT on surgical and trauma ICU patients, lactulose administration during the first 3 days after ICU admission led to a statistically significant difference in patients with bowel movements (18% in the intervention group vs. 4% in the control group, $p < 0.05$) [101]. Daily administration of lactulose reduces time to first defecation (14.5 vs. 96.0 h, $p < 0.001$), days without defecation (33.1 ± 15.7 vs. 62.3 ± 24.5, $p < 0.001$), and number of patients affected by constipation (9.1% vs. 72.7%, $p < 0.001$); moreover, daily lactulose led to a greater reduction in SOFA score at discharge (−1.907; −3.683 to 0.13; $p = 0.036$) [102].

A less recent prospective RCT compared the effectiveness of two commonly administered laxatives (PEG and lactulose) and placebo in mixed ICU (including cardiac surgical patients). Both lactulose and PEG significantly reduced time to first defecation (36.0 vs. 75.0 h for lactulose versus placebo, $p = 0.001$; 44.0 vs. 75.0 h for PEG vs. placebo, $p = 0.001$). Also, a number of patients who had defecation during the study period statistically differed when comparing lactulose and placebo (69% vs. 31%, $p = 0.001$) and PEG and placebo (74% vs. 31%, $p = 0.001$) [97].

Other pharmacological agents can help resume GI motility. Metoclopramide and erythromycin both increase gastric emptying; however, their effect on small bowel movements [103] and in patients with postoperative ileus is limited [96]. Low doses (2–2.5 mg/24 h) of neostigmine help small bowel and colon motility [103], although potentially severe cardiovascular complications are described.

Enemas can be administered when oral laxatives are contraindicated, not tolerated, or not effective.

Bowel dysfunction related to opioids can be treated by administering methylnaltrexone (oral, intravenous, or subcutaneous) or naloxone. Methylnaltrexone acts as peripheral opiates antagonist, but its molecular structure does not cross the blood-brain barrier, thus avoiding side effects such as withdrawal syndrome or inadequate analgesia [103]. Methylnaltrexone can be administered orally, subcutaneously, and intravenously, without significant side effects or effect's reduction [100].

Take-Home Messages
- Assessment of nutritional status allows identification of patients at risk for malnutrition.
- Nutrition deficits increase the risk for major outcomes (mortality and LOS) and delay wound healing and recover of patients.
- Enteral nutrition is usually preferred, since it is more physiological and less costly.

- Complications of enteral nutrition refer both to the upper and lower gastrointestinal tract and may affect the delivery of required amounts.
- Special attentions are required when administering oral and liquid drugs through nasogastric tubes, both to avoid complications and reduced effect.
- Diarrhea and constipation commonly affect ICU patients; these complications relate with major outcomes.
- Protocols can be helpful to manage enteral feeding and to uniform the approach to gastrointestinal complications.

# References

1. Marik PE. Enteral nutrition in the critically ill: myths and misconceptions. Crit Care Med. 2014;42(4):962–9. https://doi.org/10.1097/CCM.0000000000000051.
2. Lew CCh, Yandell R, Fraser RJl, Chua AP, Chong MF, Miller M. Association Between Malnutrition and Clinical Outcomes in the Intensive Care Unit: A Systematic Review. JPEN J Parenter Enteral Nutr. 2017;41(5):744–758. https://doi.org/10.1177/0148607115625638.
3. Roberts SR, Kennerly DA, Keane D, George C. Nutrition support in the intensive care unit. Adequacy, timeliness, and outcomes. Crit Care Nurse. 2003;23(6):49–57.
4. World Health Organization. BMI classifications. http://apps.who.int/bmi/index.jsp?introPage=intro_3.html. Accessed 28 Aug 2016.
5. CDC. Anthropometric reference data for children and adults: United States, 2007–2010. http://www.cdc.gov/nchs/data/series/sr_11/sr11_252.pdf. Accessed 06 Dec 2016.
6. Ruiz L, Colley JR, Hamilton PJ. Measurement of triceps skinfold thickness. An investigation of sources of variation. Br J Prev Soc Med. 1971;25(3):165–7.
7. Benítez Brito N, Suárez Llanos JP, Fuentes Ferrer M, Oliva García JG, Delgado Brito I, Pereyra-García Castro F, Caracena Castellanos N, Acevedo Rodríguez CX, Palacio Abizanda E. Relationship between mid-upper arm circumference and body mass index in inpatients. PLoS One. 2016;11(8):e0160480. https://doi.org/10.1371/journal.pone.0160480.

8. Frisancho AR. Triceps skinfold and upper arm muscle size norms for assessment of nutritional status. Am J Clin Nutr. 1974;27:1052–7.

9. Madden AM, Smith S. Body composition and morphological assessment of nutritional status in adults: a review of anthropometric variables. J Hum Nutr Diet. 2016;29(1):7–25. https://doi.org/10.1111/jhn.12278.

10. Simpson F, Early PN, Trial Investigators Group. Physical assessment and anthropometric measures for use in clinical research conducted in critically ill patient populations: an analytic observational study. JPEN J Parenter Enteral Nutr. 2015;39(3):313–21. https://doi.org/10.1177/0148607113515526.

11. McClave SA, Taylor BE, Martindale RG, Warren MM, Johnson DR, Braunschweig C, McCarthy MS, Davanos E, Rice TW, Cresci GA, Gervasio JM, Sacks GS, Roberts PR, Compher C, Society of Critical Care Medicine; American Society for Parenteral and Enteral Nutrition. Guidelines for the provision and assessment of nutrition support therapy in the adult critically ill patient: Society of Critical Care Medicine (SCCM) and American Society for Parenteral and Enteral Nutrition (a.S.P.E.N.). JPEN J Parenter Enteral Nutr. 2016;40(2):159–211. https://doi.org/10.1177/0148607115621863.

12. Kondrup J, Rasmussen HH, Hamberg O, Stanga Z, Ad Hoc ESPEN Working Group. Nutritional risk screening (NRS 2002): a new method based on an analysis of controlled clinical trials. Clin Nutr. 2003;22(3):321–36.

13. Heyland DK, Dhaliwal R, Jiang X, Day AG. Identifying critically ill patients who benefit the most from nutrition therapy: the development and initial validation of a novel risk assessment tool. Crit Care. 2011;15(6):R268. https://doi.org/10.1186/cc10546.

14. Rahman A, Hasan RM, Agarwala R, Martin C, Day AG, Heyland DK. Identifying critically-ill patients who will benefit most from nutritional therapy: further validation of the "modified NUTRIC" nutritional risk assessment tool. Clin Nutr. 2016;35(1):158–62. https://doi.org/10.1016/j.clnu.2015.01.015.

15. Coltman A, Peterson S, Roehl K, Roosevelt H, Sowa D. Use of 3 tools to assess nutrition risk in the intensive care unit. JPEN J Parenter Enteral Nutr. 2015;39(1):28–33. https://doi.org/10.1177/0148607114532135.

16. Fung EB. Estimating energy expenditure in critically ill adults and children. AACN Clin Issues. 2000;11(4):480–97.

17. Walker RN, Heuberger RA. Predictive equations for energy needs for the critically ill. Respir Care. 2009;54(4):509–21.

18. Li B, Tang S, Ma YL, Tang J, Wang B, Wang JR. Analysis of bowel sounds application status for gastrointestinal function monitoring in the intensive care unit. Crit Care Nurs Q. 2014;37(2):199–206. https://doi.org/10.1097/CNQ.0000000000000019.

19. Breum BM, Rud B, Kirkegaard T, Nordentoft T. Accuracy of abdominal auscultation for bowel obstruction. World J Gastroenterol. 2015;21(34):10018–24. https://doi.org/10.3748/wjg.v21.i34.10018.

20. Heyland DK, Cahill NE, Dhaliwal R, Sun X, Day AG, McClave SA. Impact of enteral feeding protocols on enteral nutrition delivery: results of a multicenter observational study. JPEN J Parenter Enteral Nutr. 2010;34(6):675–84. https://doi.org/10.1177/0148607110364843.

21. Choi EY, Park DA, Park J. Calorie intake of enteral nutrition and clinical outcomes in acutely critically ill patients: a meta-analysis of randomized controlled trials. JPEN J Parenter Enteral Nutr. 2015;39(3):291–300. https://doi.org/10.1177/0148607114544322.

22. de Brito-Ashurst I, Preiser JC. Diarrhea in critically ill patients: the role of enteral feeding. JPEN J Parenter Enteral Nutr. 2016;40(7):913–23. https://doi.org/10.1177/0148607116651758.

23. Pearce CB, Duncan HD. Enteral feeding. Nasogastric, nasojejunal, percutaneous endoscopic gastrostomy, or jejunostomy: its indications and limitations. Postgrad Med J. 2002;78(918):198–204.

24. Scott R, Bowling TE. Enteral tube feeding in adults. J R Coll Physicians Edinb. 2015;45(1):49–54. https://doi.org/10.4997/JRCPE.2015.112.

25. Williams NT. Medication administration through enteral feeding tubes. Am J Health Syst Pharm. 2008;65(24):2347–57. https://doi.org/10.2146/ajhp080155.

26. Alkhawaja S, Martin C, Butler RJ, Gwadry-Sridhar F. Post-pyloric versus gastric tube feeding for preventing pneumonia and improving nutritional outcomes in critically ill adults. Cochrane Database Syst Rev. 2015;8:CD008875. https://doi.org/10.1002/14651858.CD008875.pub2.

27. Taylor SJ. Confirming nasogastric feeding tube position versus the need to feed. Intensive Crit Care Nurs. 2013;29(2):59–69. https://doi.org/10.1016/j.iccn.2012.07.002.

28. Lortie MA, Charbonney E. Confirming placement of nasogastric feeding tubes. CMAJ. 2016;188(5):E96. https://doi.org/10.1503/cmaj.150609.

29. Williams TA, Leslie GD. A review of the nursing care of enteral feeding tubes in critically ill adults: part II. Intensive Crit Care Nurs. 2005;21(1):5–15. https://doi.org/10.1016/j.iccn.2004.08.003.

30. Beghetto MG, Anziliero F, Leães DM, de Mello ED. Feeding tube placement: auscultatory method and x-ray agreement. Rev Gaucha

Enferm. 2015;36(4):98–103. https://doi.org/10.1590/1983-1447.2015. 04.54700.

31. Turgay AS, Khorshid L. Effectiveness of the auscultatory and pH methods in predicting feeding tube placement. J Clin Nurs. 2010; 19(11–12):1553–9. https://doi.org/10.1111/j.1365-2702.2010.03191.x.

32. Boeykens K, Steeman E, Duysburgh I. Reliability of pH measurement and the auscultatory method to confirm the position of a nasogastric tube. Int J Nurs Stud. 2014;51(11):1427–33. https://doi.org/10.1016/j. ijnurstu.2014.03.004.

33. Bankhead R, Boullata J, Brantley S, Corkins M, Guenter P, Krenitsky J, Lyman B, Metheny NA, Mueller C, Robbins S, Wessel J, A.S.P.E.N. Board of Directors. Enteral nutrition practice recommendations. JPEN J Parenter Enteral Nutr. 2009;33(2):122–67. https://doi. org/10.1177/0148607108330314.

34. Arevalo-Manso JJ, Martinez-Sanchez P, Juarez-Martin B, Fuentes B, Ruiz-Ares G, Sanz-Cuesta BE, Parrilla-Novo P, Diez-Tejedor E. Preventing diarrhoea in enteral nutrition: the impact of the delivery set hang time. Int J Clin Pract. 2015;69(8):900–8. https://doi. org/10.1111/ijcp.12645.

35. Kuppinger DD, Rittler P, Hartl WH, Rüttinger D. Use of gastric residual volume to guide enteral nutrition in critically ill patients: a brief systematic review of clinical studies. Nutrition. 2013;29(9):1075–9. https://doi.org/10.1016/j.nut.2013.01.025.

36. Davies AR. Gastric residual volume in the ICU: can we do without measuring it? JPEN J Parenter Enteral Nutr. 2010;34(2):160–2. https:// doi.org/10.1177/0148607109357626.

37. Reintam Blaser A, Starkopf L, Deane AM, Poeze M, Starkopf J. Comparison of different definitions of feeding intolerance: a retrospective observational study. Clin Nutr. 2015;34(5):956–61. https://doi. org/10.1016/j.clnu.2014.10.006.

38. Gungabissoon U, Hacquoil K, Bains C, Irizarry M, Dukes G, Williamson R, Deane AM, Heyland DK. Prevalence, risk factors, clinical consequences, and treatment of enteral feed intolerance during critical illness. JPEN J Parenter Enteral Nutr. 2015;39(4):441–8. https://doi. org/10.1177/0148607114526450.

39. Metheny NA, Schallom L, Oliver DA, Clouse RE. Gastric residual volume and aspiration in critically ill patients receiving gastric feedings. Am J Crit Care. 2008;17(6):512–9; quiz 520

40. Montejo JC. Enteral nutrition-related gastrointestinal complications in critically ill patients: a multicenter study. The nutritional and metabolic working Group of the Spanish Society of intensive care medicine and coronary units. Crit Care Med. 1999;27(8):1447–53.

41. McClave SA, Lukan JK, Stefater JA, Lowen CC, Looney SW, Matheson PJ, Gleeson K, Spain DA. Poor validity of residual volumes as a marker for risk of aspiration in critically ill patients. Crit Care Med. 2005;33(2):324–30.

42. Juvé-Udina ME, Valls-Miró C, Carreño-Granero A, Martinez-Estalella G, Monterde-Prat D, Domingo-Felici CM, Llusa-Finestres J, Asensio-Malo G. To return or to discard? Randomised trial on gastric residual volume management. Intensive Crit Care Nurs. 2009;25(5):258–67. https://doi.org/10.1016/j.iccn.2009.06.004.

43. Marshall A, West S. Nutritional intake in the critically ill: improving practice through research. Aust Crit Care. 2004;17(1):6–8, 10-5

44. Elke G, Felbinger TW, Heyland DK. Gastric residual volume in critically ill patients: a dead marker or still alive? Nutr Clin Pract. 2015; 30(1):59–71. https://doi.org/10.1177/0884533614562841.

45. Bartlett Ellis RJ, Fuehne J. Examination of accuracy in the assessment of gastric residual volume: a simulated, controlled study. JPEN J Parenter Enteral Nutr. 2015;39(4):434–40. https://doi.org/10.1177/0148607114524230.

46. Metheny NA, Stewart J, Nuetzel G, Oliver D, Clouse RE. Effect of feeding-tube properties on residual volume measurements in tube-fed patients. JPEN J Parenter Enteral Nutr. 2005;29(3):192–7. https://doi.org/10.1177/0148607105029003192.

47. Reignier J, Mercier E, Le Gouge A, Boulain T, Desachy A, Bellec F, Clavel M, Frat JP, Plantefeve G, Quenot JP, Lascarrou JB. Clinical research in intensive care and sepsis (CRICS) Group. Effect of not monitoring residual gastric volume on risk of ventilator-associated pneumonia in adults receiving mechanical ventilation and early enteral feeding: a randomized controlled trial. JAMA. 2013;309(3):249–56. https://doi.org/10.1001/jama.2012.196377.

48. Kadamani I, Itani M, Zahran E, Taha N. Incidence of aspiration and gastrointestinal complications in critically ill patients using continuous versus bolus infusion of enteral nutrition: a pseudo-randomised controlled trial. Aust Crit Care. 2014;27(4):188–93. https://doi.org/10.1016/j.aucc.2013.12.001.

49. Montejo JC, Miñambres E, Bordejé L, Mesejo A, Acosta J, Heras A, Ferré M, Fernandez-Ortega F, Vaquerizo CI, Manzanedo R. Gastric residual volume during enteral nutrition in ICU patients: the REGANE study. Intensive Care Med. 2010;36(8):1386–93. https://doi.org/10.1007/s00134-010-1856-y.

50. Moreira TV, McQuiggan M. Methods for the assessment of gastric emptying in critically ill, enterally fed adults. Nutr Clin Pract. 2009;24(2):261–73. https://doi.org/10.1177/0884533609332176.

51. Soroksky A, Lorber J, Klinowski E, Ilgayev E, Mizrachi A, Miller A, Ben Yehuda TM, Leonov Y. A simplified approach to the management of gastric residual volumes in critically ill mechanically ventilated patients: a pilot prospective cohort study. Isr Med Assoc J. 2010;12(9):543–8.

52. Elpern EH, Stutz L, Peterson S, Gurka DP, Skipper A. Outcomes associated with enteral tube feedings in a medical intensive care unit. Am J Crit Care. 2004;13(3):221–7.

53. Steele A, Carlson KK. Nausea and vomiting: applying research to bedside practice. AACN Adv Crit Care. 2007;18(1):61–73; quiz 74-5

54. Reintam A, Parm P, Kitus R, Kern H, Starkopf J. Gastrointestinal symptoms in intensive care patients. Acta Anaesthesiol Scand. 2009; 53(3):318–24. https://doi.org/10.1111/j.1399-6576.2008.01860.x.

55. Kim H, Stotts NA, Froelicher ES, Engler MM, Porter C. Why patients in critical care do not receive adequate enteral nutrition? A review of the literature. J Crit Care. 2012;27(6):702–13. https://doi.org/10.1016/j.jcrc.2012.07.019.

56. Krishnan JA, Parce PB, Martinez A, Diette GB, Brower RG. Caloric intake in medical ICU patients: consistency of care with guidelines and relationship to clinical outcomes. Chest. 2003;124(1):297–305.

57. Reid C. Frequency of under- and overfeeding in mechanically ventilated ICU patients: causes and possible consequences. J Hum Nutr Diet. 2006;19(1):13–22. https://doi.org/10.1111/j.1365-277X.2006.00661.x.

58. Marik PE, Zaloga GP. Gastric versus post-pyloric feeding: a systematic review. Crit Care. 2003;7(3):R46–51. https://doi.org/10.1186/cc2190.

59. Kozeniecki M, McAndrew N, Patel JJ. Process-related barriers to optimizing enteral nutrition in a tertiary medical intensive care unit. Nutr Clin Pract. 2016;31(1):80–5. https://doi.org/10.1177/0884533615611845.

60. Peev MP, Yeh DD, Quraishi SA, Osler P, Chang Y, Gillis E, Albano CE, Darak S, Velmahos GC. Causes and consequences of interrupted enteral nutrition: a prospective observational study in critically ill surgical patients. JPEN J Parenter Enteral Nutr. 2015;39(1):21–7. https://doi.org/10.1177/0148607114526887.

61. O'Meara D, Mireles-Cabodevila E, Frame F, Hummell AC, Hammel J, Dweik RA, Arroliga AC. Evaluation of delivery of enteral nutrition in critically ill patients receiving mechanical ventilation. Am J Crit Care. 2008;17(1):53–61.

62. Kim H, Stotts NA, Froelicher ES, Engler MM, Porter C, Kwak H. Adequacy of early enteral nutrition in adult patients in the intensive care unit. J Clin Nurs. 2012;21(19–20):2860–9. https://doi.org/10.1111/j.1365-2702.2012.04218.x. Epub 2012 Jul 30

63. Ramakrishnan N, Daphnee DK, Ranganathan L, Bhuvaneshwari S. Critical care 24 × 7: but, why is critical nutrition interrupted? Indian J Crit Care Med. 2014;18(3):144–8. https://doi.org/10.4103/0972-5229.128704.

64. Doig GS, Simpson F, Finfer S, Delaney A, Davies AR, Mitchell I, Dobb G, Nutrition Guidelines Investigators of the ANZICS Clinical Trials Group. Effect of evidence-based feeding guidelines on mortality of critically ill adults: a cluster randomized controlled trial. JAMA. 2008;300(23):2731–41. https://doi.org/10.1001/jama.2008.826.

65. Compton F, Bojarski C, Siegmund B, van der Giet M. Use of a nutrition support protocol to increase enteral nutrition delivery in critically ill patients. Am J Crit Care. 2014;23(5):396–403. https://doi.org/10.4037/ajcc2014140.

66. Lottes Stewart M. Nutrition support protocols and their influence on the delivery of enteral nutrition: a systematic review. Worldviews Evid-Based Nurs. 2014;11(3):194–9. https://doi.org/10.1111/wvn.12036.

67. Teng R, Carlson G, Hsia J. An open-label, randomized bioavailability study with alternative methods of administration of crushed ticagrelor tablets in healthy volunteers. Int J Clin Pharmacol Ther. 2015;53(2):182–9. https://doi.org/10.5414/CP202202.

68. Klang M, McLymont V, Ng N. Osmolality, pH, and compatibility of selected oral liquid medications with an enteral nutrition product. JPEN J Parenter Enteral Nutr. 2013;37(5):689–94. https://doi.org/10.1177/0148607112471560.

69. Boullata JI. Drug administration through an enteral feeding tube. The rationale behind the guidelines. Am J Nurs. 2009;109(10):34–42; quiz 43. https://doi.org/10.1097/01.NAJ.0000361488.45094.28.

70. Matysiak-Luśnia K, Lysenko Ł. Drug administration via enteral feeding tubes in intensive therapy - terra incognita? Anaesthesiol Intensive Ther. 2014;46(4):307–11. https://doi.org/10.5603/AIT.2014.0050.

71. Phillips NM, Endacott R. Medication administration via enteral tubes: a survey of nurses' practices. J Adv Nurs. 2011;67(12):2586–92. https://doi.org/10.1111/j.1365-2648.2011.05688.x.

72. Mota ML, Barbosa IV, Studart RM, Melo EM, Lima FE, Mariano FA. Evaluation of intensivist-nurses' knowledge concerning medication administration through nasogastric and enteral tubes. Rev Lat Am Enfermagem. 2010;18(5):888–94.

73. van den Bemt PM, Cusell MB, Overbeeke PW, Trommelen M, van Dooren D, Ophorst WR, Egberts AC. Quality improvement of oral medication administration in patients with enteral feeding tubes. Qual Saf Health Care. 2006;15(1):44–7. https://doi.org/10.1136/qshc.2004.013524.

74. McPeake J, Gilmour H, MacIntosh G. The implementation of a bowel management protocol in an adult intensive care unit. Nurs Crit Care. 2011;16(5):235–42. https://doi.org/10.1111/j.1478-5153.2011.00451.x.
75. Knowles S, Lam LT, McInnes E, Elliott D, Hardy J, Middleton S. Knowledge, attitudes, beliefs and behaviour intentions for three bowel management practices in intensive care: effects of a targeted protocol implementation for nursing and medical staff. BMC Nurs. 2015;14:6. https://doi.org/10.1186/s12912-015-0056-z.
76. Knowles S, McInnes E, Elliott D, Hardy J, Middleton S. Evaluation of the implementation of a bowel management protocol in intensive care: effect on clinician practices and patient outcomes. J Clin Nurs. 2014;23(5–6):716–30. https://doi.org/10.1111/jocn.12448.
77. Ferrie S, East V. Managing diarrhoea in intensive care. Aust Crit Care. 2007;20(1):7–13.
78. Reintam Blaser A, Malbrain MLNG, Starkopf J, et al. Gastrointestinal function in intensive care patients: terminology, definitions and management. Recommendations of the ESICM Working Group on Abdominal Problems. Intensive Care Med. 2012;38(3):384–94. https://doi.org/10.1007/s00134-011-2459-y.
79. Reintam Blaser A, Deane AM, Fruhwald S. Diarrhoea in the critically ill. Curr Opin Crit Care. 2015;21(2):142–53. https://doi.org/10.1097/MCC.0000000000000188.
80. O'Donnell LJD, Heaton KW. Pseudo-diarrhea in the irritable bowel syndrome: patients' records of stool form reflect transit time while stool frequency does not. Gut. 1988;29:A1455. https://doi.org/10.1136/gut.29.10.A1429.
81. Heaton KW, Radvan J, Cripps H, Mountford RA, Braddon FE, Hughes AO. Defecation frequency and timing, and stool form in the general population: a prospective study. Gut. 1992;33(6):818–24.
82. Bishop S, Young H, Goldsmith D, Buldock D, Chin M, Bellomo R. Bowel motions in critically ill patients: a pilot observational study. Crit Care Resusc. 2010;12(3):182–5.
83. Tirlapur N, Puthucheary ZA, Cooper JA, Sanders J, Coen PG, Moonesinghe SR, Wilson AP, Mythen MG, Montgomery HE. Diarrhoea in the critically ill is common, associated with poor outcome, and rarely due to Clostridium difficile. Sci Rep. 2016;6:24691. https://doi.org/10.1038/srep24691.
84. Thibault R, Graf S, Clerc A, Delieuvin N, Heidegger CP, Pichard C. Diarrhoea in the ICU: respective contribution of feeding and antibiotics. Crit Care. 2013;17(4):R153. https://doi.org/10.1186/cc12832.
85. Baldi F, Bianco MA, Nardone G, Pilotto A, Zamparo E. Focus on acute diarrhoeal disease. World J Gastroenterol. 2009;15(27):3341–8.

86. Manzanares W, Lemieux M, Langlois PL, Wischmeyer PE. Probiotic and synbiotic therapy in critical illness: a systematic review and meta-analysis. Crit Care. 2016;19:262. https://doi.org/10.1186/s13054-016-1434-y.

87. Prat D, Messika J, Avenel A, Jacobs F, Fichet J, Lemeur M, Ricard JD, Sztrymf B. Constipation incidence and impact in medical critical care patients: importance of the definition criterion. Eur J Gastroenterol Hepatol. 2016;28(3):290–6. https://doi.org/10.1097/MEG.00000 00000000543.

88. Nguyen T, Frenette AJ, Johanson C, Maclean RD, Patel R, Simpson A, Singh A, Balchin KS, Fergusson D, Kanji S. Impaired gastrointestinal transit and its associated morbidity in the intensive care unit. J Crit Care. 2013;28(4):537.e11–7. https://doi.org/10.1016/j.jcrc.2012.12.003.

89. Nassar AP Jr, da Silva FM, de Cleva R. Constipation in intensive care unit: incidence and risk factors. J Crit Care. 2009;24(4):630.e9–12. https://doi.org/10.1016/j.jcrc.2009.03.007.

90. Fukuda S, Miyauchi T, Fujita M, Oda Y, Todani M, Kawamura Y, Kaneda K, Tsuruta R. Risk factors for late defecation and its association with the outcomes of critically ill patients: a retrospective observational study. J Intensive Care. 2016;4:33. https://doi.org/10.1186/s40560-016-0156-1.

91. Poulsen JL, Brock C, Olesen AE, Nilsson M, Drewes AM. Evolving paradigms in the treatment of opioid-induced bowel dysfunction. Ther Adv Gastroenterol. 2015;8(6):360–72. https://doi.org/10.1177/17562 83X15589526.

92. Thomas J. Opioid-induced bowel dysfunction. J Pain Symptom Manag. 2008;35:103–13. https://doi.org/10.1016/j.jpainsymman.2007.01.017.

93. van der Spoel JI, Schultz MJ, van der Voort PH, de Jonge E. Influence of severity of illness, medication and selective decontamination on defecation. Intensive Care Med. 2006;32(6):875–80. https://doi.org/10.1007/s00134-006-0175-9.

94. Vincent JL, Preiser JC. Getting critical about constipation. Pract Gastroenterol. 2015;15

95. Gacouin A, Camus C, Gros A, et al. Constipation in long- term ventilated patients: associated factors and impact on intensive care unit outcomes. Crit Care Med. 2010;38:1933–8. https://doi.org/10.1097/CCM.0b013e3181eb9236.

96. Behm B, Stollman N. Postoperative ileus: etiologies and interventions. Clin Gastroenterol Hepatol. 2003;1(2):71–80. https://doi.org/10.1053/cgh.2003.50012.

97. van der Spoel JI, Oudemans-van Straaten HM, Kuiper MA, van Roon EN, Zandstra DF, van der Voort PH. Laxation of critically ill patients with lactulose or polyethylene glycol: a two-center randomized, double-blind, placebo-controlled trial. Crit Care Med. 2007;35(12):2726–31. https://doi.org/10.1097/01.CCM.0000287526.08794.29.
98. van der Spoel JI. Oudemans-van Straaten Ubi poop, ibi evacua? HM. Crit Care Med. 2010;38(10):2064–5. https://doi.org/10.1097/CCM.0b013e3181f1789b.
99. Smonig R, Wallenhorst T, Bouju P, Letheulle J, Le Tulzo Y, Tadié JM, Gacouin A. Constipation is independently associated with delirium in critically ill ventilated patients. Intensive Care Med. 2016;42(1):126–7. https://doi.org/10.1007/s00134-015-4050-4.
100. Chappell D, Rehm M, Conzen P. Opioid-induced constipation in intensive care patients: relief in sight? Crit Care. 2008;12(4):161. https://doi.org/10.1186/cc6930.
101. Masri Y, Abubaker J, Ahmed R. Prophylactic use of laxative for constipation in critically ill patients. Ann Thorac Med. 2010;5(4):228–31. https://doi.org/10.4103/1817-1737.69113.
102. de Azevedo RP, Freitas FG, Ferreira EM, Pontes de Azevedo LC, Machado FR. Daily laxative therapy reduces organ dysfunction in mechanically ventilated patients: a phase II randomized controlled trial. Crit Care. 2015;19:329. https://doi.org/10.1186/s13054-015-1047-x.
103. Fruhwald S, Holzer P, Metzler H. Intestinal motility disturbances in intensive care patients pathogenesis and clinical impac. Intensive Care Med. 2007;33(1):36–44. https://doi.org/10.1007/s00134-006-0452-7.

# Chapter 16
# Visiting Policies in ICUs

Matteo Manici and Francesca Ghillani

## 16.1 Introduction

Intensive care units (ICUs) are highly affected by the changes in medicine that have been taking place since the start of the millennium. In ICUs, the connection between techno-scientific research, biomedical industry, professional practices, and the trajectories of life and care of patients and their families is increasingly tightening [1].

The intensive care unit was born in 1952, when the application of invasive ventilation spread as a response to the epidemic of poliomyelitis in Copenhagen. The concept has changed dramatically with the evolution of the discipline of intensive care medicine over the last 60 years, and future changes will certainly happen in the next few years [2]. In many contexts, patients and their families see ICUs as closed environments and almost completely inaccessible [3]. ICUs are probably the settings where the contrast between the increasing technological sophistication of modern medicine and its frequent failure to properly consider the human and

© Springer International Publishing AG, part of Springer Nature 2018    409
I. Comisso et al., *Nursing in Critical Care Setting*,
https://doi.org/10.1007/978-3-319-50559-6_16

relational dimensions is widely evident. For this reason, the ICU has been disparaged, reduced by the public as being "inhuman" or "high-tech" medicine [4].

In the USA in the 1960s, the discipline of medical humanities (MH)—also called "clinical humanism"—developed around the distinctions between the bonds science-technology and man-relationship. The discipline was born with the aim of avoiding the degeneration of medicine, which, at the time, was moving toward a more techno-scientific gaze.

The medical humanities cover the function of advocacy for patients, focusing on their sufferings, due to biological but also psychic and social natures of the illnesses [5].

In the MH movement, great attention is placed on the medical staff, composed by nurses, doctors, and other figures of health and social workers who operate on an interdisciplinary basis in the environment of cure. In an age of continuous expansion of the technical system of medicine, of fundamental ethical dilemmas and growing socioeconomic problems, but also of difficulties in the communication between patients, family members, and practitioners, the MH build new alliances and new models of care.

The term humanization, unlike MH, does not recall the area of study (medical and nursing) but is rather linked to the action of making more "human" (perhaps even "humble" and "gentle") the relational dynamics between patients, their families, and caregivers [6].

Humanizing care can seem, at first glance, a paradox, given that hospitals were in fact established as supportive and compassionate places of institutional care [7]. Humanization is often invoked in response to the dehumanization of ICUs, which cannot be attributed to technology alone but is especially an effect of the way in which members of staff facilitate the balance between machine and human.

The theme of humanization is certainly very wide. Indeed, humanizing the care for ICU patients entails:

- Reducing, as much as possible, biological damage and promoting the best recovery
- Enhancing the uniqueness of the person by augmenting the personal dimensions and giving meaning to the biological dimension
- Giving the patient an absolute moral value; helping to feel him/her like a human being with an intact dignity, as a consequence of the value attributed to the patient by those who have the responsibility to care [8]

The humanization of care in the ICU can be conceptually approached from the point of view of the main figures involved in the system. Namely:

- The patient, not only in terms of the obvious attention given to the reduction of the biological damage, but also as an appreciation of the uniqueness of the ill person, to whom an ontological value should be attributed. The patient's value shouldn't be subordinated to the effectiveness of the healthcare techniques or his/her personal autonomy.
- The family, in particular, the efforts that should be aimed at reducing the consequences of having a relative hospitalized in ICU and personalizing their participation in the life of the ward.
- The healthcare worker, supporting the efforts in dealing with the feelings of inadequacy and helplessness that arise when therapeutic techniques are not sufficient to reduce the biological damage or to avoid the death of the patient and always encouraging compassion for the sick, for the family members, and for themselves [8].

In more recent times, and with a view that is closer to the one expressed in this work, the "HEROIC" Bundle (Fig. 16.1) was proposed as an acronym of *Humanization to Enhance Recovery on Intensive Care* [9], divided into the chapters: "open ICU," ICU environment, communication strategies, analgesia, delirium, reorientation strategies, physiological sleep promotion,

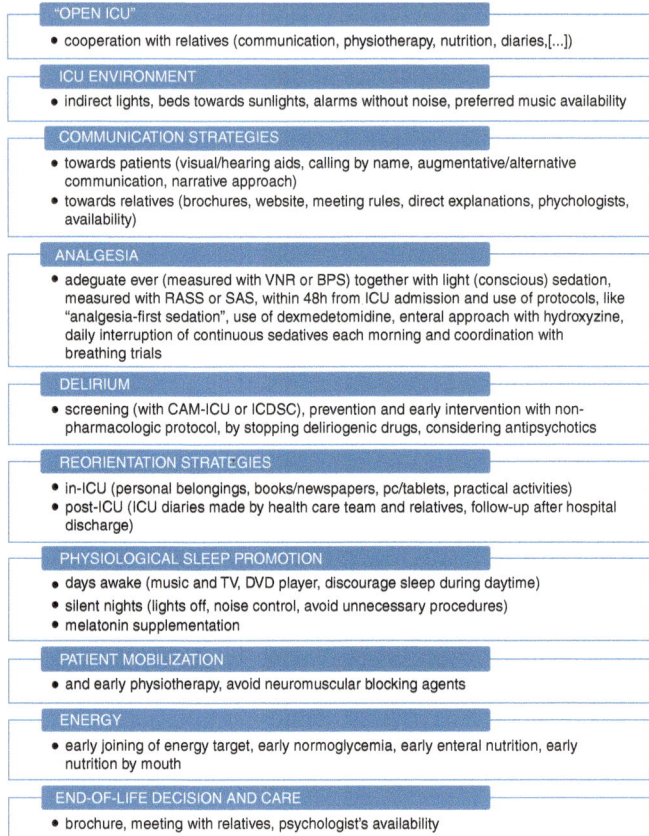

**Fig. 16.1** *Humanization to Enhance Recovery on Intensive Care* (HEROIC) Bundle (www.heroicbundle.org, accessed on 5th of May, 2016, reproduced with permission)

patient mobilization, energy, and end-of-life decision and care. Many of the topics related to this approach will be discussed in this text. Furthermore, the remainder of this chapter will be focused on the topic of "open ICU," in the European sense of the term, that is, ICU with open visiting policies.

## 16.2   Open ICU

The admission of patients to ICUs still follows a "revolving door" principle: when the patient comes in, the family is sent out [10]. The "opening" of intensive care, or rather the opening of visiting policies, is considered an important step toward the humanization of care.

The theme of the visit in the ICU has been the subject of research and debate for over 25 years [11]. A 1984 survey carried out in Ohio (USA) showed great variability in the visiting policies to ICUs in terms of duration and frequency. Most of the ICUs allowed access to only two visitors and limited the visiting time to less than 20 min. Rarely, children under the age of 12 were allowed in. Often the choices of such restrictive visiting policies were not supported by previous studies and were not in line with the current concept of "rights" of the patient [12].

About 15 years ago, Hilmar Burchardi, in his editorial in intensive care medicine entitled "Let's open the door!," affirmed the need to recognize that the ICU could be a place where high priority is given to the concept of humanity and highlighted the need to open doors that were still closed [4]. Few topics have generated such a high level of debate as the visiting policy in intensive care units. The "open" care model is different from the more traditional "intensive care with closed visiting policies" model, as the latter is characterized by access restrictions in terms of time and number of people, the use of personal protective equipment for visitors, and fragmented and limited relationships between health professionals, the patient, and the family [8]. The rationale behind the traditional "closed" model is based on the fear of family interference with the process of care as well as the idea that a more open access of visitors leads to an increased risk of infection and an augmented stress of family members. So, the patient in ICU is usually alone and separated from family members by restrictive access policies [13].

The need for and the importance of family members visiting patients admitted to the ICU has been well documented and passionately debated for many years. Nurses tend to be the main "access controllers" of visitors, although there is still little empirical knowledge of the phenomenon from the perspective of the bedside nurse [14]. Furthermore, the terminology is sometimes inconsistent: "visitation" is a generic word with many meanings. The so-called structured visit is a form of visit that imposes limits. Although these limits can be very flexible, this situation should not be confused with a completely open (or unlimited) visiting policy. The "open visit" should be distinguished from "cohabitation." In this context, cohabitation is the act of living with someone, while visits are the act of spending a period with someone. Through the application of a "visiting contract," the ICU staff creates specific agreements with visitors to meet their needs and those of patients and staff. This normally does not include an open invitation to visit the patient at any time without limits [15].

In the USA and Europe, most of ICUs poses many restrictions [16] that have been gradually decreasing over the years. In France (2000) 97% of ICUs applied visiting policies restricted to a single visit and at a designated time [17]. In Spain (2005) 94.8% of 98 ICUs investigated imposed limitations to visits [18]. In New England, USA (2007), 68% of ICUs did not adopt an open visiting policy with flexible hours [19]. In Italy, of 257 investigated ICUs (2007), only one had a non-restrictive policy on the time of the visit. 99.6% allowed access but with limitations of the visiting hours, and in five of them (2%), visitors were not allowed at all [20]. In Flanders (2007), the Dutch-speaking Belgium, 96.7% of ICUs had restrictive policies [21]. Still in Belgium (2010), visiting policies were restrictive in all of the 27 ICUs surveyed, with preassigned visiting hours spread over two or three daily time slots in 98.2% of cases [22]. In the Netherlands (2011), most of the ICUs (85.7%) had limitations [23]. In USA (2013), three kinds of restrictions (time, number of visitors, or age) persisted in 89.6% of ICUs [24].

## 16.2.1  Communication in ICU

Major features of communication in ICUs include a highly technological environment, decisions based on the interpretation of monitoring and treatment data, and the consequent development of technical skills by doctors and nurses. However, to deliver quality of care, another "step" is needed: the ability to deal with the uncertainty and anxiety of the patient and his/her family. This would be an empathetic perspective where the subjectivity and the person's symbolism are considered just as valuable as their physical symptoms [25]. Communicating means transferring information but also transferring nonverbal aspects that generate trust and satisfaction in the users of the service.

Correct information should be a basic pillar of communication in the ICU, and it must be provided in a complete and appropriate way, especially in relation to the guidelines of diagnosis, prognosis, and treatment. A study conducted by Vincent [26], who surveyed 180 users of his service, showed a good level of understanding with regard to the information received, but a series of evaluations suggested that the process of communication could be improved in order to ensure an adequate level of satisfaction. The need for more privacy during the information process emerged, to respect the dignity of patients and their families and to prevent the disclosure of sensitive information. A private place was often requested, far from people who should not be involved in the process [27].

The participation of a nurse in the information process can be useful to provide necessary clarification to the family members in order to fully understand the information provided by the doctor [26]. Clear and unambiguous communication among the staff members is crucial for the development of the dynamics of mutual understanding and respect [28]. Healthcare staff must listen and be able to respond to nonverbal cues from the patient and family members. From this point of view, increasing visiting hours can help to improve the level of understanding and acceptance of information and care received by the patients and their families [27].

Another important aspect of communication is the time required to provide family members with information that is clear, honest, and timely. The time spent with families was associated with the effectiveness of the information [29]. Fassier, in a cross-sectional study of 1 day in 90 French ICUs, measured the time spent by doctors in communication with 951 families of patients in ICUs. The average time of communication with the family was 16 min; 20% was spent clarifying the diagnosis, 20% on treatment, and 60% on illustrating the prognosis. A multivariate analysis of the results showed a factor correlated with a shorter time of communication (rooms with more than one bed) and seven factors associated with a longer time of communication: five related to the patient (surgery on the same day, high rates of organ dysfunction, coma, MV, and worsening of clinical status), and two related to the family (first contact and interview with spouse) [29].

Therefore, the central aspects of communication in ICU include the ability to receive information in an environment that offers privacy, the development of communication within the team (exceeding the medical information process and those provided by bedside nurse), and the duration of the information process.

## 16.2.2   Family Needs

Foreseeing the needs and experiences of family members is only an initial step, but it is necessary to provide appropriate care to the family and the patient. Needs can be divided into four categories: cognitive, emotional, social, and practical [30].

The need for accurate and understandable information is universal. Usually, family members wish to speak to a doctor every day for updates on their relative's condition and prognosis, and they need a nurse who can explain to them the ongoing treatment, the bed and related technology, and what they can do for the patient during visiting hours.

Family members attribute great importance to being contacted by telephone, if the condition of their loved one changes. Emotional needs of hope, reassurance, and the opportunity to be near their kin are considered fundamental. Family members always give priority to the wellness of their relative. When living through such a critical situation, family members often experience a state of confusion that leads them to reduce the time and self-care they would normally dedicate to themselves. Healthcare staff tends to underestimate the family's needs and often do not meet their requirements [30].

The needs of family members who have a relative in ICU have been investigated since the late 1970s. In 1979, Molter introduced the topic [31], and in 1983, together with Leske, he identified 45 items that could be used to measure the family needs in ICU [31]. Numerous studies have been based on this scale and have documented the needs of family members using the *Critical Care Family Needs Inventory* (CCFNI) both in its original and modified forms, which have also been translated in several languages [32–42]. Studies agree that the CCFNI is a valid diagnostic tool in the evaluation of the family needs, as it provides a systematic methodology to assess the needs of the relatives of people admitted to ICU during the period of their hospitalization [33]. The original CCFNI items [31] are shown in Table 16.1.

Wives of people admitted to ICU need to feel useful and close to their partner, although a proximity that is too close and prolonged can put family members at risk of developing pathologies correlated to the emotional load they are continually being subjected to [43].

**Table 16.1** Original Molter and Leske critical care family needs inventory [31]

| ID | Category | Need |
|----|----------|------|
| 01 | (A) | To know the expected outcome |
| 02 | (S) | To have explanations of the environment before going into the critical care unit for the first time |
| 03 | (I) | To talk to the doctor every day |
| 04 | (I) | To have specific person to call at the hospital |
| 05 | (A) | To have questions answered honestly |
| 06 | (P) | To have visiting hours changed for special conditions |
| 07 | (S) | To talk about feelings about what has happened |
| 08 | (C) | To have good food available while in the hospital |
| 09 | (S) | To have directions as to what to do at the bedside |
| 10 | (P) | To visit at any time |
| 11 | (I) | To know which staff members could give what information |
| 12 | (S) | To have friends nearby for support |
| 13 | (I) | To know why things were done for a patient |
| 14 | (A) | To feel there is hope |
| 15 | (I) | To know about the types of staff members taking care of the patient |
| 16 | (I) | To know how patient is being treated medically |
| 17 | (A) | To be assured the best possible care is being given |
| 18 | (S) | To have a place to be alone while in the hospital |
| 19 | (I) | To know exactly what is being done for patient |
| 20 | (C) | To have comfortable furniture in the waiting room |
| 21 | (C) | To feel accepted by the hospital staff |
| 22 | (S) | To have someone to help with financial problems |
| 23 | (C) | To have a telephone near the waiting room |
| 24 | (S) | To have a pastor visit |
| 25 | (S) | To talk about the possibility of the patient's death |
| 26 | (S) | To have another person with you when visiting critical care unit |
| 27 | (S) | To have someone be concerned with your health |
| 28 | (C) | To be assured it is all right to leave the hospital for a while |
| 29 | (P) | To talk to the same nurse every day |

**Table 16.1**  (continued)

| ID | Category | Need |
|----|----------|------|
| 30 | (S) | To feel it is all right to cry |
| 31 | (S) | To be told about people who could help with problems |
| 32 | (C) | To have a bathroom near the waiting room |
| 33 | (S) | To be alone at any time |
| 34 | (S) | To be told about someone to help with family problems |
| 35 | (A) | To have explanations given that are understandable |
| 36 | (P) | To have visiting hours start on time |
| 37 | (I) | To be told about chaplain services |
| 38 | (I) | To help with the patient's physical care |
| 39 | (P) | To be told about transfer plans while they are being made |
| 40 | (P) | To be called at home about changes in the condition |
| 41 | (P) | To receive information about patient once a day |
| 42 | (A) | To feel that hospital personnel care about patient |
| 43 | (A) | To know specific facts concerning patient's progress |
| 44 | (P) | To see the patient frequently |
| 45 | (P) | To have the waiting room near the patient |

Category of needs: *information* (I), *comfort* (C), *support* (S), *assurance and anxiety reduction* (A), *proximity and accessibility* (P)

Interpreting the needs of family members is not easy for healthcare professionals. A small Spanish study found that professionals overestimate the needs of family members with respect to noise, lighting, comfort, privacy, adequacy of the waiting room, and information about treatment. However, professionals mistakenly think that the family is adequately informed regarding the presence and function of technological equipment and that they know the name of the nurse who has them in charge. In other words, the satisfaction of family members was greater than supposed by the healthcare professionals who took part in the study. Both family members and healthcare professionals recognized the need to improve the comfort of the waiting room, to customize care, and to assess individual flexibility about visiting hours [44].

In Sweden Engström and Söderberg conducted a qualitative study based on interviews to describe the experiences of people whose partner had been admitted into the ICU [45]. From the thematic analysis of the content of the interviews, three themes emerged: "be present," "put oneself into the background," and "living in conditions of uncertainty." Respondents defined the experience of seeing their partner in ICU as "shocking." They found that the most important thing was to be present. Receiving confirmation of the physical integrity and dignity of the partners was also considered important, as was getting support from other family members and friends, understanding and acceptance of "what had happened," obtaining information from health professionals, and the methods of communication.

Enduring a state of deep uncertainty with respect to the outcome for the sick person was considered difficult by the respondents, who wished to maintain hope even when the prognosis was poor [45].

To conclude, people who are close to patients in ICU (be they family members, spouses, relatives, or significant others) represent one of the actors of the care and treatment process, with their own patterns of needs that must be considered. The American College of Critical Care Medicine Task Force 2004–2005 issued practical guidelines for family support in ICU, which are centered on the patient. The 43 recommendations include:

- A decision-making model
- Early and repeated conversations with the family to reduce stress and improve the consistency in communication
- Honest and culturally appropriate attitudes toward requesting the truth and in respect of informed consent
- Spiritual support
- Training for staff and debriefing moments to minimize the impact of the interactions with the family on the health of the healthcare personnel
- Presence of the family members both during duty time and critical times such as cardiopulmonary resuscitation
- Flexible visiting hours

- Friendly information methods and signage
- Family support before, during, and after death [46]

## 16.2.3   Patient Point of View

The studies about the effects of open visiting policies on patients are less numerous than those on family members. In particular, these studies are mainly observational. In this context, Fumagalli and colleagues in 2006 [47] designed a randomized pilot study to compare the complications arising from nonrestrictive visiting policies (a single visitor with frequency and hours chosen by the patient) with restrictive visiting policies (a single visitor for 30 min, twice a day). The study, which enrolled 226 users, was carried out over 2 years, alternating restrictive and nonrestrictive policies for periods of 2 months. The levels of environmental microbial contamination, sepsis, cardiovascular complications, emotional profile, and response to stress hormones were systematically detected. In people enrolled in the periods of nonrestrictive visiting policies, high levels of environmental microbial contamination were found. Despite this, the septic complications were similar in the two periods. The risk of cardiovascular complications was 50% lower in periods with nonrestrictive visiting policies. Furthermore, periods of nonrestrictive visiting policies have been associated with a large reduction in anxiety scores and a significantly lower secretion of thyroid-stimulating hormone (TSH), from admission to discharge.

In the face of the apparent advantages, for which additional studies are needed, understanding preferences of patients in regard to the visits of their families is crucial. The patients clearly identified the value of visits and specified that they were very satisfied with the flexibility of visiting hours. Flexibility is applied to positively respond to the needs of the patients and to those of their family members. The patients appreciated that having their family close was important to convey the significance of the care provided to them by the staff and indicated that the periods in which visitors should not be allowed to access the ward were those when they were unsure of the routine of the day, when they did not feel well, and when the dynamics of the family or other visitors were not optimal. The patients asked that visitors were excluded from entering the ICU in the early morning and late evening, at times when they would try to rest, when there was a diagnostic-therapeutic procedure scheduled, or when they had an opportunity to speak to the doctor [48].

## 16.2.4   Healthcare Professional Beliefs and Attitudes

In ICUs that already apply open visiting policies, the presence of relatives near the patient is perceived as normal and the absence of them causes frustration for patients. The information provided by relatives lead to the development of a truly individualized care. Nurses support relatives, providing them with information, being close to them, and trying to create a positive relationship. Relatives are important: their presence is the necessary prerequisite to critical quality nursing care and to understand the needs of patients admitted to the ICU [49]. Several studies have been conducted to investigate these dynamics. All of them originate from the models proposed by Kirchoff and Simpson [50, 51] with self-administered questionnaires for healthcare professionals working in ICUs, composed both of Likert scales and semantic differential scales that rely on the "theory of reasoned action" of Fishbein and Ajzen [52] (Fig. 16.2). According to this theory, the intention of a person, which precedes behaviors, is based on two elements: one is individual, while the other reflects social influence. The individual element is about positive or negative evaluation, i.e., the

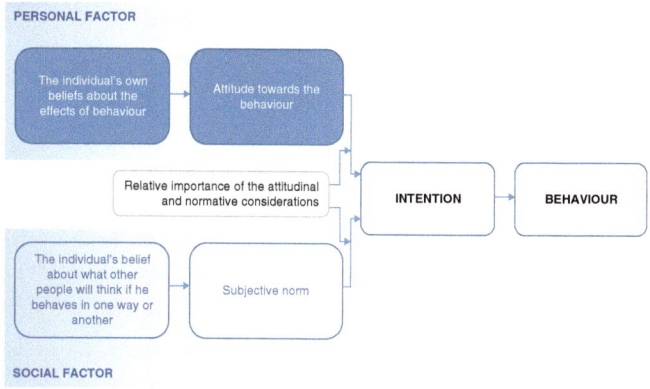

**Fig. 16.2** Operating model of Ajzen and Fishbein's theory of reasoned action [52]

attitude of the individual toward specific behaviors, called behavioral belief. The social factor is determined by the perception of social pressure that a person feels when they behave in a certain way. Several authors [21, 53, 54] identify the success of open policy initiatives of ICUs in the positive correlation between attitudes and beliefs of nurses in regard to the positive effects of the open visiting hours on patients, family members, and nurses [52].

In 2007, Berti [21] administered two different questionnaires to a large sample of nurses in the territory of Flanders: the first detected the visiting policies in 23 hospitals; the second, called *beliefs and attitudes toward visitation in the ICU* questionnaire (BAVIQ), which was structured on scales according to five levels, detected the beliefs and attitudes of nurses in relation to visiting policies in ICUs [21]. Although with some limitations, stated by the author, the study suggests that ICU nurses show slight skepticism toward open visiting policies in ICUs. The author identifies in these considerations an obstacle to those hospitals that wish to adopt open visiting policies in their ICU, in line with previous empirical experiences.

In 2008 Garrouste-Orgeas [55], in France, expanded the study not only to ICUs nurses but to a cohort of 209 patients, 149 families, and 43 healthcare workers. The study confirmed that the open visiting policy, even at 24 h, is favorably perceived by the family but induces a moderate discomfort in healthcare workers. This is particularly due to interruptions in the work, especially for nurses. Similar results were achieved by applying the BAVIQ to several samples, as performed by Melotti in 2009 [8], Biancofiore in 2010 [56], and Spreen in 2011 [23].

## 16.2.5   Visiting Hours, Number of Visits, and Number of Visitors

Restrictive visiting policies principally mean restricted visiting hours and number of visitors. Several studies have reported a varied spectrum of positions toward the issue of visiting hours. Besides many experiences of ICUs open to visitors during most of the day, there are settings where visits are allowed for less than an hour a day (Table 16.2).

More frequent visits and longer durations are likely associated with the creation of more opportunities for communication, greater individualization of care, and the implementation of a more supportive role of professionals in regard to the needs of the patient and the family.

## 16.2.6   Presence of Children Visitors

Up until recently, the needs of children visiting an adult in ICU have not been taken fully into consideration in the determination of the model of family-centered care and have not been the

**Table 16.2** Synopsys of studies for ICU visiting hours, number of visits, and number of visitors

| | | Most frequent | | | |
|---|---|---|---|---|---|
| Year | Country | Visit time | Visit number | Visitors | Reference |
| 2003 | Spain | 0.5–1 h | 2 | 1–3 | Velasco Bueno, 2005 [18] |
| 2005 | USA | 5–10 min | 1 | 2 | Farrel, 2005 [57] |
| 2006 | UK | 2.5–3 h | 1–2 | 1 | Thalanany, 2006 [58] |
| 2007 | Sweden | 1–19 h | 1–3 | 1–4 | Eriksson, 2007 [59] |
| 2008 | France | 1–2 h | 1 | 1–5 | Gaorrouste-Orgeas, 2008 [55] |
| 2008 | Italy | 1 h | 1–2 | 1–2 | Giannini, 2008 [20] |
| 2010 | UK | >4 h | 2 | – | Hunter, 2010 [60] |
| 2011 | Netherlands | 0.5–1.5 h | – | – | Spreen, 2011 [23] |
| 2012 | Netherlands | 2 h | 2 | – | Noordermeer, 2012 [61] |

subject of specific literature. However, a series of studies would be required to develop and assess the appropriate support to children visiting ICUs, to identify any potential negative effects. This approach is essential to enable training for the team and to develop and provide adequate support to meet the needs of the visiting children [62]. Papers reporting the access of children as visitors in ICUs revealed very different rules. Children aged 12 years or younger are not allowed to enter in 91% of ICUs in the USA or in 78% in the northeast of Italy [19, 63]. There is also total ban on access for children of any age in 69% of Italian ICUs, in 11% of French ICUs, and in 9% of Flemish ICUs [3, 17, 20, 22].

Children's access to ICUs is still a controversial theme. In 2006, a Swedish study revealed that most respondents were in favor of children's access to ICUs, although with some restrictions. Restrictions were linked to the severity of the patient's injuries, to the emotional environment that is considered inappropriate for a child, and to the risk of infection. Professionals think that restrictions should be stricter for children under the age of seven. Doctors and nurses have different views and motivations on this issue: this shows that the dynamics are complex, and this might be attributed to a different vision of care [28].

Some nurses in adult ICUs restrict visits of children and adolescents based on their intuition on how children might experience shock at what they might see or on the basis of the worry about not being able to control events. These prejudices are not based on evidence or on the needs of the patients [60, 64]. However, when children are allowed to visit the ICU, those who are adequately prepared have a less negative behaviors and show less emotional changes than those who are not allowed to enter [65, 66]. The ACCN recommends that visits of children and young people should be allowed in the absence of infectious diseases [67].

## 16.2.7   Family Presence During CPR and Invasive Procedures

European guidelines on resuscitation [68] favor the presence of family members during cardiopulmonary resuscitation (CPR). This practice is often discouraged by paternalistic attitudes and conjecture [69, 70]. In recent years, however, healthcare providers are increasingly offering family members the opportunity to remain present during such resuscitation maneuvers. Moreover, public opinion increasingly supports the possibility for family members to remain with their loved ones during CPR, regardless of the patient's outcome [71].

Although the trend is changing, the presence of family members during CPR remains a controversial issue. Major concerns are the potential impact of the presence of family members on the performance of resuscitation staff, the possibility that a family might experience negative emotions to develop psychological problems, and the free choice about being present or not during CPR. Possible benefits include the development of a bond with the resuscitation team, creating a much more human atmosphere than might otherwise happen when this medical practice is performed in a closed environment, and satisfaction of knowing that the loved one is in good hands.

Two European surveys, undertaken in cooperation with EfCCNa and ESPNIC Nursing, investigated the experiences and opinions of nurses working in three areas (pediatric, neonatal, and adult critical care) about the presence of family members during resuscitation [72]. These studies showed that many European critical care nurses favor the presence of family members during CPR. However, only a limited number of ICUs have codified procedures during resuscitation, including a guide to the presence of family. Consequently, the recommendation emerging from both studies is the need to conduct wider European studies on these issues.

The recommendations of the American Emergency Nursing Association and Association of Critical-Care Nurses [73, 74] suggest that the presence of family members during emergency procedures can have positive effects and that it is an opportunity that must be offered, although not necessarily mandatorily. The presence of family members at the scene of an emergency does not interfere with the performance of the staff but requires dedicated professionals to manage explanations and comfort. It is necessary that the process is encoded in a special procedure and the staff must be appropriately trained.

## 16.2.8  Visitors' Dressing and Infectious Chain

One of the most common objections to the opening of ICUs to visitors is the worry linked to possible infections. Despite the lack of empirical evidence, many healthcare professionals think that the opening of visiting policies could generate an increased risk of infections for patients [4, 20, 47]. In ICUs, both structural features and the maintenance of a clean environment are important in the fight against hospital-acquired infections [75]. It is often assumed that the transmission of microorganisms—so-called cross infection from visitors—is generated by the presence of visitors. Also, visitors are at risk of acquiring infections from the ICU environment [17].

Malacarne [76] performed an observational pilot study to test the hypothesis that family members of hospitalized people could be a pathogenic reservoir with the ability to transmit infections to patients by causing colonization or hospital infections. Visitors were required to wash their hands at the entrance and to wear a disposable coverall. They were not required to wear shoe covers, gloves, or masks. They were asked to wash their hands again upon exiting the ward. The ICU has been subjected to a health surveillance process. Visitors, for a few months, underwent nasal and hand swabs at the entrance and after hand-washing. The intersection of microorganisms in samples taken from visitors and those of health monitoring of patients showed that none of the microorganisms responsible for hospital-acquired infections had been found on the skin or in the nostrils of family members or visitors. No correlation was found between the isolated microorganisms from routine surveillance cultures of patients and those colonizing or contaminating patients' family members or other visitors. A nonrestrictive visiting policy caused greater microbial and environmental contamination but did not increase the risk of infectious complications [47]. The isolated microorganisms from patients were not the same as those transferred by the visitors, and the exposure of patients to those germs did not increase the risk of contamination when hands were properly washed at the entrance to the ICU [76]. In a "before-after" study, the main finding was that the shift from a restricted visiting policy to a partially unrestricted visiting policy was not associated with an increased rate of ICU-acquired infections [77].

The procedure of wearing disposable coveralls is often considered a "rite" by visitors (Fig. 16.3) [75] and is not supported by any

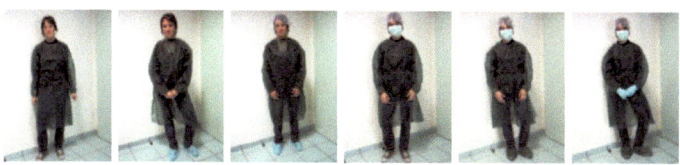

**Fig. 16.3** ICU dressing is defined by Mongardi et al., 2008 [75], "a ritual" with many "liturgical" variations

scientific evidence. In the neonatal settings, the wearing or not wearing of disposable coveralls did not affect the rate of infections related to the assistance, yet it entailed an increase in the use of resources (use of materials and involvement of healthcare professionals) [78–80]. Also in adult ICUs, the use of protective clothing (gloves, shoe covers, and masks) by visitors, although not a recommended infection control measure, is mandated in a large majority of French and Italian ICUs [17, 20]. It is surprising that hand-washing, recommended as the most important infection-prevention measure, is not required in 35% of Italian ICUs [10].

As for the visits to patients with infectious-contagious diseases or based on multiresistant bacteria, it is necessary to adopt specific measures in relation to the modes of transmission of the disease and similarly for visits to patients who have severely compromised immune systems following organ transplants, radiotherapy, or chemotherapy [75].

## 16.3   Conclusions

In the aforementioned work by Burchardi, "Let's open the door!," the experience of his team is reported as follows: "After many years of experience our intensive care staff is satisfied with an open ICU" [4]. The change requires a bit of adaptation, in particular for the nursing staff, which is usually in contact more directly with the families of patients. However, this is not the time to go backwards. It is time to recognize that ICUs should be places where humanity has high priority. It is time to open ICUs that are still closed, as all the people involved—patients, families, and the entire intensive care staff—will benefit from it. Advantages and disadvantages of an open visiting policy are summarized in Table 16.3.

ICUs must no longer be a reserved area. Welcoming families and visitors to the ICU is not a concession to the patient. Instead, through this action, healthcare professionals can recognize specific rights. Reevaluating rituals and rules of a well-established tradition can make a difference for ICU patients and their families. The complex and highly technological environment of the ICU can become a welcoming place that meets the needs of patients and families and where "Humanity is a top priority" [10]. Many and important institutional bodies representing citizens, nurses, medical doctors, and, even, governments agree. In the healthcare sector, choices and the reasons behind open visiting policies must be evaluated to assess their ethical acceptability. Table 16.4 shows the key points expressed by various scientific societies, institutions, and bioethics committees.

**Table 16.3** Advantages and disadvantages of opening a visiting policy in ICUs (inspired by Berti et al. 2007 [21])

| | Advantages of an open visiting policy | Disadvantages of an open visiting policy |
|---|---|---|
| Patient | Increased satisfaction | Poor sleep |
| | Stress reduction and increased calmness | Nurses have less time for patients |
| | Positive psychological effects | Negative psychological consequences |
| | Positive cardiovascular effects | |
| Family | Stress reduction | Family members perceive "obligation" to stay |
| | Anxiety reduction | |
| | Visits according to their needs | |
| | Better information | |
| Health professionals | Increased job satisfaction of nurses for a positive feedback from family | Ongoing evaluation of family needs |
| | The family as a support structure with increased ability to conduct health education and improve communication between families and professionals | Nurses' stress increase |
| | Improves nursing care with the possibility of finding valuable information | Adverse effects on the action of nurses (distraction, perception of discomfort, difficulty in expressing themselves freely) |

(continued)

**Table 16.3** (continued)

| | Advantages of an open visiting policy | Disadvantages of an open visiting policy |
|---|---|---|
| Health organization | | Counterproductive effects on the operating unit operation (hustle, bustle, visitors "between the feet") |
| | | Stop or postpone care procedures |

**Table 16.4** "Key points from recommendations and position statements on visiting in the ICU made by scientific societies, institutions, and committees" in Giannini et al. 2014 [10]

| Document | Country | Year | Key points |
|---|---|---|---|
| American College of Critical Care Medicine (ACCM) and Society of Critical Care Medicine (SCCM) | USA | 2007 | • Open visiting in the adult ICU allows flexibility for patients and families and is determined on a case-by-case basis<br>• Patient, family, and nurse determine the visitation schedule collectively taking into account the best interest of the patient<br>• Visiting in the PICU and NICU is open to parents and guardians 24 h a day<br>• Pets are allowed to visit the ICU if they are clean and properly immunized<br>• ICU caregivers receive training in:<br>  – Communication, conflict management, and meeting facilitation skills<br>  – Assessment of family needs and family members' stress and anxiety levels |

**Table 16.4** (continued)

| | | | |
|---|---|---|---|
| Institute for Patient- and Family- Centered Care | USA | 2010 | • Develop visiting guidelines supporting the presence of family based on patient's preferences<br>• Acknowledge the important role of families and other "partners in care" in the care process, and use language of partnership, support, and mutual respect<br>• Identify learning needs of staff to support change in practice and provide education |
| American Association of Critical-Care Nurses (AACN) | USA | 2011 | • Facilitate unrestricted access of hospitalized patients to a chosen support person (e.g., family member, friend, or trusted individual) according to patient preference<br>• Ensure a written protocol for allowing a patient's support person to be at the bedside<br>• Ensure that policies prohibit discrimination based on age, race, ethnicity, religion, culture, etc. |

(continued)

**Table 16.4** (continued)

| Document | Country | Year | Key points |
|---|---|---|---|
| British Association of Critical Care Nurses (BACCN) | UK | 2012 | • Patients should expect:<br>  – To have their privacy, dignity, and cultural beliefs recognized<br>  – The choice of whether or not to have visitors<br>  – The choice to decide who they want to visit including children and other loved ones<br>  – The choice of care assisted by their relatives<br>  – A critical care team who recognize the importance and value of visiting<br>• Relatives should have:<br>  – Access to (written) information regarding critical illness, aftercare, and support<br>  – Timely information and regular updates about the patient's condition<br>  – A comfortable and accessible waiting room<br>  – An area for private discussions with health professionals |

**Table 16.4** (continued)

| | | | |
|---|---|---|---|
| National Committee for Bioethics | Italy | 2013 | • ICU organization must promote the right of patients to have near them their family members or loved ones<br>• Patients must be consulted as to which persons they want to have near them<br>• Family members must be given the possibility of being close to the patient in ICU<br>• ICU doctors and nurses need appropriate training (communication skills, conflict management, etc.)<br>• The health authority must undertake to promote and support implementation of the "open" ICU model |

[a]Davidson et al. [81]
[b]Institute for Patient- and Family-Centered Care [82]
[c]American Association of Critical-Care Nurses [83]
[d]Gibson et al. [84]
[e]Comitato Nazionale per la Bioetica [85]

# References

1. Lusardi R. Corpi, Tecnologie e pratiche di cura. Uno studio etnografico in terapia intensiva. Milan: Franco Angeli; 2012.
2. Kelly FE, Fong K, Hirsch N, Nolan JP. Intensive care medicine is 60 years old: the history and future of the intensive care unit. Clin Med (Lond). 2014;14:376–9. https://doi.org/10.7861/clinmedicine.14-4-376.
3. Cappellini E, Bambi S, Lucchini A, Milanesio E. Open intensive care units: a global challenge for patients, relatives, and critical care teams. Dimens Crit Care Nurs. 2014;33:181–93. https://doi.org/10.1097/DCC.0000000000000052.
4. Burchardi H. Let's open the door! Intensive Care Med. 2002;28:1371–2. https://doi.org/10.1007/s00134-002-1401-8.
5. Garden R. Who speaks for whom? Health humanities and the ethics of representation. Med Humanit. 2015;41:77–80. https://doi.org/10.1136/medhum-2014-010642.
6. Dias GT, Souza JS, Barçante TA, Franco LM. Humanization of health assistance in intensive care units: a real possibility. J Nurs UFPE line. 2010;4:941–7. https://doi.org/10.5205/01012007.
7. Fave AD, Marsicano S. L'umanizzazione dell'ospedale: riflessioni ed esperienze. Milan: Franco Angeli; 2004.
8. Melotti RM, Bergonzi A, Benedetti A, Bonarelli S, Campione F, Canestrario S, et al. Progetto umanizzazione delle cure e dignità della persona in terapia intensiva della Regione Emilia-Romagna. Anestesia. Forum. 2009;2:75–82.
9. Mistraletti G. HEROIC bundle, humanization to enhance recovery on intensive care. 2016. http://www.heroicbundle.org/. Accessed 25 Sep 2016.
10. Giannini A, Garrouste-Orgeas M, Latour JM. What's new in ICU visiting policies: can we continue to keep the doors closed? Intensive Care Med. 2014;40:730–3. https://doi.org/10.1007/s00134-014-3267-y.
11. Sims JM, Miracle VA. A look at critical care visitation: the case for flexible visitation. Dimens Crit Care Nurs. 2006;25:175–80.
12. Youngner SJ, Coulton C, Welton R, Juknialis B, Jackson DL. ICU visiting policies. Crit Care Med. 1984;12:606–8.
13. Berwick DM, Kotagal M. Restricted visiting hours in ICUs: time to change. JAMA. 2004;292:736–7. https://doi.org/10.1001/jama.292.6.736.
14. Farrell MEMG. An exploration of the nature of nursing practice related to the presence of visitors in the critical care setting. Kingston: University of Rhode Island; 2002.

15. Slota M, Shearn D, Potersnak K, Haas L. Perspectives on family-centered, flexible visitation in the intensive care unit setting. Crit Care Med. 2003;31:S362–6. https://doi.org/10.1097/01.CCM.0000065276. 61814.B2.
16. Roland P, Russell J, Richards KC, Sullivan SC. Visitation in critical care: processes and outcomes of a performance improvement initiative. J Nurs Care Qual. 2001;15:18–26.
17. Quinio P, Savry C, Deghelt A, Guilloux M, Catineau J, de Tinteniac A. A multicenter survey of visiting policies in French intensive care units. Intensive Care Med. 2002;28:1389–94. https://doi.org/10.1007/s00134-002-1402-7.
18. Velasco Bueno JM, Prieto de Paula JF, Castillo Morales J, Merino Nogales N, Perea-Milla Lopez E. Organization of visits in Spanish ICU. Enferm Intensiva. 2005;16:73–83.
19. Lee MD, Friedenberg AS, Mukpo DH, Conray K, Palmisciano A, Levy MM. Visiting hours policies in New England intensive care units: strategies for improvement. Crit Care Med. 2007;35:497–501. https://doi.org/10.1097/01.CCM.0000254338.87182.AC.
20. Giannini A, Miccinesi G, Leoncino S. Visiting policies in Italian intensive care units: a nationwide survey. Intensive Care Med. 2008;34:1256–62. https://doi.org/10.1007/s00134-008-1037-4.
21. Berti D, Ferdinande P, Moons P. Beliefs and attitudes of intensive care nurses toward visits and open visiting policy. Intensive Care Med. 2007;33:1060–5. https://doi.org/10.1007/s00134-007-0599-x.
22. Vandijck DM, Labeau SO, Geerinckx CE, De Puydt E, Bolders AC, Claes B, et al. An evaluation of family-centered care services and organization of visiting policies in Belgian intensive care units: a multicenter survey. Heart Lung. 2010;39:137–46. https://doi.org/10.1016/j.hrtlng.2009.06.001.
23. Spreen AE, Schuurmans MJ. Visiting policies in the adult intensive care units: a complete survey of Dutch ICUs. Intensive Crit Care Nurs. 2011;27:27–30. https://doi.org/10.1016/j.iccn.2010.10.002.
24. Liu V, Read JL, Scruth E, Cheng E. Visitation policies and practices in US ICUs. Crit Care. 2013;17:R71. https://doi.org/10.1186/cc12677.
25. Zaforteza C, Gastaldo D, de Pedro JE, Sanchez-Cuenca P, Lastra P. The process of giving information to families of critically ill patients: a field of tension. Int J Nurs Stud. 2005;42:135–45. https://doi.org/10.1016/j.ijnurstu.2004.05.014.
26. Vincent JL. Communication in the ICU. Intensive Care Med. 1997;23:1093–8.
27. Bernat Adell MD, Tejedor López R, Sanchis Muñoz J. How well do patients' relatives evaluate and understand information provided by the intensive care unit? Enferm Intensiva. 2000;11:3–9.

28. Soderstrom IM, Saveman BI, Benzein E. Interactions between family members and staff in intensive care units--an observation and interview study. Int J Nurs Stud. 2006;43:707–16. https://doi.org/10.1016/j.ijnurstu.2005.10.005.

29. Fassier T, Darmon M, Laplace C, Chevret S, Schlemmer B, Pochard F, et al. One-day quantitative cross-sectional study of family information time in 90 intensive care units in France. Crit Care Med. 2007;35:177–83. https://doi.org/10.1097/01.CCM.0000249834.26847.BE.

30. Verhaeghe S, Defloor T, Van Zuuren F, Duijnstee M, Grypdonck M. The needs and experiences of family members of adult patients in an intensive care unit: a review of the literature. J Clin Nurs. 2005;14:501–9. https://doi.org/10.1111/j.1365-2702.2004.01081.x.

31. Molter NC, Leske JS. Critical care family needs inventory. Unpublished manuscript. 1983.

32. Bandari R, Heravi-Karimooi M, Rejeh N, Montazeri A, Zayeri F, Mirmohammadkhani M, et al. Psychometric properties of the Persian version of the Critical Care Family Needs Inventory. J Nurs Res. 2014;22:259–67. https://doi.org/10.1097/jnr.0000000000000057.

33. Bijttebier P, Delva D, Vanoost S, Bobbaers H, Lauwers P, Vertommen H. Reliability and validity of the Critical Care Family Needs Inventory in a Dutch-speaking Belgian sample. Heart Lung. 2000;29:278–86. https://doi.org/10.1067/mhl.2000.107918.

34. Chien WT, Ip WY, Lee IY. Psychometric properties of a Chinese version of the critical care family needs inventory. Res Nurs Health. 2005;28:474–87. https://doi.org/10.1002/nur.20103.

35. Coutu-Wakulczyk G, Chartier L. French validation of the critical care family needs inventory. Heart Lung. 1990;19:192–6.

36. Gomez-Martiinez S, Arnal RB, Julia BG. The short version of Critical Care Family Needs Inventory (CCFNI): adaptation and validation for a Spanish sample. An Sist Sanit Navar. 2011;34:349–61.

37. Harrington L. An evaluation of validity, reliability, and readability of the Critical Care Family Needs Inventory. Heart Lung. 1992;21:199–200.

38. Leske JS. Internal psychometric properties of the Critical Care Family Needs Inventory. Heart Lung. 1991;20:236–44.

39. Lopez-Fagin L. Critical Care Family Needs Inventory: a cognitive research utilization approach. Crit Care Nurse. 1995;15:23–6.

40. Macey BA, Bouman CC. An evaluation of validity, reliability, and readability of the Critical Care Family Needs Inventory. Heart Lung. 1991;20:398–403.

41. Padilla Fortunatti CF. Most important needs of family members of critical patients in light of the critical care family needs inventory. Invest

Educ Enferm. 2014;32:306–16. https://doi.org/10.1590/S0120-53072014000200013.

42. Redley B, Beanland C. Revising the critical care family needs inventory for the emergency department. J Adv Nurs. 2004;45:95–104.

43. Eldredge D. Helping at the bedside: spouses' preferences for helping critically ill patients. Res Nurs Health. 2004;27:307–21. https://doi.org/10.1002/nur.20033.

44. Santana Cabrera L, Sanchez Palacios M, Hernandez Medina E, Garcia Martul M, Eugenio Ronaina P, VillanuevaOrtiz A. Needs of the family of intensive care patients: perception of the family and the professional. Med Intensiva. 2007;31:273–80.

45. Engstrom A, Soderberg S. The experiences of partners of critically ill persons in an intensive care unit. Intensive Crit Care Nurs. 2004;20:299–308. https://doi.org/10.1016/j.iccn.2004.05.009.

46. Davidson JE, Powers K, Hedayat KM, Tieszen M, Kon AA, Shepard E, et al. Clinical practice guidelines for support of the family in the patient-centered intensive care unit: American College of Critical Care Medicine Task Force 2004-2005. Crit Care Med. 2007;35:605–22. https://doi.org/10.1097/01.CCM.0000254067.14607.EB.

47. Fumagalli S, Boncinelli L, Lo Nostro A, Valoti P, Baldereschi G, Di Bari M, et al. Reduced cardiocirculatory complications with unrestrictive visiting policy in an intensive care unit: results from a pilot, randomized trial. Circulation. 2006;113:946–52. https://doi.org/10.1161/CIRCULATIONAHA.105.572537.

48. Gonzalez CE, Carroll DL, Elliott JS, Fitzgerald PA, Vallent HJ. Visiting preferences of patients in the intensive care unit and in a complex care medical unit. Am J Crit Care. 2004;13:194–8.

49. Engström A, Söderberg S. Close relatives in intensive care from the perspective of critical care nurses. J Clin Nurs. 2007;16:1651. https://doi.org/10.1111/j.1365-2702.2005.01520.x.

50. Kirchhoff KT, Pugh E, Calame RM, Reynolds N. Nurses' beliefs and attitudes toward visiting in adult critical care settings. Am J Crit Care. 1993;2:238–45.

51. Simpson T, Wilson D, Mucken N, Martin S, West E, Guinn N. Implementation and evaluation of a liberalized visiting policy. Am J Crit Care. 1996;5:420–6.

52. Ajzen I, Fishbein M. Understanding attitudes and predicting social behavior. Upper Saddle River: Prentice-Hall; 1980.

53. Marco Landa L, Bermejillo Eguia I, Garayalde Fernandez de Pinedo N, Sarrate Adot I, Margall Coscojuela MA, Asiain Erro MC. Opinions and attitudes of intensive care nurses on the effect of open visits on patients, family members, and nurses. Enferm Intensiva. 2000;11:107–17.

54. Marco L, Bermejillo I, Garayalde N, Sarrate I, Margall MA, Asiain MC. Intensive care nurses' beliefs and attitudes towards the effect of open visiting on patients, family and nurses. Nurs Crit Care. 2006;11:33–41.

55. Garrouste-Orgeas M, Philippart F, Timsit JF, Diaw F, Willems V, Tabah A, et al. Perceptions of a 24-hour visiting policy in the intensive care unit. Crit Care Med. 2008;36:30–5. https://doi.org/10.1097/01.CCM.0000295310.29099.F8.

56. Biancofiore G, Bindi LM, Barsotti E, Menichini S, Baldini S. Open intensive care units: a regional survey about the beliefs and attitudes of health care professionals. Minerva Anestesiol. 2010;76:93–9.

57. Farrell ME, Joseph DH, Schwartz-Barcott D. Visiting hours in the ICU: finding the balance among patient, visitor and staff needs. Nurs Forum. 2005;40:18–28. https://doi.org/10.1111/j.1744-6198.2005.00001.x.

58. Thalanany MM, Mugford M, Mitchell-Inwang C. Visiting adult patients in intensive care: the importance of relatives' travel and time costs. Intensive Crit Care Nurs. 2006;22:40–8. https://doi.org/10.1016/j.iccn.2005.10.004.

59. Eriksson T, Bergbom I. Visits to intensive care unit patients--frequency, duration and impact on outcome. Nurs Crit Care. 2007;12:20–6. https://doi.org/10.1111/j.1478-5153.2006.00196.x.

60. Hunter JD, Goddard C, Rothwell M, Ketharaju S, Cooper H. A survey of intensive care unit visiting policies in the United Kingdom. Anaesthesia. 2010;65:1101–5. https://doi.org/10.1111/j.1365-2044.2010.06506.x.

61. Noordermeer K, Rijpstra TA, Newhall D, Pelle AJM, Van der Meer NJM. Visiting policies in the adult intensive care units in the Netherlands: survey among ICU directors. ISRN Critical.

62. Clarke C, Harrison D. The needs of children visiting on adult intensive care units: a review of the literature and recommendations for practice. J Adv Nurs. 2001;34:61–8.

63. Anzoletti AB, Buja A, Bortolusso V, Zampieron A. Access to intensive care units: a survey in North-East Italy. Intensive Crit Care Nurs. 2008;24:366–74. https://doi.org/10.1016/j.iccn.2008.04.004.

64. Smith L, Medves J, Harrison MB, Tranmer J, Waytuck B. The impact of hospital visiting hour policies on pediatric and adult patients and their visitors. JBI Libr Syst Rev. 2009;7:38–79. https://doi.org/10.11124/jbisrir-2009-181.

65. Plowright C. Visiting practices in hospitals. Nurs Crit Care. 2007;12:61–3. https://doi.org/10.1111/j.1478-5153.2007.00218.x.

66. Kean S. Children and young people visiting an adult intensive care unit. J Adv Nurs. 2010;66:868–77. https://doi.org/10.1111/j.1365-2648.2009.05252.x.

67. Practice Alert ACCN. Family Presence: visitation in the Adult ICU. Crit Care Nurse. 2012;32:76–8.

68. Baskett PJ, Steen PA, Bossaert L, European Resuscitation Council. European Resuscitation Council guidelines for resuscitation 2005. Section 8. The ethics of resuscitation and end-of-life decisions. Resuscitation. 2005;67:S171–80. https://doi.org/10.1016/j.resuscitation.2005.10.005.

69. Walker WM. Do relatives have a right to witness resuscitation? J Clin Nurs. 1999;8:625–30.

70. Boyd R. Witnessed resuscitation by relatives. Resuscitation. 2000;43:171–6.

71. Mazer MA, Cox LA, Capon JA. The public's attitude and perception concerning witnessed cardiopulmonary resuscitation. Crit Care Med. 2006;34:2925–8. https://doi.org/10.1097/01.CCM.0000247720.99299.77.

72. Fulbrook P, Albarran JW, Latour JM. A European survey of critical care nurses' attitudes and experiences of having family members present during cardiopulmonary resuscitation. Int J Nurs Stud. 2005;42:557–68. https://doi.org/10.1016/j.ijnurstu.2004.09.012.

73. Egging D, Crowley M, Arruda T, Proehl J, Walker-Cillo G, Papa A, et al. Emergency nursing resource: family presence during invasive procedures and resuscitation in the emergency department. J Emerg Nurs. 2011;37:469–73. https://doi.org/10.1016/j.jen.2011.04.012.

74. AACN Practice Alert. Family presence during resuscitation and invasive procedures. Crit Care Nurse. 2016;36:e11–4. https://doi.org/10.4037/ccn2016980.

75. Mongardi M, Melotti R, Sonetti S, Moro ML. Il rito della "vestizione" per l'accesso dei visitatori nelle Unità di Terapia Intensiva: revisione della letteratura ed indicazioni operative. Scenario. 2008;25:30–4.

76. Malacarne P, Pini S, De Feo N. Relationship between pathogenic and colonizing microorganisms detected in intensive care unit patients and in their family members and visitors. Infect Control Hosp Epidemiol. 2008;29:679–81. https://doi.org/10.1086/588703.

77. Malacarne P, Corini M, Petri D. Health care-associated infections and visiting policy in an intensive care unit. Am J Infect Control. 2011;39:898–900. https://doi.org/10.1016/j.ajic.2011.02.018.

78. Eason S. Are cover gowns necessary in the NICU for parents and visitors? Neonatal Netw. 1995;14:50.

79. Webster J, Pritchard MA. Gowning by attendants and visitors in new born nurseries for prevention of neonatal morbidity and mortality. Cochrane Database Syst Rev. 2003;3:CD003670. https://doi.org/10.1002/14651858.CD003670.

80. Kostiuk N, Ramachandran C. Does gowning prevent infection in the NICU? Can Nurse. 2003;99:20–3.

81. Davidson JE, Powers K, Hedayat KM, Tieszen M, Kon AA, Shepard E, et al. Clinical practice guidelines for support of the family in the patient- centered intensive care unit: American College of Critical Care Medicine Task Force 2004–2005. Crit Care Med 2007;35:605–22.

82. Institute for Patient- and Family- Centered Care. Changing hospital "visiting" policies and practices: support family presence and participation. 2010. http://www.ipfcc.org/resources/visiting.pdf. Accessed 12 Feb 2017.

83. American Association of Critical Care Nurses. Family presence: visitation in the adult ICU. 2011. http://www.aacn.org/WD/practice/docs/practicealerts/family-visitation-adult-icu-practicealert.pdf. Accessed 29 Dec 2016.

84. Gibson V, Plowright C, Collins T, Dawson D, Evans S, Gibb P, et al. Position statement on visiting in adult critical care units in the UK. Nurs Crit Care 2012;17:213–8.

85. Comitato Nazionale per la Bioetica. Terapia intensiva "aperta" alle visite dei familiari. 2013. http://bioetica.governo.it/media/170725/p112_2013_terapia-intensiva-aperta_it.pdf. Accessed 20 Dec 2016.

# Part IV
# Future Perspectives in Intensive Care Nursing

# Chapter 17
# A Systemic Approach: ABCDEF Bundle

**Matteo Manici, Alessandra Negro, and Stefano Bambi**

## 17.1 Introduction

Aristotle said, "the whole is greater than the sum of its parts." *A care bundle* is a little set (3–5) of evidence-based interventions, behaviors, and/or practices, aimed at a specific category of patients and care settings, to improve the outcomes. The base of *bundle* concept is to apply jointly and correctly its single parts, improving the quality and outcome of healthcare processes with larger effects than those obtained if every strategy is implemented separately [1].

Since 1996 many studies have questioned: how can we reduce tube time and days of MV? How can we reduce ICU LOS? How can we reduce hospital LOS? How can we improve patients' survival rates? The answers were found in some practices as light level of sedation, protocol-led weaning from MV, spontaneous breathing trials, delirium prevention and management, and early mobility. The evolution of ABCDEF begun in the middle of the 1990s and is summarized in Table 17.1.

© Springer International Publishing AG, part of Springer Nature 2018     445
I. Comisso et al., *Nursing in Critical Care Setting*,
https://doi.org/10.1007/978-3-319-50559-6_17

**Table 17.1** Evolution of ABCDEF concept

| Year | Concept | Authors | Outcomes/messages |
|------|---------|---------|-------------------|
| 1996 | SBT protocol | Ely et al. [2] | −1.5 days MV |
| 2000 | SAT—daily sedative interruption | Kress et al. [3] | −2 days MV<br>−3.5 days ICU LOS |
| 2001 | CAM-ICU validated | Ely et al. [4] | Delirium prevalence 87% |
| 2002 | Sedation-analgesia guideline revision | Jacobi et al. [5] | |
| 2004 | ICU delirium mortality risk | Ely et al. [6] | 10% per day of delirium |
| 2005 | SAT and targeted sedation | Breen et al. [7] | −2.2 days MV |
| 2006 | Analgesia/sedation protocol titrated to BPS and RASS | Chanques et al. [8] | −21% pain<br>−17% agitation<br>−2.2 days MV<br>−50% infection rates |
| 2007 | Feasibility, safety of early mobilization in MV respiratory ICU patients | Bailey et al. [9] | |
| 2008 | SAT + SBT = ABC (awakening and breathing controlled trial) | Girard et al. [10] | −3 days MV<br>−4 days ICU and hospital LOS<br>−32% risk of death |
| 2008 | ABC + EM | Morris et al. [11] | −1.4 days ICU LOS<br>−3.3 days hospital LOS |
| 2010 | ABCDE protocol proposed | Vasilevskis et al. [12] | |
| 2010 | Duration of ICU delirium predicts long-term cognitive dysfunction | Girard et al. [13] | |

**Table 17.1**  (continued)

| Year | Concept | Authors | Outcomes/messages |
|------|---------|---------|-------------------|
| 2011 | Confirmation of ABCDE bundle as organizational approaches to improve the management of mechanically ventilated patients | Morandi et al. [14] | |
| 2013 | Revised PAD guidelines | Barr et al. [15] | |
| 2015 | Systematic review of strategies for delirium | Trogrlić et al. [16] | Strategies targeting ICU delirium assessment and prevention and treatment and integrated within PAD or ABCDE bundle have the potential to improve clinical outcomes |

The single studies aiming to implement specific practices should be seen as "improvement vectors" with different intensities, but having coordinated directions and orientations to a common goal. This target is the improvement of "hard" outcomes in ICU patients: morbidity and mortality rate reduction.

Therefore, the evidence-based *ABCDE bundle* is an integrated, systemic, and interdisciplinary approach to the management of MV patients. Spontaneous awakening and breathing trials have been combined into *awake and breathing coordination*, with the aim to reduce the duration of mechanical ventilation and ICU and hospital LOS and improve the survival rates. *Delirium monitoring* improves the recognition of this disorder, but data on pharmacologic treatment are conflicting. *Early mobility and exercise* may reduce physical dysfunction and delirium rates [14].

Many institutions have expressed the concept of ABCDE bundle (or ABCDEF bundle, if we insert also the family involvement in patient's care) in different practice guidelines. The main models are those released by the American Association of Critical-Care Nurses (ACCN) [17] and Society of Critical Care Medicine (SCCM) [18] (Table 17.2).

The following paragraphs describe the ABCDEF bundle as a mix of two different approaches, highlighting the main topics of each one.

## 17.2   Assess and Manage Pain

Adult ICU patients routinely experience pain, both at rest and during routine care such as turning or endotracheal suctioning. Lack of treatment of pain can result in many complications including delirium, while assessing pain is associated with better outcomes and lower use of sedative and hypnotic agents [19].

Pain is a concept already explored in Chap. 2 and well defined by pain, agitation, and delirium guidelines [15]. It should be routinely monitored in all adult ICU patients. Self-report scales are considered the "gold standard," and pain can be assessed in patients unable to communicate through the BPS or CPOT [20].

It is suggested that analgesia-first sedation should be used in MV adult ICU patients.

There's only one GRADE A1 PAD recommendation about pain management, concerning use of gabapentin or carbamazepine in addition to intravenous opioids, for treatment of neuropathic pain. The other recommendations are based on weak strength of evidence.

**Table 17.2** ACCN vs. SCCM model of ABCDE(F) bundle [17, 18]

| ACCN | Element | SCCM |
|---|---|---|
| **Awakening and breathing trial coordination** | A | **Assess, prevent, and manage pain** |
| Oversedation and undersedation can lead to prolonged ventilator times for patients. | | Recognize pain and find tools for its assessment, treatment, and prevention |
| *This "ABC" bundle component addresses daily* | B | **Both SAT and SBT** |
| *spontaneous awakening trials (sedation vacation)* | | Both spontaneous awakening trials and |
| *and spontaneous breathing trials to promote early* | | spontaneous breathing trails |
| *weaning and extubation* | C | **Choice of analgesia and sedation** |
| | | Recognize the importance of defining the depth of sedation, choosing the right medication |
| **Delirium assessment and management** | D | **Delirium: assess, prevent, and manage** |
| All of our patients are susceptible to developing delirium, often undetected and untreated in many patients, potentially leading to a host of negative long-term consequences. | | Recognize delirium risk factors and find tools for its assessment, treatment and prevention |
| *This "D" bundle component addresses early* | | |
| *identification and management of patients with* | | |
| *delirium* | | |

(continued)

**Table 17.2** (continued)

| ACCN | Element | SCCM |
|------|---------|------|
| **Early exercise and progressive mobility** | E | **Early mobility and exercise ICU** |
| All patients with prolonged bedrest or immobility are prone to developing muscle weakness and atrophy, which can lead to a longer hospital stay and long-term muscle dysfunction. | | Early mobility involves more than changing the patient's position |
| *This "E" bundle component provides guidance for enabling patients to become progressively more active and, possibly, walk while intubated* | | |
| | F | **Family engagement and empowerment** |
| | | Involving the family in patient care can help recovery |

## 17.3   Both Spontaneous Awakening Trial and Spontaneous Breathing Trial

The daily interruption of sedative administration (whether given by infusion or bolus doses) is combined with daily spontaneous breathing trials in the awakening and breathing controlled (ABC). A randomized controlled trial comparing a daily SAT + SBT protocol against a usual sedation + daily SBT approach showed a significant decrease in the 28-day and 1-year mortality in the intervention groups [10]. This set of interventions also significantly reduced the number of days on MV with a concomitant lessening in the LOS (4 days difference), when compared to SBT alone [10]. Lastly, although a higher proportion of patients in the intervention group self-extubated (10 vs. 4%, $p = 0.03$), the reintubation rates were not statistically different (3% against 2%, $p = 0.47$), showing that SAT + SBT was not less safe than traditional care [10].

The clinical practice guidelines for the management of pain, agitation, and delirium in adult patients in the intensive care unit recommend either daily sedation interruption or a light target level of sedation should be routinely used in mechanically ventilated adult ICU patients [21].

Both awakening and breathing trials are preceded by a safety screening to determine the possibility to stop sedatives and then to disconnect mechanical ventilation. The success of the trials is confirmed through a list of failure criteria. Many protocols for SAT-SBT are available in the web sites of hospitals and professional associations. An example of SAT/SBT strategies is synthesized in Fig. 17.1.

The American approach to SBT is performed using one of three breathing or ventilator modes reported in Table 17.3 [22]. The European approach is softer, acting a gradual weaning from ventilator supports, passing from PSV to T-piece, through CPAP systems. All methods/modes work without a clear superiority of no one [23].

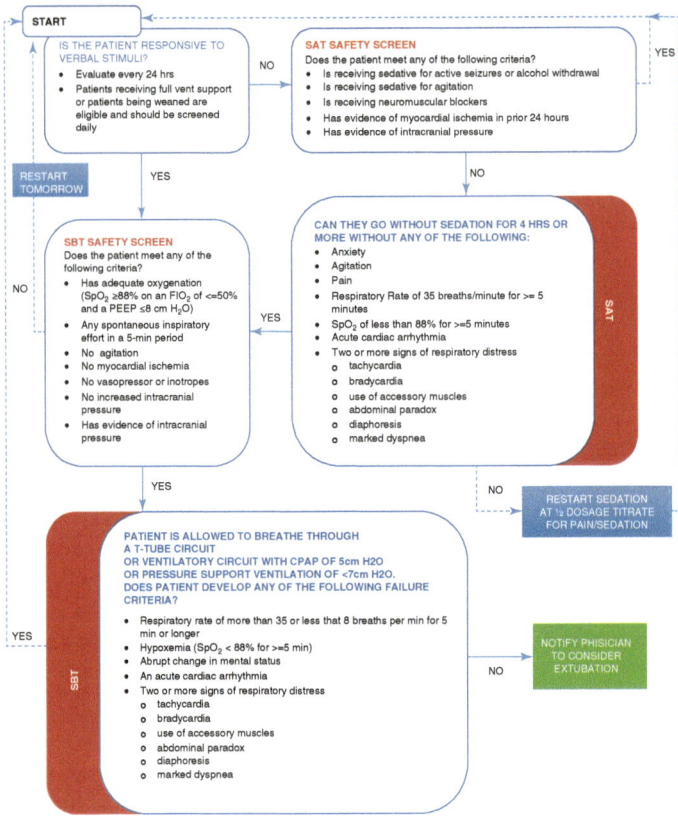

**Fig. 17.1** Spontaneous breathing trial (SBT) example of protocol adapted from Girard 2008 [10]

**Table 17.3** SBT methods/ventilator modes

| "American approach" Ventilator discontinuation: Stopping ventilator if unnecessary and placing | Breathing or ventilator methods/modes | "European approach" Weaning from ventilator: Reducing ventilator support by |
|---|---|---|
| In | PSV <7 cmH$_2$O, with or without PEEP | Progressive reduction PSV |
| Or in | CPAP 5 cmH$_2$O | Progressive reduction PEEP |
| Or in | T-piece (FiO$_2$ pre-SBT) | |

## 17.4  Coordination and Communication

ABCDEF bundle necessarily needs a multi-professional team to be implemented. Usually, in the USA, the team is composed of nurses, physicians, respiratory therapists, pharmacists, and physical therapists, while in the European ICUs, frequently the team is made up only by physicians and nurses.

Effective communication and teamwork are important non-technical skills that every component of the ICU team needs to develop [21].

The value of effective teamwork for the provision of safe, high-quality care in fast-paced and unpredictable environments, such as intensive care units, has been increasingly recognized [24].

The PAD guidelines recommend to implement an interdisciplinary ICU team approach that includes provider education, preprinted and/or computerized protocols and order forms, and quality ICU rounds checklists. This approach aims to facilitate the use of pain, agitation, and delirium management guidelines and protocols in adult ICUs [15].

Several barriers to the implementation process of the ABCDE bundle were identified in literature.

The ABCDEF bundle requires coordinated care and timing among the different professionals as well as effective communication. In many circumstances, this would be best achieved via a process of multidisciplinary rounds. Formalizing the process of interdisciplinary rounds proved to be a key element to both improving interprofessional communication and improving ABCDE compliance [25].

Balas et al. found that the biggest problem about coordination of care was related to the lack of consistent interdisciplinary rounds. Also, when the rounds did occur, ABCDE bundle-related interventions and outcomes were rarely discussed [25].

A systematic review identified several best practices for ICU patient care rounds to increase providers' satisfaction, reduce rounding time, and improve patients' outcomes [26]. These included:

- Interprofessional rounds (physician, nurse, and pharmacist at minimum)
- Standardized practices
- Defined roles for all participants
- Use of structured tools
- Reduced time spent on nonessential activities
- Minimized interruptions
- Development and documentation of daily goals
- Choice of the best location for the rounds (bedside vs. conference room) to optimize patient-centeredness and efficiency
- Establishment of an open and collaborative discussion environment

## 17.5   Delirium Assessment, Prevention, and Management

Delirium is a concept already being explored in Chap. 2, defined as a disturbance of consciousness with inattention, accompanied by a change in cognitive status, or perceptual disturbance that develops over a short period of time (hours to days) and fluctuates over time.

The implementation strategies to improve ICU clinicians' ability to effectively assess, prevent, and treat delirium and their effects on clinical outcomes were summarized in a recent literature review [16]. The authors concluded that multicomponent implementation including delirium-oriented interventions in critically ill patients can be useful [16]. Many studies reported improvements of both process outcomes (delirium screening adherence and knowledge) and clinical outcomes (short-term mortality and ICU LOS). Among the mentioned evidence-based interventions, early and progressive mobilization was the only intervention able to improve both delirium and clinical outcomes [16, 27].

Risk factors for delirium vary from patient to patient in ICU, and thus an individualized delirium prevention strategy should be sought. Nonetheless, three main risk factors are widespread in ICU settings: sedatives, immobility, and sleep disruption. These are often the result of clinical practice habits in most ICUs that should be changed focusing on delirium prevention. The delirium "preventive" strategies may be of benefit even in patients who have already developed this syndrome via their effect on duration of delirium [28]. The ABCDEF bundle combines the efforts to prevent delirium with the power to remind the importance of a patient- and family-centered care.

## 17.6 Early Mobilization

Early mobilization is a concept already explored in Chap. 5. A high proportion of survivors of critical illness suffer from significant physical, cognitive, and psychological disabilities. Profound neuromuscular weakness secondary to critical illness, prolonged bed rest, and immobility leads to impaired physical function. Physical impairment affects approximately 50% of

ICU patients, with at least half of discharged patients unable to return to premorbid levels of activity [29].

Cognitive impairment, including reduced executive function, memory, language, and attention, is widespread [30]. Evidence suggests that mobilization mitigates the physical, cognitive, and psychological complications of critical illness.

Mobilization has also been linked to decreased time on the ventilator [31], decreased LOS [32], and improved functional outcomes [33]. The mobilization of ICU patients is safe and feasible [34].

Serious adverse events following session of physical and occupational therapy in ICU patients are rarely reported, and only 4% of the sessions were interrupted for patient's instability (mainly due to asynchronies with mechanical ventilation) [27].

However, ICU patients are typically perceived as being too sick to tolerate activity. As a result they often have limited exposure to physical rehabilitation.

Protocols have been developed to describe and implement a safe and feasible early mobility practice, especially in the American context. In Europe where there is a frequent lack of physiotherapists dedicated to ICUs, nurses become protagonists in the implementation and guide of the mobilization of ICU patients. Tools, such as those represented in Table 17.4 , can be useful to assist nurses in implementing mobility programs. Patients admitted to ICU should be evaluated within the first 8 h and every day for a safety screening (neurological, respiratory, and hemodynamic assessment) and then be included in the mobility protocol.

## 17.7   Family Engagement

The term "family" refers to persons related in any way (not only biologically but also legally or emotionally) to patients.

**Table 17.4** Example of early mobilization protocol [35]

| | | | | | Walking |
|---|---|---|---|---|---|
| | | | | Out of bed twice a day | Out of bed twice a day |
| | | | Dangling twice a day | Dangling twice a day | Dangling twice a day |
| | | HOB 80° X 30' + At least once a shift | HOB 80° X 30' + At least once a shift | HOB 80° X 30' + At least once a shift | HOB 80° X 30' + At least once a shift |
| | HOB 60° X 30 min At least once a shift | HOB 60° X 30 min At least once a shift | HOB 60° X 30 min At least once a shift | HOB 60° X 30 min At least once a shift | HOB 60° X 30 min At least once a shift |
| HOB 30-45° + Lateral decubitus min once a shift | HOB 30-45° + Lateral decubitus min once a shift | HOB 30-45° + Lateral decubitus min once a shift | HOB 30-45° + Lateral decubitus min once a shift | HOB 30-45° + Lateral decubitus min once a shift | HOB 30-45° + Lateral decubitus min once a shift |
| Level 1 | Level 2 | Level 3 | Level 4 | Level 5 | Level 6 |
| RASS   -5 | -4 | -3 | -2 | -1 | 0 |
| SAS   1 | 1 | 3 | 3 | 3 | 4 |
| Consider, if possible | Transcutaneous electrical muscle stimulation (TEMS) | | | | |
| | | Consider, if possible | Passive Cycle ergometer | | |
| | | | | Consider, if possible | Passive Cycle ergometer |

Sedation max

Unrestricted visitation and participation of a significant others (i.e., *family* as defined by the patient) can improve the safety of care and enhance patient and family satisfaction. This is especially true in ICU, where patients are usually intubated and cannot independently express their will. Unrestricted visitation from significant others can improve communication, facilitate a better understanding of the patient, advance patient- and family-centered care, and enhance staff satisfaction [36].

Family engagement comprises not only the interesting debate about visitation hours but more importantly how to involve significant others in the care of patients. McAdam et al. identified five roles that families take in the care of patients that were at high risk for dying in the ICU setting. These roles were [37]:

- To be an active presence for the patient, who facilitates communication and offers important personal and clinical information about the patient
- To be a protector and provide a feeling of safety for the patient by watching over them and advocate for him/her
- To act as historian, who provides much needed information about the patient
- To act as facilitator, to maintain relationships with other family members, friends, and coworkers
- To act as a coach providing motivation and inner strength
- To act as a voluntary caregiver aiding to accomplish the actual physical care of the patient and providing intimacy and caring touch

Some advantages of the family's participation were the perception of a greater sense of control and satisfaction with care. The disadvantages were family fatigue, guilt if the loved one does not do well, and additional work for the healthcare providers due to frequent interactions [37].

In 2016, the American Association of Critical-Care Nurses published an alert entitled "Family Visitation in Adult Critical-Care Unit Practice," stating that children supervised by an adult family member are welcome as visitors in ICU [36]. There are no age restrictions. Although younger children may be unable to remain with the patient for long periods of time, contact with these children can be significant to the patient. They need to be prepared for the hospital environment and the family member's illness as appropriate. Their behavior should be monitored by a responsible adult and the staff nurse to ensure a safe and restful environment for the patient and a positive and appropriate experience for children.

ICUs are encouraged to draft policies and procedures to create an optimal environment meeting the needs of patients, families, and healthcare workers.

## 17.8   Conclusion

Multicomponent implementation programs with strategies targeting ICU delirium assessment, prevention, and treatment and integrated within ABCDEF bundle have the potential to improve clinical outcomes [16].

A recent pre-post study showed statistically significant improvements of all patients' outcomes related to the implementation of every single component of ABCDE bundle in ICU and at the same time an unchanged safety profile if compared with the pre-ABCDE bundle period in terms of accidental extubations, self-extubations, and reintubation rates [38]. There was also a reduction of the percent of ICU time in physical restraints post-ABCDE bundle period, even if not significant (6.9 vs. 12.7%, $p = 0.29$) [38].

However, the most encouraging results are from a recent large prospective cohort study about the implementation of PAD guidelines via ABCDE bundle on 6064 ICU patients [40]. If implemented all the interventions included in the bundle, there was a hospital survival OR of 1.07 (95% CI, 1.04–1.11; $p < 0.001$) for every rise of 10% in total bundle compliance. The patients' hospital survival OR was 1.15 (95% CI, 1.09–1.22; $p < 0.001$) for every rise of 10% in partial bundle compliance [39]. These results show that the efforts of ICU team in implementing this complex set of interventions can be widely paid back with better patients' outcomes.

There is also the need to develop adequate education and training programs to overcome potential resistance to change. At the same time, ABCDE bundle implementation is necessary in establishing a monitoring system about the affection of these interventions on the patients' "hard" outcomes.

The vision of the future about the ABCDEF philosophical approach is well drawn by E. Wes Ely, since he stated that this kind of approach shifts the healthcare workers' attention from the technological aspects of ICUs to a more "human connection" [40]. This holistic vision includes the respect of human dignity and the personal values of patients, during their stay in ICU, with an early use of palliative care to guarantee a respectable process of dying in patients that can't survive to their critically illness [40].

# References

1. Resar R, Pronovost P, Haraden C, Simmonds T, Rainey T, Nolan T. Using a bundle approach to improve ventilator care processes and reduce ventilator-associated pneumonia. Jt Comm J Qual Patient Saf. 2005;31:243–8.
2. Ely EW, Baker AM, Dunagan DP, Burke HL, Smith AC, Kelly PT, et al. Effect on the duration of mechanical ventilation of identifying

patients capable of breathing spontaneously. N Engl J Med. 1996;335:1864–9. https://doi.org/10.1056/NEJM199612193352502.

3. Kress JP, Pohlman AS, O'Connor MF, Hall JB. Daily interruption of sedative infusions in critically ill patients undergoing mechanical ventilation. N Engl J Med. 2000;342:1471–7. https://doi.org/10.1056/NEJM200005183422002.

4. Ely EW, Margolin R, Francis J, May L, Truman B, Dittus R, et al. Evaluation of delirium in critically ill patients: validation of the Confusion Assessment Method for the Intensive Care Unit (CAM-ICU). Crit Care Med. 2001;29:1370–9.

5. Jacobi J, Fraser GL, Coursin DB, Riker RR, Fontaine D, Wittbrodt ET, et al. Clinical practice guidelines for the sustained use of sedatives and analgesics in the critically ill adult. Crit Care Med. 2002;30:119–41.

6. Ely EW, Shintani A, Truman B, Speroff T, Gordon SM, Harrell FE Jr, et al. Delirium as a predictor of mortality in mechanically ventilated patients in the intensive care unit. JAMA. 2004;291:1753–62. https://doi.org/10.1001/jama.291.14.1753.

7. Breen D, Karabinis A, Malbrain M, Morais R, Albrecht S, Jarnvig IL, et al. Decreased duration of mechanical ventilation when comparing analgesia-based sedation using remifentanil with standard hypnotic-based sedation for up to 10 days in intensive care unit patients: a randomised trial. Crit Care. 2005;9:R200–10. https://doi.org/10.1186/cc3495.

8. Chanques G, Jaber S, Barbotte E, Violet S, Sebbane M, Perrigault PF, et al. Impact of systematic evaluation of pain and agitation in an intensive care unit. Crit Care Med. 2006;34:1691–9. https://doi.org/10.1097/01.CCM.0000218416.62457.56.

9. Bailey P, Thomsen GE, Spuhler VJ, Blair R, Jewkes J, Bezdjian L, et al. Early activity is feasible and safe in respiratory failure patients. Crit Care Med. 2007;35:139–45. https://doi.org/10.1097/01.CCM.0000251130.69568.87.

10. Girard TD, Kress JP, Fuchs BD, Thomason JW, Schweickert WD, Pun BT, et al. Efficacy and safety of a paired sedation and ventilator weaning protocol for mechanically ventilated patients in intensive care (awakening and breathing controlled trial): a randomised controlled trial. Lancet. 2008;371:126–34. https://doi.org/10.1016/S0140-6736(08)60105-1.

11. Morris PE, Goad A, Thompson C, Taylor K, Harry B, Passmore L, et al. Early intensive care unit mobility therapy in the treatment of acute respiratory failure. Crit Care Med. 2008;36:2238–43. https://doi.org/10.1097/CCM.0b013e318180b90e.

12. Vasilevskis EE, Ely EW, Speroff T, Pun BT, Boehm L, Dittus RS. Reducing iatrogenic risks: ICU-acquired delirium and weakness-crossing the quality chasm. Chest. 2010;138:1224–33. https://doi.org/10.1378/chest.10-0466.

13. Girard TD, Jackson JC, Pandharipande PP, Pun BT, Thompson JL, Shintani AK, et al. Delirium as a predictor of long-term cognitive impairment in survivors of critical illness. Crit Care Med. 2010;38:1513–20. https://doi.org/10.1097/CCM.0b013e47be1.

14. Morandi A, Brummel NE, Ely EW. Sedation, delirium and mechanical ventilation: the 'ABCDE' approach. Curr Opin Crit Care. 2011;17:43–9. https://doi.org/10.1097/MCC.0b013e3283427243.

15. Barr J, Fraser GL, Puntillo K, Ely EW, Gelinas C, Dasta JF, et al. Clinical practice guidelines for the management of pain, agitation, and delirium in adult patients in the intensive care unit. Crit Care Med. 2013;41:263–306. https://doi.org/10.1097/CCM.0b013e3182783b72.

16. Trogrlić Z, Van der Jagt M, Bakker J, Balas MC, Ely EW, Van der Voort PHJ, et al. A systematic review of implementation strategies for assessment, prevention, and management of ICU delirium and their effect on clinical outcomes. Crit Care. 2015;19:157. https://doi.org/10.1186/s13054-015-0886-9.

17. ACCN - American Association of Critical-Care Nursing. Implementing the ABCDE Bundle at the bedside. 2014. http://www.aacn.org/wd/practice/content/actionpak/withlinks-abcde-toolkit.pcms?menu=practice. Accessed 16 Sep 2016.

18. SCCN - Society of Critical-Care Medicine. ABCDEF Bundle. 2015. http://www.iculiberation.org/Bundles/Pages/default.aspx. Accessed on 16 Sep 2016.

19. Payen JF, Bosson JL, Chanques G, Mantz J, Labarere J, Investigators DOLOREA. Pain assessment is associated with decreased duration of mechanical ventilation in the intensive care unit: a post hoc analysis of the DOLOREA study. Anesthesiology. 2009;111:1308–16. https://doi.org/10.1097/ALN.0b013e3181c0d4f0.

20. Vazquez M, Pardavila MI, Lucia M, Aguado Y, Margall MA, Asiain MC. Pain assessment in turning procedures for patients with invasive mechanical ventilation. Nurs Crit Care. 2011;16:178–85. https://doi.org/10.1111/j.1478-5153.2011.00436.x.

21. Reader T, Flin R, Lauche K, Cuthbertson BH. Non-technical skills in the intensive care unit. Br J Anaesth. 2006;96:551–9. https://doi.org/10.1093/bja/ael067.

22. MacIntyre NR. Evidence-based assessments in the ventilator discontinuation process. Respir Care. 2012;57:1611–8. https://doi.org/10.4187/respcare.02055.

23. Cabello B, Thille AW, Roche-Campo F, Brochard L, Gómez FJ, Mancebo J. Physiological comparison of three spontaneous breathing trials in difficult-to-wean patients. Intensive Care Med. 2010;36:1171–9. https://doi.org/10.1007/s00134-010-1870-0.

24. Dietz AS, Pronovost PJ, Mendez-Tellez PA, Wyskiel R, Marsteller JA, Thompson DA, et al. A systematic review of teamwork in the intensive care unit: what do we know about teamwork, team tasks, and improvement strategies? J Crit Care. 2014;29:908–14. https://doi.org/10.1016/j.jcrc.2014.05.025.

25. Balas M, Buckingham R, Braley T, Saldi S, Vasilevskis EE. Extending the ABCDE bundle to the post-intensive care unit setting. J Gerontol Nurs. 2013;39:39–51. https://doi.org/10.3928/00989134-20130530-06.

26. Lane D, Ferri M, Lemaire J, McLaughlin K, Stelfox HT. A systematic review of evidence-informed practices for patient care rounds in the ICU*. Crit Care Med. 2013;41:2015–29. https://doi.org/10.1097/CCM.0b013e31828a435f.

27. Schweickert WD, Pohlman MC, Pohlman AS, Nigos C, Pawlik AJ, Esbrook CL, et al. Early physical and occupational therapy in mechanically ventilated, critically ill patients: a randomised controlled trial. Lancet. 2009;373:1874–82. https://doi.org/10.1016/S0140-6736(09)60658-9.

28. Brummel NE, Girard TD. Preventing delirium in the intensive care unit. Crit Care Clin. 2013;29:51–65. https://doi.org/10.1016/j.ccc.2012.10.007.

29. Adler J, Malone D. Early mobilization in the intensive care unit: a systematic review. Cardiopulm Phys Ther J. 2012;23:5–13.

30. Desai SV, Law TJ, Needham DM. Long-term complications of critical care. Crit Care Med. 2011;39:371–9. https://doi.org/10.1097/CCM.0b013e3181fd66e5.

31. Hanekom S, Louw QA, Coetzee AR. Implementation of a protocol facilitates evidence-based physiotherapy practice in intensive care units. Physiotherapy. 2013;99:139–45. https://doi.org/10.1016/j.physio.2012.05.005.

32. Kayambu G, Boots R, Paratz J. Physical therapy for the critically ill in the ICU: a systematic review and meta-analysis. Crit Care Med. 2013;41:1543–54. https://doi.org/10.1097/CCM.0b013e31827ca637.

33. Leditschke IA, Green M, Irvine J, Bissett B, Mitchell IA. What are the barriers to mobilizing intensive care patients? Cardiopulm Phys Ther J. 2012;23:26–9.

34. Li Z, Peng X, Zhu B, Zhang Y, Xi X. Active mobilization for mechanically ventilated patients: a systematic review. Arch Phys Med Rehabil. 2013;94:551–61. https://doi.org/10.1016/j.apmr.2012.10.023.

35. Hodgson CL, Berney S, Harrold M, Saxena M, Bellomo R. Early patient mobilization in the ICU. Crit Care. 2013;17:207. https://doi.org/10.1186/cc11820.

36. ACCN - American Association of Critical-Care Nursing. Family Presence: Visitation in the adult ICU. 2016. http://www.aacn.org/wd/practice/content/practicealerts/family-visitation-icu-practice-alert.pcms?menu=practice. Accessed 16 Sep 2016.

37. McAdam JL, Arai S, Puntillo KA. Unrecognized contributions of families in the intensive care unit. Intensive Care Med. 2008;34:1097–101. https://doi.org/10.1007/s00134-008-1066-z.

38. Balas MC, Vasilevskis EE, Olsen KM, Schmid KK, Shostrom V, Cohen MZ, et al. Effectiveness and safety of the awakening and breathing coordination, delirium monitoring/management, and early exercise/mobility bundle. Crit Care Med. 2014;42:1024–36. https://doi.org/10.1097/CCM.0000000000000129.

39. Barnes-Daly MA, Phillips G, Ely EW. Improving hospital survival and reducing brain dysfunction at seven California community hospitals: implementing PAD guidelines via the ABCDEF bundle in 6,064 patients. Crit Care Med. 2017;45:171–8. https://doi.org/10.1097/CCM.0000000000002149.

40. Ely EW. The ABCDEF bundle: science and philosophy of how ICU liberation serves patients and families. Crit Care Med. 2017;45:321–30. https://doi.org/10.1097/CCM.0000000000002175.

# Chapter 18
# Nurse Staffing Levels: Skill Mix and Nursing Care Hours Per Patient Day

**Alberto Lucchini, Michele Pirovano, Christian De Felippis, and Irene Comisso**

## 18.1 Introduction

Nursing workload (patient care commitment) is a relevant part of the nursing care routine, significantly affecting the quality of care and the goals of nursing care plans. As a term, "nursing workload" (NW) has often been used in scientific literature, but frequently without a real reference background [1]. Many authors throughout the years have suggested possible definitions, according to development of the nursing professional's role and nursing theoretical principles. In the past, NW concept was just patient-related tasks (nursing care and bedside activities) in connection with the time spent to carry out these activities. Recently, the same NW concept has been reviewed including the time spent by nurses to perform non-patient-related tasks (or bedside cares) such as continuing educations, clinical updates, and management processes [2]. Several authors have outlined that NW concept is not merely based on the physical efforts to perform nursing care, but as a comprehensive part of high-dependency patient care, it should consider the

© Springer International Publishing AG, part of Springer Nature 2018
I. Comisso et al., *Nursing in Critical Care Setting*,
https://doi.org/10.1007/978-3-319-50559-6_18

reflection process, urging time of maneuvers, and the related emotional involvement [3].

Lately also nursing managers and researchers have shown interest about new potential ways to define and measure NW concept. Researchers have investigated the relationship between clinical data and the events in order to improve quality and safety; on the other hand, nurse management is motivated and focused to find out tools and strategies able to promote the best use of nurse staff resources.

Most of the time, the existing relationship between financial budget cost, limited resources, and clinical/staff achievements has been analyzed by scientific literature. It is well recognized that there is a direct relation between patient's outcomes and nursing staff levels: (understaffing with) high level of NW score produces an increase of mortality rate [4, 5], potential complications, and adverse events [6, 7]. From a nursing staff perspective, it could lead to potential job decline due to frustration or professional burnout phenomenon [4, 8, 9].

However, it is crucial to bear in mind that nursing staff represents the largest amount of professionals inside hospitals, and from a personnel-budget point of view, it remains one of the main cost items [2]. So, planning and matching the right amount of nurse staffing is a key point to provide the best cost-effective quality and safety of care.

Introducing tools to measure the NW can help in supporting the decision-making process with the latest evidence available, thus getting the best resources' efficiency. Nevertheless, understanding and evaluating the NW concept appears to be complex and difficult [10].

Patient-specific nursing care, severity of illness, complexity of techniques, and the wide range of fields where nursing care is provided show only a part of the issues involved in the NW's evaluating process. Several methods and tools have been developed according to specific features and approaches related to specific fields of work.

In the critical care setting, it is essential to evaluate the intensity of care, in order to provide adequate levels of care for high-dependency patients and to justify the high costs of human and technological investments. Since the early 1970s, inside ICUs, tools and procedures were tested and improved according to the evolution of clinical, technological, and organizational dimensions and the evolving nursing role. The new contest of limited financial resources for health-care providers requires to correctly estimate the right amount of nursing staff through correct tools.

When comparing all the available options in literature, the nursing activities score (NAS) seems to be the most useful tool across European ICUs [11–15] and worldwide [16].

## 18.2   Nursing Activities Score (NAS)

NAS [1] was developed on a basic principle: nursing care is not defined only by the gravity of illness and therapeutic procedures. This tool was realized from the basics of TISS 28 score [17]. Compared to TISS 28, NAS' authors have pointed out the real-time evaluation of this tool, expression of the time taken to administer ICU's patient care. NAS' score is made up of 13 main areas (parts), split into 23 items (Table 18.1), able to describe patient-related and non-patient-related works, administrative tasks, and level of patient's dependency as well. The resulting score, worked out by percentage, represents the total amount of time required to deliver nursing care. A NAS score of 100% corresponds to one nurse dedicated to a single patient over 24 h (nurse-to-patient ratio 1:1 equal to 1440 min of nurs-

**Table 18.1** Nursing activities score: interventions and attributed weights

| Basic activities | Score |
|---|---|
| **1. Monitoring and titration** | |
| **1.a Hourly vital signs, regular registration, and calculation of fluid balance.** Patients who require **NORMAL** monitoring, according to the ICU routine application of assessment scales (pain, RASS, Glasgow), and water balance control (including nasogastric and nasoenteral tubes) and who do not need frequent alterations in treatment, therapy, or monitoring intensification. Assisted oral feeding | 4.5 |
| **1.b Present at bedside and continuous observation or active for 2 h or more in any shift, for reasons of safety, severity, or therapy, such as noninvasive mechanical ventilation, weaning procedures, restlessness, mental disorientation, prone position, donation procedures, preparation and administration of fluids and/or medication, and assisting specific procedures.** Patients who require intensified monitoring (MORE THAN NORMAL) due to alterations in the clinical condition, hemodynamic instability, oliguria, bleeding, dyspnea, fever, alteration in the level of consciousness, measurements in the assessment scales higher than the ICU standard, measurement of central venous pressure, invasive arterial pressure, intra-abdominal pressure, use of sedatives or long-term use of insulin, ventilator support, noninvasive mechanical ventilation or alteration of the ventilator parameters, preparation of fluids, and emergency medication. Patient is stable after the therapeutic behavior adopted. Immediate postoperative care after cardiac surgery or major surgery, where the patient remains stable. Invasive procedures with intercurrences. Extubation without intercurrences. Assisted oral feedings that demand more time than normal | 12.1 |

**Table 18.1**   (continued)

| Basic activities | Score |
|---|---|
| **1.c Present at bedside and active for 4 h or more in any shift for reasons of safety, severity, or therapy, such as those examples above (1b).** Critical patients who require MUCH MORE THAN NORMAL monitoring, in at least one shift in 24 h, without stabilization after the therapeutic interventions were adopted, require continuous nursing presence. Alterations described in the "MORE THAN NORMAL" category, however, with a greater frequency and the need for interventions. Hemodialysis with intercurrence, requiring nursing intervention (when hemodialysis is performed by ICU staff). Unstable patients in immediate postoperative care after cardiac surgery or major surgery | 19.6 |
| **2. Laboratory: Biochemical and microbiological investigations.** Patients submitted to any biochemical or microbiological exam, regardless of the quantity, performed at bedside by a nursing professional, including capillary glucose. For example, HGT, glycosuria, tracing cultures, and blood gas analysis, among others. This item should not be scored if the laboratory collector or physician performs the collection | 4.3 |
| **3. Medication.** Vasoactive drugs excluded. Patients who received any type of medication, regardless of the route and dose. Vasoactive drugs will be scored in a specific item (item 12) | 5.6 |
| **4. Hygiene procedures. Performing hygiene procedures such as dressing of wounds and intravascular catheters, changing linen, washing patient, incontinence, vomiting, burns, leaking wounds, complex surgical dressing with irrigation, special procedures (e.g., barrier nursing, cross-infection related, room cleaning following infections, staff hygiene) and especially obese patients, etc.** | |
| 4.a **Normal.** Patients who were submitted, in **NORMAL** frequency (ICU routine), to one of the hygiene procedures mentioned above in at least one shift in 24 h. Also including dressings closed in vascular catheter once a day | 4.1 |

(continued)

**Table 18.1** (continued)

| Basic activities | Score |
|---|---|
| 4.b **The performance of hygiene procedures took more than 2 h in any shift.** Patients who were submitted, in **MORE THAN NORMAL** frequency, to one of the hygiene procedures mentioned above in at least one shift in 24 h. Vascular catheter dressing twice a day, medium dressing for pressure ulcer, dressing a surgical incision twice a day, medium dressing (with suture dehiscence), changing linen twice in 24 h, washing of unstable patients by three professionals, body hygiene twice per shift. Fecal incontinence three times a day. Patients in isolation | 16.5 |
| 4.c **The performance of hygiene procedures took more than 4 h in any shift.** Patients who were submitted, in **MUCH MORE THAN NORMAL** frequency, to one of the hygiene procedures mentioned above in at least one shift in 24 h. Extensive, complex, open cavity dressing for ≥three times a day | 20.0 |
| 5. **Care of drains: All (except gastric tube).** Patients with any type of drain or tube with the aim of draining. Including long-term catheter, external ventricular drain (EVD), and thorax drain, among others. EXCLUDING gastric tubes (nasogastric, nasoenteral, gastrostomies, and others), which should be considered in item 1 or 21 | 1.8 |
| 6. **Mobilization and positioning. Including procedures such as turning the patient, mobilization of the patient, moving from bed to chair, and team lifting (e.g., immobile patient, traction, prone position)** | |
| 6.a **Performing procedure(s) up to 3 times per 24 h.** Patients who require mobilization and positioning up to three times in 24 h | 5.5 |
| 6.b **Performing procedures(s) more frequently than 3 times per 24 h, or with 2 nurses—any frequency.** Patients who require mobilization and positioning, as described in item 6, which have been performed more than three times in 24 h or by two members of the nursing staff in at least one shift in 24 h | 12.4 |

**Table 18.1**  (continued)

| Basic activities | Score |
|---|---|
| 6.c **Performing procedure with three or more nurses—any frequency.** Complex mobilization and positioning as per the procedure described in item 6, which have been performed by three or more members of the nursing staff, in any frequency, in at least one of the shifts in 24 h | 17.0 |
| 7.0 **Support and care of relatives and patient**. Including procedures such as telephone calls, interviews, and counseling. Often, the support and care of either relatives or patient allow staff to continue with other nursing activities (e.g., communication with patients during hygiene procedures, communication with relatives while present at bedside and observing patient) | |
| 7.a **Support and care of either relatives or patient requiring full dedication for about 1 h in any shift such as explaining clinical condition and how to deal with pain and distress and difficult family circumstances**. This item receives a score when guidance or instructions are given to patients and/or their families, providing emotional support with full dedication of a nurse from the staff, with **NORMAL** duration, according to the routine established in the unit, in at least one shift in 24 h | 4.0 |
| 7.b **Support and care of either relatives or patient requiring full dedication for 3 h or more such as explaining clinical condition and how to deal with pain and distress and difficult family circumstances.** This item receives a score when guidance or instructions are given to patients and/or their families, providing emotional support with full dedication of a nurse from the staff, with **MORE THAN NORMAL** duration, according to the routine established in the unit, in at least one shift in 24 h | 32.0 |
| 8. **Administrative and managerial tasks** | |
| 8.a **Performing routine tasks such as processing of clinical data, ordering examinations, and professional exchange of information (e.g., ward rounds).** Including records performed as nursing process and/or shift change, multidisciplinary rounds, or administrative and managerial tasks related to patients, with **NORMAL** duration | 4.2 |

(continued)

**Table 18.1** (continued)

| Basic activities | Score |
|---|---|
| 8.b **Performing administrative and managerial tasks requiring full dedication for about 2 h in any shift such as research activities, protocols in use, admission, and discharge procedures**. Including records performed as part of nursing process and/or shift change, multidisciplinary rounds, or administrative and managerial tasks related to patients, with **MORE THAN NORMAL** duration. Admission of patients in immediate postoperative period, unstable patients who require more extensive records. Need for providing materials and equipment. Assembly of the hemodialysis machine, application of protocols such as ECLS, transplantation, and others. When the nurse needs help from a colleague to perform his/her activities. For example, the nurse continues assisting a patient and a colleague takes over the administrative tasks | 23.2 |
| 8.c **Performing administrative and managerial tasks requiring full dedication for about 4 h or more of the time in any shift such as death and organ donation procedures and coordination with other disciplines.** Including any administrative and managerial task related to the patient, with **MUCH MORE THAN NORMAL** duration, according to the routine established in the unit. Critical, unstable patients who require intense records. Detailed shift change records, multidisciplinary rounds, organization of special materials and equipment for patient care, surgical procedures at bedside, protocols such as transplantation, ECLS, ventricular assist devices, and teaching and supervising education/training | 30.0 |
| **Ventilatory support** | |
| 9. **Respiratory support. Any form of mechanical ventilation/ assisted ventilation with or without positive end-expiratory pressure, with or without muscle relaxants; spontaneous breathing with positive end-expiratory pressure (e.g., CPAP or BiPAP), with or without endotracheal tube; and supplementary oxygen by any method.** Patients making use of any respiratory support, from nasal catheter to mechanical ventilation | 1.4 |

**Table 18.1** (continued)

| Basic activities | Score |
|---|---|
| 10. **Care of artificial airways**. Endotracheal tube or tracheostomy cannula. Patients making use of orotracheal or nasotracheal tube or tracheostomy | 1.8 |
| 11. **Treatment for improving lung function. Lung physiotherapy, incentive spirometry, inhalation therapy, and intratracheal suctioning.** Patients who underwent treatment to improve their pulmonary function, performed in any frequency by the nursing staff. Aspiration with open or closed system and nebulization | 4.4 |
| **Cardiovascular support** | |
| 12. **Vasoactive medication, irrespective of type or dose.** Patients who have received any vasoactive medication, regardless of the type and dose and who need intensive monitoring in their endovenous use: sodium nitroprusside, vasopressin, prostaglandin, norepinephrine, epinephrine, dopamine, dopexamine, dobutamine, isoproterenol, phenylephrine, nitroglycerin, and clonidine hydrochloride. Metoprolol and propranolol (beta blockers) should be scored | 1.2 |
| 13. **Intravenous replacement of large fluid losses. Fluid administration > 3 l/m2/day, irrespective of type of fluid administered.** Patients who have received fluid replacement greater than 4.5 liters of solution per day, irrespective of the type of fluid administered | 2.5 |
| 14. **Left atrium monitoring. Pulmonary artery catheter with or without cardiac output measurement.** Patients making use of pulmonary artery catheter (Swan-Ganz catheter). Including the use of cardiac pacemaker, intra-aortic balloon pumping, cardiac output monitoring, extracorporeal life support (ECLS), and ventricular assist devices | 1.7 |
| 15. **Cardiopulmonary resuscitation after arrest: in the past 24 h (single precordial thump not included). Patients who suffered a heart problem and were submitted to cardiopulmonary resuscitation, independently of the environment where the cardiac arrest took place. This item should be scored only once in 24 h** | 7.1 |

(continued)

**Table 18.1** (continued)

| Basic activities | Score |
|---|---|
| **Renal support** | |
| **16. Hemofiltration techniques. Dialysis techniques.** Patients who have received any type of intermittent or continuous dialytic procedure | 7.7 |
| **17. Quantitative urine output measurement (e.g., by indwelling urinary catheter).** Patients who require diuresis control, in milliliters, with or without any type of urinary device | 7.0 |
| **Neurological support** | |
| **18. Measurement of intracranial pressure.** Patients submitted to intracranial pressure monitoring, jugular bulb catheter, or microdialysis. Do consider this item if the patient has external ventricular drainage and assessment of ICP | 1.6 |
| **Metabolic support** | |
| **19. Treatment of complicated metabolic acidosis/alkalosis.** Patients who made use of specific medication to adjust metabolic acidosis or alkalosis, such as administration of sodium bicarbonate in continuous or bolus infusion. Respiratory acidosis and alkalosis should not be scored in this item, and neither should ventilator correction. The item considers those conditions requiring the permanent presence of a nurse for monitoring severe physiological deregulation and for titrating (fine-tuning) the therapy in acute conditions. During hemofiltration, if correction is necessary, additional score is indicated | 1.3 |
| **20. Intravenous hyperalimentation.** Patients who receive central or peripheral venous infusion of parenteral nutrition | 2.8 |
| **21. Enteral feeding. Through gastric tube or other gastrointestinal routes (e.g., jejunostomy).** Patients who receive enteral feeding through tubes, by any route of the gastrointestinal tract. Measurement of aspiration/retention included | 1.3 |

**Table 18.1** (continued)

| Basic activities | Score |
|---|---|
| **Specific interventions** | |
| **22. Specific intervention(s) in the intensive care unit. Endotracheal intubation, insertion of pacemaker, cardioversion, endoscopies, emergency surgery in the past 24 h, and gastric lavage. Routine interventions without direct consequences for the clinical condition of the patient, such as X-rays, echography, electrocardiogram, dressing, or insertion of venous or arterial catheters, are not included.** Patients submitted to a diagnostic or therapeutic intervention listed above in the ICU. Specific procedures performed in the unit and which require active intervention of the staff can be considered in this item, including the insertion of venous or arterial catheters and spinal puncture. Procedures performed by the nurse, such as passing a relief or indwelling urinary catheter, a nasoenteral or gastric tube, or a peripherally inserted central catheter (PICC) and installation of intra-abdominal pressure, among others, that might be particularly complex and require more nursing time for their execution can also be considered | 2.8 |
| **23. Specific interventions outside the intensive care unit. Surgery or diagnostic procedures.** Patients who require diagnostic or therapeutic interventions performed outside the ICU. For example, tomography, radionuclide imaging, magnetic resonance, hemodynamics (take or pick up a patient), surgical procedures (take or pick up a patient), patient transfer to any hospitalization unit or discharge, and sending the body to the morgue | 1.9 |

ing care). The NAS average value for an ICU will determine the level of workload of the nursing staff.

This validation study involved 15 countries, 99 ICUs from Europe, the North American region, and Australia. In the first stage, a survey was submitted to ICU nurses and doctors, to find out what kind of items should have been considered; after this step, a wide validation process was performed. Research was focused on two main targets: to evaluate the relationship between TISS-28 and NAS and to analyze the way of employ of nursing care timing in the ICU setting (comparison of each item versus total score). The time spent to deliver nursing care was investigated by a registration method and then classified depending on (1) the amount of time to deliver patient-related care; (2) non-patient-related activities, e.g., management tasks; (3) supporting the staff's requirements; and (4) every kind of activity not previously mentioned.

According to point (1), collection of data has shown as follows: using 6.451 data that were collected (2041 patients recruited), the average TISS-28 value was 26.9 (SD ± 9.9), with median value (the middle of the distribution) of 27, whereas mean NAS value was 56 (SD ±17.5), with median value of 54. The correlation TISS-28-NAS was 0.56 ($r = 0.56$–$p < 0.001$).

With reference to point (2), results have shown as follows: the tool's reliability to describe/define NW was 81% of the total amount of time spent to deliver nursing care, while the 11% of it was referred to non-patient-care-related activities, 6% was referred to personal activities, and only 2% wasn't recognized by the aforementioned categories.

A literature review [18] outlined that NAS score has been investigated on different levels of dependency (ITU, HDU) and different fields (adult, pediatric, neonatal), despite the tool being tailored for adults only. So far, the use of NAS in ICU for its accuracy is supported by scientific literature [14, 19]. In the last decade, NAS became the first choice to evaluate and analyze NW inside ICUs; however, Goncalves et al. outlined several limitations due to potential misinterpretations of the items [20]. Table 18.2 summarizes the results concerning the mean values of NAS in the studies of the past 10 years.

**Table 18.2** Key studies on nursing workload

| Author, year | Pts | NAS sheets | Setting (type of ICU) | NAS (MD ± SD) | Ideal N/P ratio (NAS/100) |
|---|---|---|---|---|---|
| Adell et al. [21] | 250 | 1880 | GICU | 41(13) | 0.4 |
| Altafin et al. [19] | 437 | ns | GICU | 75(9) | 0.7 |
| Camuci et al. [22] | 50 | 1221 | Burns ICU | 70(ns) | 0.7 |
| Carmona-Monge et al. [23] | 103 | 941 | GICU | 55(15) | 0.5 |
| Carmona-Monge et al. [24] | 563 | 5704 | MICU | 53(ns) | 0.5 |
| Oliveira et al. [25] | 190 | ns | GICU | 58(3) | 0.6 |
| Nogueira De Souza et al. [26] | 600 | ns | GICU | 68 and 53 | 0.7 and 0.5 |
| Debergh et al. [27] | 155 | 1280 | GICU, PICU | 55 | 0.5 |
| Lucchini et al. [12] | 250 | ns | GICU | 76 (15) | 0.7 |
| Lucchini et al. [7] | 240 | ns | GICU | 82 (9) | 0.8 |
| Lucchini et al. [28] | 200 | ns | GICU | 74 (9) | 0.7 |
| Lucchini et al. [14] | 5856 | 28,390 | GICU, CICU, NICU | 66 (2) | 0.7 |
| Lucchini et al. [29] | 7588 | | GICU, CICU, NICU | 62(19) | 0.6 |
| Nogueira et al. [30] | 200 | 200 | Trauma ICU | 71 (17) | 0.7 |
| Padilha et al. [31] | 200 | 200 | GICU, NICU | 73 (14) | 0.7 |
| Padilha et al. [32] | 68 | 690 | GICU | 64 (2) | 0.6 |
| Queijo et al. [33] | 100 | ns | GICU, CICU, NICU | 65 (7) | 0.7 |
| Stafseth et al. [13] | 235 | ns | GICU | 96 (22) | 0.9 |

*CICU* cardiosurgical intensive care unit, *GICU* general intensive care unit, *MICU* medical intensive care unit, *NICU* neurosurgical intensive care unit, *PICU* pediatric intensive care unit

## 18.3 Determining Factors in ICU Nursing Workload

Available studies evaluated the possible determinants of the NW in the ICU. The main factors can be summarized as follows:

- Sociodemographic characteristics
- Clinical features
- Therapeutic treatments
- Clinical trials

Tables 18.3 and 18.4 summarize the impact of these factors on the NW.

**Table 18.3** Sociodemographic characteristics and nursing workloads

| Author, year | Factors related to the NW | Factors NOT related to the NW | Sample/ surveys | ICU type |
|---|---|---|---|---|
| Altafin et al. [19] | | Age ($p = 0.754$) Gender ($p = 0.68$) | | M/S ICU |
| Nogueira et al. [26] | | Age ($p = 0.749$) | $n = 187$ | CICU |
| Nogueira et al. [30] | ↑ Male gender ($p = 0.033$) | | $n = 200$ | GICU |
| Lucchini et al. [14] | ↑ Age 0–10 ($p < 0.05$, children have a higher NAS) | | $n = 5856$ | GICU, CICU |
| Queijo et al. [33] | ↓ Inverse correlation with age ($p = 0.035$) | | $n = 100$ | NICU |

*M/S ICU* medical/surgical intensive care unit, *CICU* cardiosurgical intensive care unit, *GICU* general intensive care unit, *MICU* medical intensive care unit, *NICU* neurosurgical intensive care unit

**Table 18.4** Determinants of nursing workload in ICU, quantitative studies

| Author, year | Factors related to the NW | Factors NOT related to the NW | Sample/ surveys | ICU type |
|---|---|---|---|---|
| Altafin et al. [19] | ↑ Death ($p = 0.001$) ↑ APACHE II ($< 0.001$), and SOFA ($p < 0.001$) ↓ LOS ($p < 0.001$) | Septic shock ($p = 0.085$) | $n = 437$ | GICU |
| Carmona-Monge et al. [24] | ↓  Acute coronary syndrome versus ARDS and septic shock | | $n = 536$ | GICU |
| Oliveira et al. [25] | ↑ LOS, ($p = 0.036$) ↓ SAPS III ($r = -0.441$), and SOFA ($r = -0.168$)↑ Occurrence of complications ($p < 0.001$) | | $n = 287$ | CICU |
| de Souza Nogueira et al. [26] | ↑ APACHE II ($p = 0.004$); ↑ Acute lung injury ($p = 0.005$), ↑ Number of the body parts with injury ($p = 0.020$) | | $n = 200$ | GICU |

(continued)

**Table 18.4** (continued)

| Author, year | Factors related to the NW | Factors NOT related to the NW | Sample/ surveys | ICU type |
|---|---|---|---|---|
| Lucchini et al. [28] | ↑ CPAP >10 cm $H_2O$ and PEEP >10 ($p = 0.01$) <br> ↑ Non invasive ventilation and invasive ventilation ($p < 0.0001$) | | $n = 200$ | GICU |
| Lucchini et al. [14] | ↑ Patient death versus alive ($p < 0.001$) <br> ↑ECMO ($p < 0.05$) <br> ↑ LOS ($p < 0.003$) | Sedation level SAPS II and III | $n = 5856$ | GICU, NICU, CICU |
| Queijo et al. [35] | ↑ Death ($P = 0.038$) <br> ↑ SAPSII ($p = 0.29$, $P = 0.000$) | | $n = 100$ | NICU |

*CICU,* cardiosurgical intensive care unit; *GICU,* general intensive care unit; *MICU,* medical intensive care unit; *NICU,* neurosurgical intensive care unit

## 18.4 ESICM (European Society of Intensive Care Medicine) Recommendations on Basic Nursing Requirements for ICU Units [34]

### 18.4.1 Head Nurse

The nursing staff is managed by a dedicated, full-time head nurse, who is responsible for the functioning and quality of the nursing care. The head nurse should have extensive experience in intensive care nursing and should be supported by at least one deputy head nurse able to replace him (her). The head nurse should ensure the continuing education of the nursing staff. Head nurses and deputy head nurses should not normally be expected to participate in routine nursing activities. The head nurse works in collaboration with the medical director, and together they provide policies and protocols and directives and support to the team.

## 18.4.2  Nurses

Intensive care nurses are registered nursing personnel, formally trained in intensive care medicine and emergency medicine. A specific program should be available to assure a minimum of competencies among the nursing staff. An experienced nurse (head nurse or a dedicated nurse) is in charge of education and evaluation of the competencies of the nurses. In the near future, a specific curriculum for ICU nurses should be available. In addition to clinical expertise, some nurses may develop specific skills (e.g., human resource management, equipment, research, teaching new nurses) and assume the responsibility for this aspect of unit management. Staff meetings together with physicians, nurses, and AHCP must be regularly organized in order to carry out the following [34–35]:

- Discuss difficult cases and address ethical issues.
- Present new equipment.
- Discuss protocols.
- Share information and discuss organization of the ICU.
- Provide continuous education.

The number of intensive care nurses necessary to provide appropriate care and observation is calculated according to the levels of care (LOCs) in the ICU.

## 18.4.3    Levels of Care (LOCs) [38–41]

### 18.4.3.1    Level of Care III (Highest)

LOC III represents patients with multiple (two or more) acute vital organ failure of an immediate life-threatening character. These patients depend on pharmacological as well as device-related organ support such as hemodynamic support, respiratory assistance, or renal replacement therapy.

### 18.4.3.2    Level of Care II

LOC II represents patients requiring monitoring and pharmacological and/or device-related support (e.g., hemodynamic support, respiratory assistance, renal replacement therapy) of only one acutely failing vital organ system with a life-threatening character.

### 18.4.3.3    Level of Care I (Lowest)

LOC I patients experience signs of organ dysfunction necessitating continuous monitoring and minor pharmacological or device-related support. These patients are at risk of developing one or more acute organ failures. This category includes patients recovering from one or more acute vital organ failures but whose condition is too unstable or when the nursing workload is too high/complex to be managed on a regular ward (Tables 18.3–18.5).

For these different LOCs, the following minimum nurse-to-patient ratios are considered to be appropriate (Table 18.6) [34]:

**Table 18.5**  Nursing workload and clinical pathways

| Author, year | Factors related to NW | Sample | ICU type |
|---|---|---|---|
| Altafin et al. [19] | ↑ Urgent surgery versus elective surgery and medical type ($p = 0.014$) | $n = 437$ | GICU |
| Debergh et al. [27] | ↑ PICU versus MICU ($p = 0.042$) | $n = 225$ | PICU, GICU |
| Lucchini et al. [14] | ↑ GICU versus NICU & CICU ($p < 0.001$) | $n = 7588$ | GICU, NICU, CICU |

*CICU* cardiosurgical intensive care unit, *GICU* general intensive care unit, *MICU* medical intensive care unit, *NICU* neurosurgical intensive care unit, *PICU* pediatric intensive care unit

**Table 18.6**  LOC and suggested nurse-to-patient ratio

| LOC | Nurse-to-patient ratio | Nursing FTE per ICU bed |
|---|---|---|
| III | 1/1 | 6 |
| II | 1/2 | 3 |
| I | 1/3 | 2 |

*LOC* level of care, *FTE* full time equivalent

## 18.5   Conclusions

The endless improvements of hospital strategies in order to provide the highest cost-effective quality of care in the intensive care setting justify the use of evaluating tools for NW supporting the management in the allotment process of limited resources. The aim of this literature's review was to identify the available tools and describe the key factors of NW concept.

The NAS appears to be a precise tool for this task according to several studies [14, 19], although others [16, 23] have underpinned limitations related to misinterpretations of several items that affect feasibility and reliability to describe nursing work inside ICUs.

Data available from the last 6 years have pointed out a lack of knowledge about the intensity of nursing workload. Crucial factors able to affect NW are related to the severity of illness (e.g., respiratory distress), advanced therapies (e.g., ECMO support-advanced ventilatory strategies), and ICU LOS. Further investigations are needed to reinforce scientific evidence and longitudinal data analysis desirable in order to evaluate potential changes about determinant factors. Nearly 100% of this data review were performed inside ICUs; therefore, enhancing the use of NAS in different aspects of critical care fields appears as mandatory.

The regular daily use of NAS, especially for ICUs with eight or more bed spaces, is able to match the proper LOC, and then it becomes possible to match the variable nurse staffing requirements, modifying the nurse-to-patient ratio based on a proper evaluation of NW.

Take-Home Messages
- NAS has been applied in clinical settings in various types of ICUs.
- The NAS tool is a valuable tool, and its pervasiveness and degree of implementation worldwide indicate its relevance.
- The analysis of the results indicates that NAS was used to test several variables that fall into the structure category (mainly age, sex, and severity of illness), but few variables are related to process.
- With regard to outcome, the most frequently tested variables were mortality and LOS, which are not nurse-sensitive outcomes.

# References

1. Alghamdi MG. Nursing workload: a concept analysis. J Nurs Manag. 2016;24:449–57. https://doi.org/10.1111/jonm.12354.
2. Morris R, MacNeela P, Scott A, Treacy P, Hyde A. Reconsidering the conceptualization of nursing workload: literature review. J Adv Nurs. 2007;57:463–71. https://doi.org/10.1111/j.1365-2648.2006.04134.x.

3. Carayon P, Alvarado CJ. Workload and patient safety among critical care nurses. Crit Care Clin N Am. 2007;19:121–9. https://doi.org/10.1016/j.ccell.2007.02.001.

4. Tarnow-Mordi W, Hau C. Hospital mortality in relation to staff workload: a 4 year study in an adult intensive care unit. Lancet. 2000;356:185–9.

5. Neuraz A, Guérin C, Payet C, Polazzi S, Aubrun F, Dailler F, et al. Patient mortality is associated with staff resources and workload in the ICU: a multicenter observational study. Crit Care Med. 2015;43:1587–94. https://doi.org/10.1097/CCM.0000000000001015.

6. Daud-Gallotti RM, Costa SF, Guimarães T, Padilha KG, Inoue EN, Vasconcelos TN, et al. Nursing workload as a risk factor for healthcare associated infections in ICU: a prospective study. PLoS One. 2012;7:e52342. https://doi.org/10.1371/journal.pone.0052342.

7. Lucchini A, Peruta M, Canella R, Elli S, Sanvito G, De Angelis C. Number of nurses and adverse events: the results of a study. Assist Inferm Ric. 2011;30:172–9. https://doi.org/10.1702/1007.10955.

8. Aiken LH, Clarke SP, Sloane DM. Hospital nurse staffing and patient mortality, nurse burnout, and job dissatisfaction. JAMA. 2002;288:1987–93.

9. Patterson J. The effect of nurse to patient ratios. Nurs Times. 2011;107:22–5.

10. Twigg D, Duffield C. A review of workload measures: a context for a new staffing methodology in Western Australia. Int J Nurs Stud. 2009;46:132–40. https://doi.org/10.1016/j.ijnurstu.2008.08.005.

11. Miranda DR, Nap R, de Rijk A, Schaufeli W, Iapichino G, TISS Working Group. Nursing activities score. Therapeutic intervention scoring system. Crit Care Med. 2003;31:374–82. https://doi.org/10.1097/01.CCM.0000045567.78801.CC.

12. Lucchini A, Chinello V, Lollo V, De Filippis C, Schena M, Elli S, et al. The implementation of NEMS and NAS systems to assess the nursing staffing levels in a polyvalent intensive care unit. Assist Inferm Ric. 2008;27:18–26.

13. Stafseth SK, Solms D, Bredal IS. The characterization of workload and nursing staff allocation in intensive care units: a descriptive study using the nursing activities score for first time in Norway. Intensive Crit Care Nurs. 2011;27:290–4. https://doi.org/10.1016/j.iccn.2011.07.003.

14. Lucchini A, De Felippis C, Elli S, Schifano L, Rolla F, Pegoraro F, et al. Nursing activities score (NAS): 5 years of experience in the intensive care units of an Italian university hospital. Intensive Crit Care Nurs. 2014;30:152–8. https://doi.org/10.1016/j.iccn.2013.10.004.

15. Padilha KG, Stafseth S, Solms D, Hoogendoom M, Monge FJ,

Gomaa OH, et al. Nursing activities score: an updated guideline for its application in the intensive care unit. Rev Esc Enferm USP. 2015;49:131–7. https://doi.org/10.1590/S0080-623420150000700019.

16. Palese A, Comisso I, Burra M, Di Taranto PP, Peressoni L, Mattiussi E, et al. Nursing activity score for estimating nursing care need in intensive care units: findings from a face and content validity study. J Nurs Manag. 2016;24:549–59. https://doi.org/10.1111/jonm.12357.

17. Miranda DR, de Rijk A, Schaufeli W. Simplified Therapeutic Intervention Scoring System: the TISS-28 items--results from a multicenter study. Crit Care Med. 1996;24:64–73.

18. Lachance J, Douville F, Dallaire C, Padilha KG, Gallani MC. The use of the nursing activities score in clinical settings: an integrative review. Rev Esc Enferm USP. 2015;49:147–56. https://doi.org/10.1590/S0080-623420150000700021.

19. Altafin JA, Grion CM, Tanita MT, Festti J, Cardoso LT, Veiga CF, et al. Nursing activities score and workload in the intensive care unit of a university hospital. Rev Bras Ter Intensiva. 2014;26:292–8.

20. Gonçalves LA, Padilha KG, Cardoso Sousa RM. Nursing activities score (NAS): a proposal for practical application in intensive care units. Intensive Crit Care Nurs. 2007;23:355–61. https://doi.org/10.1016/j.iccn.2007.04.009.

21. Adell AB, Campos RA, Rey MCB, Rochera ES, Munoz JS, Canuto MS, et al. Nursing Activity Score (NAS). Nuestra experiencia con un sistema de computo de cargas de enfermaria basado en tiempos. Enferm Intensiva. 2005;16:164–73.

22. Camuci MB, Martins JT, Cardeli AAM, Cruz Robazzi ML. Nursing activities score: nursing work load in a burns intensive care unit. Rev Latino Am Enfermagem. 2014;22:325–31. https://doi.org/10.1590/0104-1169.3193.2419.

23. Carmona-Monge FJ, Jara-Pérez A, Quiros-Herranz C, Rollan-Rodriguez G, Cerrillo-Gonzalez I, García-Gómez S, et al. Assessment of nursing workload in three groups of patients in a Spanish ICU using the nursing activities scores scale. Rev Esc Enferm USP. 2013;47:335–40.

24. Carmona-Monge FJ, Uranga IU, Gomez SG, Herranz CQ, Bengoetxea MB, Unanue GE, et al. Usage analysis of the nursing activities score in two Spanish ICUS. Rev Esc Enferm USP. 2013;47:1108–16. https://doi.org/10.1590/S0080-623420130000500014.

25. Oliveira LB, Rodrigues AR, Püschel VA, Silva FA, Conceição SL, Béda LB, Fidelis B, et al. Assessment of workload in the postoperative period of cardiac surgery according to the nursing activities score. Rev Esc Enferm USP. 2015;49:80–6. https://doi.org/10.1590/S0080-623420150000700012.

26. Nogueira Lde S, Koike KM, Sardinha DS, Padilha KG, de Sousa RM. Nursing workload in public and private intensive care units. Rev Bras Ter Intensiva. 2013;25:225–32. https://doi.org/10.5935/0103-507X.20130039.
27. Debergh DP, Myny D, Van Herzeele I, Van Maele G, Reis Miranda D, Colardyn F. Measuring the nursing workload per shift in the ICU. Intensive Care Med. 2012;38:1438–44. https://doi.org/10.1007/s00134-012-2648-3.
28. Lucchini A, Elli S, Bambi S, Foti G, Fumagalli R. Invasive and non-invasive ventilation: impact on nursing workload. Assist Inferm Ric. 2013;32:124–31. https://doi.org/10.1702/1338.14853.
29. Lucchini A, Elli S, Bambi S, Becattini G, Vanini S, Piantanida C, et al. Nursing activities score: differences in nursing workload in three intensive care units. Assist Inferm Ric. 2015;34:6–14. https://doi.org/10.1702/1812.19744.
30. Nogueira LDS, Domingues CDA, Poggetti RS, Sousa RMC. Nursing workload in intensive care unit trauma patients: analysis of associated factors. PLoS One. 2014;9:e112125. https://doi.org/10.1371/journal.pone.0112125.
31. Padilha KG, de Sousa RMC, Queijo AF, Mendes AM, Miranda DR. Nursing Activities Score in the intensive care unit: analysis of the related factors. Intensive Crit Care Nurs. 2008;24:197–204. https://doi.org/10.1016/j.iccn.2007.09.004.
32. Padilha KG, Sousa RM, Garcia PC, Bento ST, Finardi EM, Hatarashi RH. Nursing workload and staff allocation in an intensive care unit: a pilot study according to Nursing Activities Score (NAS). Intensive Crit Care Nurs. 2010;26:108–13. https://doi.org/10.1016/j.iccn.2009.12.002.
33. Queijo AF, Martins RS, Andolhe R, Oliveira EM, Barbosa RL, Padilha KG. Nursing workload in neurological intensive care units: cross-sectional study. Intensive Crit Care Nurs. 2013;29:112–6. https://doi.org/10.1016/j.iccn.2012.08.001.
34. Valentin A, Ferdinande P, ESICM Working Group on Quality Improvement. Recommendations on basic requirements for intensive care units: structural and organizational aspects. Intensive Care Med. 2011;37:1575–8. https://doi.org/10.1007/s00134-011-2300-7.
35. Schmalenberg C, Kramer M. Types of intensive care units with the healthiest, most productive work environments. Am J Crit Care. 2007;16:458–68.
36. Gurses AP, Carayon P. Performance obstacles of intensive care nurses. Nurs Res. 2007;56:185–94. https://doi.org/10.1097/01.NNR.0000270028.75112.00.
37. Dawson S, Runk JA. Right patient? Right bed? A question of appropriateness. AACN Clin Issues. 2000;11:375–85.

38. Pirret AM. Utilizing TISS to differentiate between intensive care and high-dependency patients and to identify nursing skill requirements. Intensive Crit Care Nurs. 2000;18:19–26.
39. Iapichino G, Radrizzani D, Rossi C, Pezzi A, Anghileri A, Boffelli S, et al. Proposal of a flexible structural organizing model for the intensive care units. Minerva Anestesiol. 2007;73:501–6.
40. Wild C, Narath M. Evaluating and planning ICUs: methods and approaches to differentiate between need and demand. Health Policy. 2005;71:289–301. https://doi.org/10.1016/j.healthpol.2003.12.020.
41. Moreno R, Reis MD. Nursing staff in intensive care in Europe: the mismatch between planning and practice. Chest. 1998;113:752–8.

# Chapter 19
# Evolution of Intensive Care Unit Nursing

Stefano Bambi

## 19.1 Introduction

Recently, Professor Jean-Louis Vincent (along with other luminaries in the field of intensive and critical care medicine), has published articles that consider the history and perspectives of intensive care medicine and intensive care units (ICUs) [1–3].

The fields of critical care medicine (CCM) and critical care nursing arose to provide special treatment and care for the most severely ill hospital patients [2]. These patients need high levels of surveillance, intensive nursing care, and biomedical technology to support and monitor their vital functions and failed organs/systems. This type of care is carried out in ICUs, which are specific spaces, separated from other hospital areas, set up to receive critically ill patients and provide highly specialized medical and nursing competences and skills [2, 4].

However, in the past 30 years, despite the increasing amount of research in CCM, major therapeutic progress does not seem to have been made in the field [1]. The reduction of mortality achieved in ICUs is due essentially to improvements in supportive care and in the relevant technologies [5].

© Springer International Publishing AG, part of Springer Nature 2018    489
I. Comisso et al., *Nursing in Critical Care Setting*,
https://doi.org/10.1007/978-3-319-50559-6_19

Some therapeutic progress has been shown in the following fields [1]:

- Protective strategies for mechanical ventilation in acute respiratory distress syndrome (ARDS)
- Increasing employment of noninvasive ventilation (NIV)
- Reduction of (long-term) sedation use
- Enteral nutrition preferred to parenteral nutrition
- Less invasive monitoring systems
- Reduction in blood transfusions
- Reduction in anti-arrhythmic medications
- Greater attention to the use of antibiotic drugs
- Early and active patient mobilization.

However, greater steps have been made in the process of care, including all the healthcare professionals involved with the critically ill patients, the environment, the "interpretation" and organization of the work [1]. Such achievements that can positively affect patient outcomes are [1, 2]:

- Multidisciplinary outcome-oriented teamwork. The ICU staff now goes beyond critical care nurses and doctors, and includes physiotherapists, pharmacists, infectious disease consultants, nutritionists, and psychologists.
- Implementation of protocols for weaning of patients from mechanical ventilation; sedation; nutrition; glucose control; vasopressor and electrolyte-targeted infusion; patient positioning; and early mobilization/ambulation.
- Processes of cure and care driven by the "time is tissue" motto (early diagnosis and treatment of critical illnesses produces better patients outcomes).
- Utilization of continuous renal replacement therapy (CRRT) to better manage the intake and removal of fluids during the hyperacute phase of critical illnesses and the later phases, in which there can be the need to remove fluids.

- Early mobilization of patients to prevent ventilator-associated pneumonia (VAP), deep vein thrombosis (DVT), pressure ulcer (PU), and delirium.
- Increased utilization of clinical risk management tools (incident-reporting systems, morbidity and mortality reviews, and audits).
- Humanization of ICU scenarios through open visiting policies and ethical approaches to the issue of end-of-life (EOL) care.
- More awareness of the limited (or even absent) evidence for the effectiveness of many therapeutic and interventional options now used in the ICU (e.g., albumin, pulmonary artery catheter, tight glycemic control, dopamine).
- More awareness of the need to prevent cross-infections and device-related infections.
- Implementation of the concept of an in-hospital medical emergency team and an outreach team philosophy.
- Greater understanding of the role of intra-abdominal hypertension and compartment syndrome in multi-organ failure and patient outcomes.
- Establishment of multicenter and international patient registries for specific pathologies (e.g., trauma, cardiac arrest, etc.), in order to improve quality assurance programs and benchmarking.

Technology has made great contributions to the availability of monitoring and interventional options, together with providing higher standards of safety for patients, being user-friendly, and, in some cases, with devices being smaller and lighter in weight than in the past [2].

What about the future of ICUs? Vincent [2] envisions increases in the number of ICU beds relative to the number of hospital beds in other areas, even in a scenario of decreasing costs. The shortage of intensivists could be "compensated" for by computerized or nurse-driven clinical protocols, but the nursing workload would then increase, and nursing staff numbers should be adequate to deal with this increase [2].

More multicenter and international trials will be performed to test drugs and treatments, offering greater evidences to use in CCM [3]. Furthermore, pharmacological treatments for critically ill patients should be improved through strategies such as [5]:

- Selecting samples for research in critically ill populations, taking into account biological and clinical variables
- Promoting the early administration of drugs during the initial manifestations of diseases and also before the admission of patients to the ICU
- Performing phase 2 trials to test new generic drugs
- Implementing cell-based therapies and therapies that will enhance the resolution of organ failure.

Organizational strategies should involve the use of inclusive models, concentrating ICU personnel in a few large units, and promoting the concept of centralization to improve patient outcomes and to provide flexible management of healthcare workers [2]. Extracorporeal organ support technologies will be improved [1].

Information technology should cover all the bureaucratic aspects of healthcare work, improving handover, drug prescriptions, and data collection with a network consisting of patient monitoring systems, point-of-care systems, clinical records, and charts [2]. In addition, computerized systems could provide real-time calculation of staffing needs, based on the nursing workload and patient risk prediction and stratification, improving triage for ICU admission and discharge [4].

This kind of progress could be time-saving and prevent mistakes, and it could also leave more time for doctors and nurses to care for their patients at the bedside [2]. Multidisciplinary rounds should become the norm. Patient follow-up post-ICU stay could become the source of valuable information employed to direct interventions that recover the patient's quality of residual life and improve the quality of care in the ICU [2].

A better continuum of care between the pre-hospital phase, the emergency care phase, the ICU phase, and the post-ICU phase should be implemented. At the same time, adequate data collection and analysis models are needed, to accurately evaluate the effectiveness of interventions delivered to patients in the whole healthcare path of the critical illness [1].

In addition, policies should be drafted to manage increasing demands for critical care beds in the event of maxi-emergencies [3].

Discussing future perspectives in critical care nursing is not a simple issue. However, four main lines of discussion can be addressed: priorities in critical care nursing research, holistic care and humanization of care issues, specific populations of ICU patients requiring competent and expert nursing care, and ICU nurses' preparedness during outbreaks of emerging infectious diseases. Across (and beyond) all the above considerations, this chapter will provide an overview of current and more meaningful issues for critical care nursing, noting the areas that require particular consideration and further investigation.

## 19.2 Priorities in Critical Care Nursing Research

Nursing research plays a central role in scientific production, increasing the disciplinary body of knowledge. The main problems related to research in critical care settings are related to the small sample numbers and the large number of variables that are difficult to control. Moreover, research findings are not simple to retrieve. Hence, some large nursing associations, such as the American Association of Critical-Care Nurses (AACN) and the European Federation of Critical Care Nurses Associations (EFCCNA), have promoted the identification of priorities in nursing research and are developing international networks to support multicenter designed studies.

According to an American professional task force, priorities in critical care nursing research should be oriented toward [6]:

- Development of methods for fast recognition of acute patients at high risk of rapid deterioration
- Minimally invasive organ support technologies
- New approaches to enhance patient comfort while reducing changes of consciousness
- Effective process and outcome measurements for critical illness research and palliative and EOL care.

The areas of nursing interest in healthcare service research should cover [6]:

- Strategies to improve communication and coordination of care
- Tools, processes, and programs to promote knowledge transfer and implementation
- Factors related to an effective learning environment
- Strategies for the application of clinical risk management concepts and methods
- Assessment of the distressing effects of interventions on the patient and their family.

On the European side, the EFCCNA, through a Delphi study design, has identified 52 research topics in 12 different domains [7]. The priorities of nursing research in critical care settings noted in that study mainly cover patient safety issues, the impact of evidence-based practice (EBP) and the workforce on patients' outcomes, the comfort/well-being of patients and relatives, and the impact of EOL care on staff and their practice [7]. The five research topics with the highest ranking scores were [7]:

- Interventions to reduce nosocomial infections in the ICU
- Pain management and pain assessment

- Exploration of the extent of anxiety, fear, and stress in ICU patients, and strategies to reduce their occurrence
- Prevalence and prevention of critical incidents in the ICU (medication errors, adverse events)
- Impact of the ICU nurse-patient ratio on patient outcomes.

Some authors have also proposed new strategies to increase effectiveness in the production and local dissemination of scientific knowledge, reducing the distance between researchers and clinicians. Such strategies involve the "tripartite model," based on synergy among universities, hospitals, and single hospital wards [8].

## 19.3 Open Intensive Care Units

The American College of Critical Care Medicine guidelines for support of the family in the patient-centered ICU rely on the concept that relatives are essential resources for patients' health [9]. These guidelines refer to major concepts such as "flexibility," "single-case basis evaluation," and "open ICU" [9]. The open ICU philosophy is based on the reduction/elimination of temporal (liberalization of visiting policies), physical (overcoming the imposed barriers to physical contact between relatives and patients), and relational restrictions (trust-based relationship between ICU staff and families) [10, 11]. This progressive change of view toward a "holistic" approach to the cure and the care of the patient-family as a whole, greatly challenges ICU staff [12]. Some authors promote open visiting policies as a standard, as well as promoting the adoption of patient-centered outcomes (not only survival) [13].

Evidence on the influence of programs for the implementation of open ICUs on patient mortality, length of stay (LOS), infection risk, and the mental health of patients and their relatives is currently lacking, and the influence of such programs needs to be investigated [12]. Further, the efforts of ICU teams to improve the relationship climate inside the ICU will require addressing according to the indications arising from the research results.

Recently, some authors have hypothesized that open ICU programs and the presence of family members during cardiopulmonary resuscitation could also play a role in reducing the rates of opposition to organ donation [14, 15]. More studies are needed to confirm this hypothesis, introducing important scenarios with potential lifesaving effects for future ICU patients [14, 15].

## 19.4   Animal-Assisted Therapy

Animal-assisted therapy (AAT) is defined as "the use of human-animal bond to attenuate stress and improve mood" [16]. AAT works on the interaction between humans and pets, with the aim to reduce stress and feelings of isolation and depression [16]. Areas of AAT implementation range from simple social well-being to the improvement of language or motor functions [16]. Dogs are the most frequent animals used for AAT, although rabbits and cats can also be employed, under the guidance of specially trained teams. Adequate procedures that address hygiene guidelines, times of use, and safety measures are needed [16].

Although the introduction of AAT inside ICUs has been referred to in the literature since the early 1990s [17] and finds enthusiasm among staff nurses [18], experience on its implementation in ICUs is very limited.

A preliminary randomized controlled trial (RCT) conducted on 76 adult patients with advanced heart failure in the ICU showed reductions of cardiopulmonary pressure, neurohormone levels, and anxiety during the visitation of a dog and a volunteer [19].

Another pilot RCT study, performed on 40 children (aged between 3 and 17 years), showed that the employment of dog visitations in the immediate postoperative period after general surgery facilitated the recovery of vigilance and activity after anesthesia and significantly reduced the perception of pain [20].

This fascinating adjunctive therapy needs to be the target of more scientific research, to expand the areas of implementation and produce better evidence of its effectiveness than that currently available.

## 19.5  Work Environment Climate and Relationship Dynamics in the Intensive Care Unit

Working in an ICU is not a simple matter [21]. The ICU work environment is complex, as a result of three different determinants involved: the physical environment, emotional environment, and professional environment [21].

The physical environment is often challenging for healthcare professionals, generating stress. Unfavorable (artificial) lighting, frequent irritating noises (e.g., monitor and device alarms), clumsily placed equipment, narrow patient units, and overcrowding are the main workplace stressors generated by the physical environment [21]. Human factor engineering is a discipline that can provide some solutions to these difficulties, improving work conditions for all members of the ICU staff [21].

The emotional environment in the ICU is well portrayed by the metaphor of "a continuous hot and cold shower" [21]. The emotional stress for healthcare workers is very high, owing to the high mortality and disability rates, the need for making fast life-or-death decisions, and the need to balance the effort to save lives with the realistic limits of technologies and medical/nursing sciences [21]. These elements can easily lead to feelings of frustration, exhaustion, and (sometimes) anger, in the personnel, particularly in critical care nurses, because they are the professionals who are always on the frontline at the patient's bedside [21]. Anger, in particular, is an emotion that needs to be adequately addressed before it develops into hostility, aggression, and violence [22]. Some studies have reported that about a quarter of workers in the United States experience anger in the workplace [22]. It is important for staff to recognize their own trigger points for anger, and to prevent negative feelings and their escalation; strategies that can be used for this are [22]:

- Be constructive and practice open listening.
- Identify the signs and causes of anger.
- Use calming techniques.
- Maintain eye contact with the person who has triggered the anger and express genuine concern.
- Try to understand elements that could resolve the anger.

The recent widespread implementation of the "open ICU" concept has exposed nurses to additional emotional stressors arising from the family's feelings and needs, because the relatives spend more time in ICU, at the patient's bedside. The consequent physical and emotional stress can cause depersonalization and/or avoidance behaviors, exhaustion, burnout, and higher turnover rates in ICU personnel [21]. Some proposed solutions rely on teamwork learning programs (with the focus on interprofessional relationships). Educational interventions and workshops aiming to provide psychological stress management tools and improve interpersonal social and communication skills have also been recommended [21].

Concerning the professional environment, work satisfaction seems to be the key to the adequate development and expression of positive potential in healthcare professionals. To increase work satisfaction, the ICU environment should promote group cohesion, effective communication, autonomy, and supportive management [21]. When teamwork is not effective, synergistic, and harmonious, burnout and errors can easily arise. Burnout is a syndrome characterized by absenteeism, fatigue, reduced personal commitment, and low job satisfaction levels.

Team training programs and, above all, reduced staff workload can be effective in increasing work satisfaction levels, preventing the above-mentioned negative consequences [21].

It has been found that most ICU staff share the same definition of interprofessional work, that includes concepts as "shared team identity, clarity, interdependence, integration, and shared responsibility." [23] Nevertheless, except for critical events, the most common work interactions developed in the ICU are synthesized as collaboration (interactions related to specific questions), coordination (working in parallel), and networking (acquiring skills and expertise, and consultations with others) [23].

Nurses and other ICU team members are often frustrated by doctors not listening to them [23].

It has been reported that the only event in which an ICU staff acts as a team is during an emergency code. Such behavior is well known in crisis resource management, but this behavior fails to be shown in daily practice and workflows [24, 25].

Therefore, the only way for the multidisciplinary ICU team to achieve better outcomes is to develop a high level of trust, improve communication and discussion, and share clear and structured clinical and organizational information [25].

Currently, some authors recommend that future research be focused on the mechanisms that drive learning and interactions in the ICU team, seen through the "magnifying lens" provided by the social sciences (organizational behavior, anthropology, and network science), taking into account that the composition of the ICU team can vary largely from one shift to another [4].

During the past 10 years, the AACN has recognized the positive influence of healthy work environments on nursing staff outcomes and retention [26]. The AACN has identified and promoted six standard elements that define a work environment as "healthy": "skilled communication," "true collaboration," "effective decision-making," "appropriate staffing," "meaningful recognition," and "authentic leadership" [26]. Despite the efforts of the AACN to disseminate these standards and improve nursing workplace environments, the results of two surveys, performed 7 years apart, showed only a marginal improvement in communication [27].

When ICU nurses were surveyed in regard to the elements that provided them with work satisfaction, they responded that the main elements were related to nursing unit management; the relationships with and the organization of medical staff; rostering practices; nurses roles in ICU patient care; and general relationships in the workplace [28].

Nurses and physicians are the two main professionals driving the workflows inside the ICU. The relationships between the two professional groups are influenced by three components of the ICU workplace environment, their specific roles, differences in expected patient outcomes, and levels of stress and workloads. Therefore, conflicts between these two professional groups are not rare. However, to better understand this phenomenon, it is necessary to differentiate vertical conflicts (nurses-doctors) from internal conflicts among nurses (horizontal conflicts).

### 19.5.1   Vertical Conflicts

A large multicenter study reported that 33% of conflicts within the ICU team were nurse-physician conflicts, being the most common types of struggles within the ICU team [29]. Hostility and lack of communication were the main causes of the conflicts [29]. Most conflicts arise around two main issues: EOL decisions and communication matters [30]. Conflicts about EOL decisions are one of the most important causes of moral distress in nursing staff, with profound effects on the workplace climate [30]. Disagreement with postoperative goals of care is another important cause of conflict between physicians and nurses [30]. The need to keep relatives adequately informed about patients' conditions can also cause some tension between ICU staff nurses and doctors [30].

Further, many nurse-physician conflicts emerge from procedural factors (related to team processes), organizational factors (related to the local unit or hospital), contextual factors (legal, social, and cultural features), relational factors (variables influencing the social relationship) [31], and, probably, anthropological factors (the idea of nursing as an oppressed discipline) [32].

A simple but effective intervention to improve communication between ICU nurses and doctors could be the introduction of a multidisciplinary daily round and daily planning of activities, to share objectives and desired clinical outcomes [30, 31]. After a conflict has happened, the best strategy is to try first to resolve the problems with the individuals, taking the discussion back to the real subject of the conflict (often the patient or the organizational problem) and depersonalizing the situation [30]. Unprofessional, offensive, or unsuitable behaviors should not be tolerated by a team that has common shared values and should be referred to the internal disciplinary authority [30].

## 19.5.2 Horizontal Violence Among Nurses

To really understand the "internal world" of the "nurses' tribe" in depth (these anthropological terms can be used to describe the characteristics of nurses' relationships), one has to observe nurses' particular positive and negative internal relationship dynamics. Nurses colleagues show strong bonds, forged by the unique, intense, and emotional challenges shared daily at their patients' bedsides. The shared experiences of their patients' pain, suffering, and death, as well as shared experiences of hope and healing, can bond nurses to their colleagues at deeper levels than those seen in other professions. But, similarly to the strong attachments between nursing colleagues, internal conflicts among nurses can be fierce. Horizontal violence (HV) is one of the terms used for behaviors ranging from verbal and emotional abuse to physical violence perpetrated by workers against their peers inside an organization [33]. The reported prevalence rate of this phenomenon among nurses ranges widely, from 5.7 [34] to 79.1% [33] and is associated with important psychosocial [35] and professional consequences. Symptoms of posttraumatic stress disorder (PTSD) have been reported in nurses, and high rates of job leaving are recorded in those with shorter lengths of service [36]. Moreover, some authors suppose that there may be a relationship between HV and patient safety, owing to changes in the flows of clinical information among nurses [37].

Various researchers have advanced explanations for the origin and development of HV. The "oppressed group behavior theory" [38], interpersonal, intrapersonal, evolutionary, and biological models offer different views about the emergence of this phenomenon [39], but, currently, none of these models has been completely validated. The key elements of these theories and models are [40, 41]:

- "Lack of self-esteem"
- "Generational and hierarchical abuses"
- "Actor-observer effect"
- "Nursing as an oppressed discipline"
- "Working practices depriving rights/privileges"
- "Aggression leading to aggression" and "development of cliques".

Despite the high rates of the HV phenomenon and the perceived relevance of its effects by nurses, the solutions proposed have been limited to position statements [42] and guidelines

[43] released by some nurses associations, as well as ideas on team building [44] and self-esteem augmentation [45, 46], education programs, and an educational tool-kit to identify and resolve workplace bullying and harassment [47]. Interventional studies of solutions (e.g. the implementation of zero tolerance policies [48]) are lacking. Hence, there is a need to focus nursing research on HV prevention, because it is difficult to eradicate the problem once it becomes part of the structure of a group.

## 19.6    Challenging Patient Populations in Intensive Care Units

During the delivery of care, critical care nurses should pay attention to the particular features appropriate to specific patient populations, as shown in the framework summarized in Fig. 19.1.

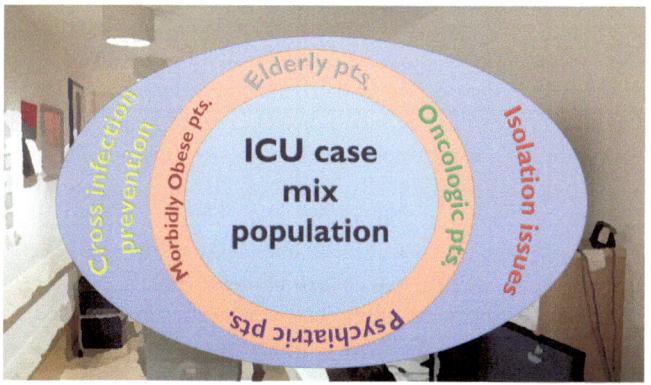

**Fig. 19.1** Challenging intensive care unit (ICU) patient populations

## 19.6.1   Morbidly Obese Patients

Recent epidemiological data has shown that about 2.1 billion people worldwide are obese (i.e., have a body mass index [BMI] higher than 25 kg/m$^2$), with an increasing trend [49]. The fight against this harmful condition requires powerful prevention programs, and such programs need political commitment [49].

Morbid obesity (BMI >40 kg/m$^2$) is a condition affecting about 6.6% of the United States population (data from 2010) [50]. Morbid obesity is often associated with potential complications in the ICU, such as difficult airways and/or ventilation, and challenging peripheral and central venous access [50]. Frequent comorbidities are obstructive sleep apnea, diabetes, insulin resistance, low levels of vitamin D, hyperlipidemia, and hypertension [51].

Moreover, respiratory and cardiovascular impairments can be frequent, both seen with a chronic inflammatory state. In particular, the respiration of these patients can be affected by increased work of breathing and chest wall resistance and high chest wall resistance, increased intra-abdominal pressure, $CO_2$ production, and oxygen consumption, and the possibility of muscle weakness [51]. Cardiovascular impairment can be caused by increasing levels of circulating blood or $CO_2$, risk of heart failure and dysrhythmias, hypertrophy, and other myocardial structural alterations [51]. Additionally, hypercoagulability and late wound healing can be expressions of metabolic changes due to obesity [51]. Lastly, the pharmacokinetic and pharmacodynamic characteristics of most drugs can change in these patients [50].

Currently the association between higher BMI class and patient outcomes in ICUs is still controversial ("obesity paradox") and requires more accurate comparisons between the obese BMI classes and "normal" BMI subjects [52, 53]. However, BMI calculation alone is not sufficient to stratify patients, since it does not take into account differences in body composition (adipose tissue, lean tissue, body fluids) [52].

From the logistical and nursing care points of view, morbidly obese patients present challenges for bed and stretcher weight limits and dimensions, and for patient repositioning and transfers. Standard hospital beds can bear weights of up to 150–170 kg, but morbidly obese patients are often beyond these body weight limits [54]. Sometimes radiological examinations cannot be performed, owing to the limits of radiological stretchers. Standard radiology beds can hold weights of 158–204 kg, while in patients over these weight limits, the performance of a computerized tomography (CT) scan or magnetic resonance imaging (MRI) can require special equipment (beds bearing a weight of up to 306 kg for CT and up to 248 kg for MRI) [54].

All this information is useful for planning the nursing and medical care of these patients, considering the complex physio-pathological, logistical, and safety factors that characterize their stay in critical care units.

Airway management can be very difficult. The "ear-to-sternal notch positioning" (so-called ramped position) can improve the management of intubation in these patients, when there is no suspicion of cervical spine injury. This position can be obtained by rolling layers of bedsheets under the patient's shoulders, until the back elevation reaches the desired alignment [54].

Ventilation can be improved using the "beach chair" position or anti-Trendelenburg position at 45°. These solutions allow better diaphragmatic excursion and prevent the risk of micro-inhalation. In morbidly obese patients, the supine position and Trendelenburg must be avoided because of the risk of "obesity supine death syndrome" [54]. During mechanical ventilation (MV), tidal volume according to ideal body weight (IBW) should be used, since the size of the lungs does not depend on the real body weight of the patient. Also, for these patients the limit of 30 $cmH_2O$ for plateau pressure has to be respected to prevent ventilator-associated lung injury [54].

It is sometimes difficult to insert vascular catheters in morbidly obese patients. Echocardiographic insertion techniques are greatly limited owing to the large stratification of adipose tissue [54]. So arterial and venous catheters are often maintained in place for a longer time than recommended, exposing patients to a high risk of infection and other kinds of complications [53].

Hypocaloric nutrition is indicated in obese patients. In the higher BMI classes, the aim is to reach 60–70% of the patient's energy requirements. Protein supply in patients with BMI $\geq 40$ should be $\geq 2.5$ g/kg of IBW, except for those with renal failure [53].

Some pharmacological considerations should also be taken into account. Reduced peak serum levels and increased clearance time can be recorded for lipophilic drugs [54]. The doses of highly lipophilic medications should be calculated according to the real weight, while the doses of minimally lipophilic medications should be calculated according to the IBW. Increased creatinine clearance in obese patients can reduce the levels of medications excreted by the kidneys [54]. Altered absorption through intramuscular, intradermal, and subcutaneous pathways is typical in obese patients [54].

Beyond preventing the deterioration of vital and organ functions, nursing care has to be directed toward the provision of adequate staff numbers, special beds, and equipment to facilitate patients' repositioning and early mobilization, with particular attention paid to the development of "traditional" PU and device-related PU [53].

Finally, during their clinical practice, critical care nurses need to pay attention to aspects related to the emotional support needed by obese patients and the social stigma they experience, as obesity still has a negative social connotation. Indeed, some stereotypes and prejudices portray obese persons as being short-tempered and nasty [54]. Verbal and emotional abuse of obese patients perpetrated by healthcare workers has been reported in the literature; it is mandatory for healthcare workers to avoid behaviors that blame patients who are unable to control their unhealthy or excessive eating habits [54].

## 19.6.2  Elderly Patients

The percentage of the world's population aged over 60 years has increased from 8% in 1950 to 12% in 2013, and in 2050 the percentage is projected to be up to 21%, with a large proportion of people over 70 years old [55].

Older people (aged over 80 years) admitted to ICUs are the subject of complex ethical debates related to poor outcomes and the poor quality of residual life after intensive care [56]. Moreover, interest in financial issues has emerged in recent years (especially owing to the worldwide economic crisis), since medical costs rise exponentially in people older than 50 years [56]. Another factor is that, in any kind of patient, deciding to withdraw treatment and organ support is surely more difficult than deciding to apply some kind of advance care directive (such as "do not resuscitate", or do "not intubate" orders). Therefore, discussions about the ways to offer and employ intensive care support in elderly patients are influenced by ethical, cultural, and political variables, and such discussions are far from ended [57].

In a recent Canadian multicenter prospective cohort study, conducted by Heyland et al. [58] on patients ≥80 years old admitted to 22 ICUs, the mortality rate in the ICU was 22% and the in-hospital mortality was 35%. Patients died at a median of 10 days after ICU admission. No predictors for prolonged time of intensive care support were found by the authors [58]. Frailty indexes or advance care directives had little influence on the decision to limit life-support measures [58]. Many other studies have shown a mortality trend of over 50% 1 to 2 years after hospital discharge in very old ICU patients [55]. Heyland et al. [59], studying recovery after a critical illness in patients aged ≥80 years, found that 26% of the surviving patients achieved physical recovery 12 months after hospital admission. Physical recovery was significantly associated with younger age, lower acute physiology and chronic health evaluation II (APACHE II) score, lower Charlson comorbidity score, and a lower frailty index [59].

Comorbidities in older patients probably play an important role in survival rates and quality of life (QOL) after intensive care [55]. To improve the care of these frail patients, professional integration between intensivists and geriatricians is recommended [55].

More research in older patients is needed to explore care, life-sustaining therapies, EOL problems, ICU effectiveness, and QOL after a critical illness [55].

Critical care nursing in older patients should take into account these patients' comorbidities, with the frequent presence of chronic diseases such as diabetes, chronic obstructive pulmonary disease, congestive heart failure, and end-stage renal disease. Another typical complication seen in this population is "geriatric syndromes," including PUs, incontinence, falls, functional decline, and delirium [60]. The other big issue in the aging population is the concept of frailty. Frailty, a condition that arises owing to reduced physiological and sensorial/cognitive reserves, typically in older people, plays an important role in the occurrence of adverse events and outcomes [59].

Some authors, in discussing the consequences of nursing care in critically ill older patients, have pointed out new challenges, such as environmental modifications, the need for education and training in healthcare staff, changes in their own professional attitudes, and collaboration with experts in geriatrics [61]. Functional assessment and awareness of existing medications are two key elements on which a nursing care plan should be based, also providing an "after ICU perspective" to critical care nursing [61].

Critical care nursing assessment of vulnerability in frail elderly patients should be multidimensional [62]. Physiological assessment is directed toward the patients' sensorial status, level of mobility, and chronic pathologies. Psychological assessment should focus on the identification of cognitive changes, dementia, and psychiatric conditions. Lastly, an evaluation of social conditions and social supports is needed [62].

The data collected can help critical care nurses to plan adequate strategies for the prevention of complications and for the support of older patients in the ICU and to draft personalized discharge planning [62]. Common negative events that should be prevented in these patients are falls, abuse, malnutrition, hypothermia, depression, fear, low levels of self-care, and loss of autonomy [62].

## 19.6.3  Patients with Psychiatric Disorders and Consequent Emergencies

Historically, the presence of psychiatric disorders in ICU patients was not well recognized or well managed [63]. Only in recent times has this trend been reversed. The most frequent psychiatric clinical problems in ICU patients are delirium, anxiety-panic-agitation loop, depression, psychosis, and persecution ideation [63, 64]. The causes of these problems are mainly metabolic and electrolyte disorders, infections, head injuries, withdrawal syndromes, and vascular conditions [63].

The high level of stress during an ICU stay can itself be the source of a patient's psychological impairment [64].

According to some authors, certain environmental variables trigger the establishment of these conditions. High sound levels and loud noises, lack of sleep and rest, impairment of circadian rhythms, procedure-related pain, and in intubated patients, the impossibility of speaking, are typical features of the ICU environment [63].

Care efforts should be oriented toward [63, 64]:

- Maintaining patients in single ICUs.
- Guaranteeing low levels of technological noise and quiet voices.

- Providing calendars, clocks, and other tools for patients' time and space orientation.
- Improving the quality of the patient's sleep and rest and reducing light levels at night.
- Promoting relatives' visitations and contact with patients.
- Establishing an empathetic relationship with patients (and their relatives).

Early physical rehabilitation plays a fundamental role in the prevention of conditions such as delirium [65].

For patients who survive after ICU admission and a hospital stay, PTSD symptoms are frequent and very disturbing [64].

However, except for delirium, the other psychiatric disorders noted above are rarely considered by staff nurses in the ICU.

Nurses have to be aware of the importance of promptly recognizing psychiatric emergencies, which can sometimes be deadly [66]. Psychiatric emergencies can be related to overdoses of psychotropic medications, but are not limited to overdosing [66]. In fact, the withdrawal or interruption of drug treatment can be the cause of a psychiatric emergency [66]. Delirium, drug toxicity, uncontrolled schizophrenia, agitation, and suicidal attempts are typical psychiatric emergencies [66]. Common psychiatric emergencies in the ICU are agitated delirium, overdose of psychiatric medication, neuroleptic malignant syndrome, and serotonin syndrome [65].

Often non-specific signs and symptoms, such as tachycardia, diarrhea, fever, and seizure, can hinder the rapid recognition of these emergencies [66].

Almost all of the above-mentioned psychiatric emergencies in the ICU require treatment with specific medications, and quick action by nurses [65].

### 19.6.4 Oncology Patients

Although deaths caused by oncological illnesses have diminished since the 1990s, cancer is still the second most common cause of death, after heart illnesses, accounting for 20% of deaths in the United States [67]. Recent estimates from Europe, for 2012, indicated 3.45 million new cases of cancer and 1.75 million deaths caused by the disease [68].

ICU admission criteria for patients with cancer have changed over the years, from an approach excluding "do not resuscitate" patients to offering the chance to recover from an acute on chronic event owing to the illness or the toxic effects of pharmacological treatments [69].

Traditional oncology emergencies requiring ICU treatment are currently treated in oncology or medical-surgical units [70]. These emergencies, owing to the illness or its therapy, are, mainly, tumor lysis syndrome, superior vena cava syndrome, and malignant spinal cord compression [70]. Currently, oncological complications requiring assessment and support in the ICU are cardiac and respiratory failure, severe bleeding and coagulopathies, and sepsis [70]. Specifically, these complications can be pneumonia, venous thromboembolism, ARDS, pulmonary toxicity associated with chemotherapy and radiation, malignant pericardial effusions, heart failure, dysrhythmias, prolonged QT syndrome, gastrointestinal bleeding, disseminated intravascular coagulation, sepsis, and hypersensitivity reactions [70].

Admitting cancer patients to the ICU makes sense for improving short-term survival rates after a critical care illness [71]. Furthermore, some recent general achievements and progress in ICU use support the admission of these patients; such items are: more "open" admission policies, NIV, diagnostic strategies in acute respiratory failure, treatment of acute renal failure, blood component transfusion policies, diagnostic strategies in neurological complications, and treatment of organ failure in macrophage-activation syndrome [71].

However, cancer patients can also die in the ICU. The QOL of oncology patients who die in an ICU seems to be worse than that of patients who die in a hospice or at home [67]. Moreover, relatives of oncology patients who have died in an ICU can be affected by symptoms of PTSD [67].

One big challenge to the implementation of high-quality EOL care in the ICU is to incorporate palliative care early in the care plan [67]. Palliative care aims to relieve symptoms and pain related to the treatment and the illness and to take into account the spiritual and psychological spheres of the patient and his/her relatives, independently of the severity and progression of the illness [67].

There are some hindrances to the implementation of EOL care in the ICU [67]:

- Mission of the ICU (lifesaving and restoring patients' QOL)
- Culture of the ICU (death-denying and difficult-to-manage communication on prognosis)
- Goals of the ICU (technology-oriented to implement life-support treatment, relegating the holistic approach to a low priority)
- Environment of the ICU (an open space is a more frequent architectural configuration than a single patient rooms unit)
- Competing priorities for nurses' time (dying patients considered a low priority; difficulties in managing the relatives' needs and requests for information about their loved ones).

A key element in EOL care in the ICU is the nursing management of symptoms of discomfort and pain. Often these patients are treated with all the organ support that the ICU can offer (MV, hemodynamic pharmacological support, CRRT, artificial nutrition, etc.) [67]. Moreover, large numbers of invasive devices are often in place, causing procedural pain, discomfort, and delirium. The most frequent symptoms presented in these patients are dyspnea and pain [67].

The withdrawal or withholding of organ- or life-support treatments is complex, and often a long time is required for making the decision, with the involvement of the patient, the healthcare professionals, and relatives (as proxy decision-makers) [67]. At the same time, there are important implications of such decisions, related to ethical debates and influenced by religion, national culture, and national laws.

However, the key to the successful implementation of oncology patient care in the ICU can only be a real commitment to interprofessional collaboration among nurses, doctors, palliative care and oncology specialists, cultural-linguistic mediators, and spiritual care providers [69]. Without adequate information, meaningful collaboration, and realistic goals of care for the patients, the risk of moral distress for critical care nurses is quite elevated [72].

## 19.7 Infectious Diseases in the ICU: Challenging Critical Care Nursing in an Isolation Setting

In the past 15 years, disease outbreaks have often overwhelmed the attention of healthcare workers and ICU teams. The outbreaks were: severe acute respiratory syndrome coronavirus (SARS-CoV) (2002–2003), avian influenza H5N1 (2004 and later), pandemic influenza A (H1N1) (2009), the Middle East respiratory syndrome coronavirus MERS-CoV) (2012 and later), and Ebola virus disease (2014–2015) [73].

An outbreak is defined as "a sudden increase in incidence compared with the "normal" morbidity rates for any certain disease in a given area" [74]. The consequences of the "sudden" features of an outbreak can be disruptive, causing chaos, panic, and insecurity. Increasing levels of stress and anxiety related to work can be experienced by healthcare personnel. In some extreme cases, inadequate preparedness for a disease outbreak can lead to hospital closure [74].

The term "outbreak" can also refer to the cross-transmission of multiresistant microorganisms inside hospital wards (e.g., *Acinetobacter baumannii* and *Clostridium difficile*), as well as referring to pandemic or epidemic diseases (e.g., SARS, H1N1).

Some examples of strategies to improve ICU infection control for multiresistant microorganisms, such as *Klebsiella pneumoniae* and *A. baumannii*, are [74, 75]:

- Handwashing, the first and most important intervention to prevent the spread of infectious disease [75].
- Daily surveillance cultures for all patients
- Strict surveillance of housekeeping, since the average proportion of surfaces and objects that will be disinfected in a patient's room is not more than 50% [76]
- 24-h scheduled briefings with the ICU and infection control teams
- Isolation procedures as soon as infection or contamination is suspected
- Early discharge of ICU patients
- Contaminated patients to be cared for in cohorts by designated nursing staff, with additional nurses to increase the workforce
- Particular attention to be paid to hospital surfaces, such as room door handles, and items that are transported by colonized persons, such as sterile packaging, mops, fabrics, plastics, pens, keyboards and monitors, stethoscopes, and telephones, because microorganisms easily contaminate such surfaces. In 65% of nurses caring for an infected patient, gowns or uniforms are contaminated, and in 42% of healthcare staff caring for a contaminated patient, their gloves are contaminated without the staff member having touched the contaminated patient [76].
- Closure of ICU beds, to improve the nurse-to-patient ratio.

In the case of a highly diffusive airborne infectious disease, such as H1N1, successful strategies for infection control in the ICU include [74]:

- Additional training for nurses on mechanical ventilation management
- Increasing ICU staffing, calling back the critical care nurses who previously worked in the ICU

- Weekly tracheal aspirate cultures and nasopharyngeal swabs for the early detection of patients who no longer need isolation and discharging these patients from the ICU
- Isolating patients through cohorts or private isolation rooms. Evidence suggests that transfer from semiprivate to private rooms alone can decrease hospital-acquired infection rates by up to 45% [76]
- Strengthening of collaboration levels among members of the ICU team
- Educating relatives about healthy hygienic behaviors to prevent the spread of the infection.

## 19.7.1 Issues Related to Standards and Precautions Related to Disease Transmission

Reaction to a disease outbreak in the ICU must be twofold: increasing the competencies and skills of the ICU staff in disease management and implementation of safety measures to contain the spread of the infection, as well as implementing adequate isolation procedures [74].

Education and training about infection control for critical care nurses should include [74]:

- Training modules about the fundamentals of quarantine and isolation, routes of infection transmission, and infectious disease prevention and control
- Basic pediatric intensive care protocols
- High-fidelity simulation of the management of high-risk and complex scenarios
- Debriefing and teach-back models
- Certification of the successful completion of education, and annual recertification.

However, the key to reaching a safe and optimal care setting depends on the availability of a robust hospital epidemiology program [77].

Many microorganisms responsible for recent outbreaks of viral infections can be deadly, not only for patients (even when they receive the best care) but also for the healthcare staff.

For infectious diseases transmitted through respiratory droplets, the ICU is a high-risk setting, owing to the performance of aerosol-generating procedures (suctioning, intubation, NIV, and bronchoscopy). Patients needing multiple procedures pose a high risk of contamination for healthcare staff [77].

The Ebola virus outbreak has set a new standard of infection control precautions (maximum isolation). Together with contact, droplet, and airborne precautions (Table 19.1), the need to prevent accidental exposure of all body surfaces emerged, with the provision of adequate protective clothing. Furthermore, a dedicated staff member, present as a trained observer, directly puts on and takes off the protective clothing and equipment from the care personnel to reduce the risk of mistakes and self-contamination [77].

Lastly, suitable protocols are needed to disinfect the care environment and to manage infected waste, and, in some cases, the architectural design of hospital areas has been modified [77].

**Table 19.1** Isolation precautions for airborne diseases [80]

| | |
|---|---|
| Isolation mode | Single room |
| | Negative pressure |
| | 6–12 Air exchanges per hour |
| | High Efficiency Particulate Air (HEPA) filtration |
| | Door maintained continuously closed |
| | Isolation sign on door |
| Staff members | N95, using high-level particulate respirator masks |
| | Education on use of respirator mask, fit testing, and checking the seal |
| | Healthcare worker medicine service scheduled controls |
| Patient | Surgical mask is mandatory if patient leaves the isolation room |

Currently, the employment of full protective body suits and powered air-purifying respirators is mandatory for the care of patients infected by Ebola, MERS-CoV, and SARS-CoV [77]. This kind of equipment requires high standards of training and periodic retraining [77]. Achieving an optimal level of proficiency in donning and removing the personal protective equipment for this kind of infective threat is critical. Studies have been performed comparing the effectiveness of different training programs for the management of full protective body suits [78]. However, there are still debates about the actual adequacy and effectiveness of the protective equipment used in the prevention of Ebola transmission [79].

The special training should be conducted while the critical care nurse is performing invasive procedures typical of critical care settings: intubation, MV (closed-system endotracheal tube suctioning and placement of a bacterial filter on the expiratory side of the ventilator circuit) [80], venous access introduction (ultrasound guided), CRRT, and bedside imaging, with the nurse using the full protective equipment in a high-containment unit (negative-pressure room) under biosafety level 3–4 isolation conditions [77]. Working inside a high-containment unit requires the nurses to place their own safety before the patient's needs, to move slowly, to pay great attention to sharp objects, and always to think before acting [81]. All the nursing care and procedures should be performed in pairs: one nurse cares for the patient and the other checks for breaches in personal protective equipment, disinfects the environment, and manages the waste appropriately, covering all the containers to avoid splashing [81]. Training programs also have to cover some important psychological features of this kind of nursing care: fatigue, fear, a sense of impotence, and the social consequences of the risks the nurses are exposed to.

In regard to the prevention of disease transmission, each institution should draft protocols for the management of laboratory tests, the handling of biological specimens, and imaging testing. Surgery and specialist consultations should also be considered in the safety management procedures. Lastly, the healthcare teams that will provide care for these high risk infected patients should be previously assigned, on either a voluntary or an obligatory basis [77].

## Take-Home Messages

- In future ICUs will probably see increases in the number of ICU beds relative to the number of beds in the rest of the hospital and the staff shortages could be "compensated by" computerized and/or nurse-driven clinical protocols. More multicenter and international trials will need to be performed, and pharmacological treatments for critically ill patients should be improved through various strategies.
- Priorities in critical care nursing research are: the development of methods for the rapid recognition of acute illness in high-risk patients; new approaches to enhancing patient comfort while reducing changes of consciousness; effective process and outcome measurements for critical illness research and palliative and EOL care; focus on patient safety issues; the impact of EBP and the workforce on patient outcomes; the comfort/well-being of patients and their relatives; the impact of EOL care on staff and nursing practice.
- Critical care nursing should, in particular, take into account the special needs of different patient populations, such as oncology patients, elderly patients, morbidly obese patients, and psychiatric patients admitted to the ICU.
- Forthcoming and highly challenging issues for ICU nurses are those related to critical care management during outbreaks of emerging infectious diseases.

## References

1. Vincent JL, Singer M, Marini JJ, Moreno R, Levy M, Matthay MA, et al. Thirty years of critical care medicine. Crit Care. 2010;14:311. https://doi.org/10.1186/cc8979.

2. Vincent JL. Critical care – where have we been and where are we going? Crit Care. 2013;17:S2. https://doi.org/10.1186/cc11500.
3. Vincent JL, Singer M. Critical care: advances and future perspectives. Lancet. 2010;376:1354–61. https://doi.org/10.1016/S0140-6736(10)60575-2.
4. Costa DK, Kahn JM. Organizing critical care for the 21st century. JAMA. 2016;315:751–2. https://doi.org/10.1001/jama.2016.0974.
5. Matthay MA, Liu KD. New strategies for effective therapeutics in critically ill patients. JAMA. 2016;315(8):747. https://doi.org/10.1001/jama.2016.0661.
6. Deutschman CS, Ahrens T, Cairns CB, Sessler CN, Parsons PE, Critical Care Societies Collaborative/USCIITG Task Force on Critical Care Research. Multisociety task force for critical care research: key issues and recommendations. Am J Respir Crit Care Med. 2012;185:96–102. https://doi.org/10.1164/rccm.201110-1848ST.
7. Blackwood B, Albarran JW, Latour JM. Research priorities of adult intensive care nurses in 20 European countries: a Delphi study. J Adv Nurs. 2011;67:550–62. https://doi.org/10.1111/j.1365-2648.2010.05512.x.
8. Giusti GD. The priorities in the nurse research in critical care. Scenario. 2015;32:3.
9. Davidson JE, Powers K, Hedayat KM, Tieszen M, Kon AA, Shepard E, et al. Clinical practice guidelines for support of the family in the patient-centered intensive care unit: American College of Critical Care Medicine Task Force 2004-2005. Crit Care Med. 2007;35:605–22. https://doi.org/10.1097/01.CCM.0000254067.14607.EB.
10. Giannini A. Open intensive care units: the case in favour. Minerva Anestesiol. 2007;73:299–305.
11. Giannini A. The "open" ICU: not just a question of time. Minerva Anestesiol. 2010;76:89–90.
12. Cappellini E, Bambi S, Lucchini A, Milanesio E. Open intensive care units: a global challenge for patients, relatives, and critical care teams. Dimens Crit Care Nurs. 2014;33:181–93. https://doi.org/10.1097/DCC.0000000000000052.
13. Cabrini L, Landoni G, Antonelli M, Bellomo R, Colombo S, Negro A, et al. Critical care in the near future: patient-centered, beyond space and time boundaries. Minerva Anestesiol. 2016;82:599–604.
14. Peris A, Bambi S. Family presence during cardiopulmonary resuscitation could make more natural organ donation. Int Emerg Nurs. 2014;22:234. https://doi.org/10.1016/j.ienj.2013.04.002.
15. Bambi S, Bombardi M, Bonizzoli M, Migliaccio ML, Giovannoni L, Minardi A, et al. Open visiting policies in intensive care units may not

affect consent to organ donation. Br J Anaesth. 2015;115:142–3. https://doi.org/10.1093/bja/aev179.

16. Tracy MF, Chlan L. Nonpharmacological interventions to manage common symptoms in patients receiving mechanical ventilation. Crit Care Nurse. 2011;31:19–28. https://doi.org/10.4037/ccn2011653.

17. Martin S. What criteria should be used for pet therapy in critical care? Are you aware of any hospitals doing this? Crit Care Nurse. 1993;13:74.

18. Cole KM, Gawlinski A. Animal-assisted therapy in the intensive care unit. A staff nurse's dream comes true. Nurs Clin North Am. 1995;30: 529–37.

19. Cole KM, Gawlinski A, Steers N, Kotlerman J. Animal-assisted therapy in patients hospitalized with heart failure. Am J Crit Care. 2007; 16:575–85.

20. Calcaterra V, Veggiotti P, Palestrini C, De Giorgis V, Raschetti R, Tumminelli M, et al. Post-operative benefits of animal-assisted therapy in pediatric surgery: a randomised study. PLoS One. 2015;10:e0125813. https://doi.org/10.1371/journal.pone.0125813.eCollection 2015.

21. Alameddine M, Dainty KN, Deber R, Sibbald WJ. The intensive care unit work environment: current challenges and recommendations for the future. J Crit Care. 2009;24:243–8. https://doi.org/10.1016/j.jcrc.2008.03.038.

22. Miracle VA. Suggestions for handling anger in the workplace. Dimens Crit Care Nurs. 2013;32:125–7. https://doi.org/10.1097/DCC.0b013e318286477e.

23. Alexanian JA, Kitto S, Rak KJ, Reeves S. Beyond the team: understanding interprofessional work in two north American ICUs. Crit Care Med. 2015;43:1880–6. https://doi.org/10.1097/CCM.0000000000001136.

24. Parker MM. Teamwork in the ICU-do we practice what we preach? Crit Care Med. 2016;44:254–5. https://doi.org/10.1097/CCM.0000000000001524.

25. Kelso LA. Teamwork in the ICU: from training camp to the super bowl. Crit Care Med. 2015;43:2026–7. https://doi.org/10.1097/CCM.0000000000001177.

26. Blake N. The nurse leader's role in supporting healthy work environments. AACN Adv Crit Care. 2015;26:201–3. https://doi.org/10.1097/NCI.0000000000000089.

27. Blake N. The healthy work environment standards: ten years later. AACN Adv Crit Care. 2015;26:97–8. https://doi.org/10.1097/NCI.0000000000000078.

28. Darvas JA, Hawkins LG. What makes a good intensive care unit: a nursing perspective. Aust Crit Care. 2002;15:77–82.

29. Azoulay E, Timsit JF, Sprung CL, Soares M, Rusinová K, Lafabrie A, et al. Prevalence and factors of intensive care unit conflicts: the conflicus study. Am J Respir Crit Care Med. 2009;180:853–60. https://doi.org/10.1164/rccm.200810-1614OC.

30. Grant M. Resolving communication challenges in the intensive care unit. AACN Adv Crit Care. 2015;26:123–30. https://doi.org/10.1097/NCI.0000000000000076.

31. Hartog CS, Benbenishty J. Understanding nurse-physician conflicts in the ICU. Intensive Care Med. 2015;41:331–3. https://doi.org/10.1007/s00134-014-3517-z.

32. Bambi S, Mattiussi E, Giusti GD, Lucchini A, Manici M, Comisso I. The strange and conflicting world of nursing. Intensive Care Med. 2015;41:1372–3. https://doi.org/10.1007/s00134-015-3843-9.

33. Bambi S, Becattini G, Giusti GD, Mezzetti A, Guazzini A, Lumini E. Lateral hostilities among nurses employed in intensive care units, emergency departments, operating rooms, and emergency medical services. A national survey in Italy. Dimens Crit Care Nurs. 2014;33:347–54. https://doi.org/10.1097/DCC.0000000000000077.

34. Camerino D, Estryn-Behar M, Conway PM, van Der Heijden BIJ, Hasselhorn H. Work-related factors and violence among nursing staff in the European NEXT study: a longitudinal cohort study. Int J Nurs Stud. 2008;45:35–50.

35. Moayed FA, Daraiseh N, Shell R, Salem S. Workplace bullying: a systematic review of risk factors and outcomes. Theor Issues Ergon. 2006;7:311–27.

36. Vessey JA, Demarco RF, Gaffney DA, Budin WC. Bullying of staff registered nurses in the workplace: a preliminary study for developing personal and organizational strategies for the transformation of hostile to healthy workplace environments. J Prof Nurs. 2009;25:299–306. https://doi.org/10.1016/j.profnurs.2009.01.022.

37. Purpora C, Blegen MA. Horizontal violence and the quality and safety of patient care: a conceptual model. Nurs Res Pract. 2012;306948. https://doi.org/10.1155/2012/306948.

38. Roberts SJ. Oppressed group behavior: implications for nursing. ANS Adv Nurs Sci. 1983;5:21–30.

39. Vessey JA, De Marco R, Di Fazio R. Bullying, harassment, and horizontal violence in the nursing workforce. The state of the science. Annu Rev Nurs Res. 2010;28:133–57.

40. Roberts SJ, Demarco R, Griffin M. The effect of oppressed group behaviours on the culture of the nursing workplace: a review of the evidence and interventions for change. J Nurs Manag. 2009;17:288–93.

41. Brinkert R. A literature review of conflict communication causes, costs, benefits and interventions in nursing. J Nurs Manag. 2010;18:145–56. https://doi.org/10.1111/j.1365-2834.2010.01061.x.

42. The Joint Commission. Behaviors that undermine a culture of safety. Sentinel Event Alert. Issue 40. 2008. https://www.jointcommission.org/assets/1/18/SEA_40.PDF. Accessed 15 Feb 2016.

43. American Association of Critical Nurses (AACN). Standards for establishing and sustaining healthy work environments. A journey to excellence. Executive Summary. AACN. 2005. http://www.aacn.org/wd/hwe/docs/execsum.pdf. Accessed on 15 Feb 2016.

44. Barrett A, Piatek C, Korber S, Padula C. Lessons learned from a lateral violence and team-building intervention. Nurs Adm Q. 2009;33:342–51. https://doi.org/10.1097/NAQ.0b013e3181b9de0b.

45. Deltsidou A. Undergraduate nursing students' level of assertiveness in Greece: a questionnaire survey. Nurse Educ Pract. 2009;9:322–30. https://doi.org/10.1016/j.nepr.2008.08.002.

46. Begley CM, White P. Irish nursing students' changing self-esteem and fear of negative evaluation during their preregistration programme. J Adv Nurs. 2003;42:390–401.

47. Royal College of Nursing (RCN). Dealing with bullying and harassment at work—a guide for RCN members. 2015, Revised December 2005. http://www2.rcn.org.uk/__data/assets/pdf_file/0009/643482/Bullying-at-work-short.pdf. Accessed 15 Feb 2016.

48. Dimarino TJ. Eliminating lateral violence in the ambulatory setting: one center's strategies. AORN J. 2011;93:583–8. https://doi.org/10.1016/j.aorn.2010.10.019.

49. Kleinert S, Horton R. Rethinking and reframing obesity. Lancet. 2015;385:2326–8. https://doi.org/10.1016/S0140-6736(15)60163-5.

50. Jones SB. Preface: obesity. Int Anesthesiol Clin. 2013;51:xi–xii. https://doi.org/10.1097/AIA.0b013e3182988c98.

51. Koba P. Identifying obstacles for the obese trauma patient. J Trauma Nurs. 2016;23:45–8. https://doi.org/10.1097/JTN.0000000000000178.

52. Erstad BL. Obesity in critical illness: what weight or why weight? Crit Care Med. 2012;40:1657–9. https://doi.org/10.1097/CCM.0b013e3182411720.

53. Shearer E. Critical care management of obese patients. Int Anesthesiol Clin. 2013;51:164–78. https://doi.org/10.1097/AIA.0b013e31829813a8.

54. Bambi S, Ruggeri M, Becattini G, Lumini E. Bariatric patients in emergency department: a challenge for nursing care. Scenario. 2013;30:4–15.

55. Flaatten H, Garrouste-Orgeas M. The very old ICU patient: a never-ending story. Intensive Care Med. 2015;41:1996–8. https://doi.org/10.1007/s00134-015-4052-2.

56. Crippen DW. Very elderly patients in the ICU: should there be a line in the sand? Crit Care Med. 2015;43:1527–8. https://doi.org/10.1097/CCM.0000000000001044.

57. Zivot JB. Elder care in the ICU: spin bravely? Crit Care Med. 2015;43:1526–7. https://doi.org/10.1097/CCM.0000000000001055.

58. Heyland D, Cook D, Bagshaw SM, Garland A, Stelfox HT, Mehta S, et al. The very elderly admitted to ICU: a quality finish? Crit Care Med. 2015;43:1352–60. https://doi.org/10.1097/CCM.0000000000001024.

59. Heyland DK, Garland A, Bagshaw SM, Cook D, Rockwood K, Stelfox HT, et al. Recovery after critical illness in patients aged 80 years or older: a multi-center prospective observational cohort study. Intensive Care Med. 2015;41:1911–20. https://doi.org/10.1007/s00134-015-4028-2.

60. Stevens CL, Torke AM. Geriatric trauma: a clinical and ethical review. J Trauma Nurs. 2016;23:36–41. https://doi.org/10.1097/JTN.0000000000000179.

61. Deeny P. Care of older people in critical care: the hidden side of the moon. Intensive Crit Care Nurs. 2005;21:325–7. https://doi.org/10.1016/j.iccn.2005.09.005.

62. Hardin SR. Vulnerability of older patients in critical care. Crit Care Nurse. 2015;35:55–61. https://doi.org/10.4037/ccn2015995.

63. Ampélas JF, Pochard F, Consoli SM. Psychiatric disorders in intensive care units. Encéphale. 2002;28:191–9.

64. Pochard F. Psychiatric issues during and after intensive care (ICU) stays. Bull Acad Natl Med. 2011;195:377–85.

65. Bienvenu OJ, Neufeld KJ, Needham DM. Treatment of four psychiatric emergencies in the intensive care unit. Crit Care Med. 2012;40:2662–70. https://doi.org/10.1097/CCM.0b013e31825ae0f8.

66. New AM, Nelson S, Leung JG. Psychiatric emergencies in the intensive care unit. AACN Adv Crit Care. 2015;26:285–93. https://doi.org/10.1097/NCI.0000000000000104.

67. Brennan CW, Prince-Paul M, Wiencek CA. Providing a "good death" for oncology patients during the final hours of life in the intensive care unit. AACN Adv Crit Care. 2011;22:379–96. https://doi.org/10.1097/NCI.0b013e31823100dc.

68. Ferlay J, Steliarova-Foucher E, Lortet-Tieulent J, Rosso S, Coebergh JW, Comber H, et al. Cancer incidence and mortality patterns in Europe: estimates for 40 countries in 2012. Eur J Cancer. 2013;49:1374–403. https://doi.org/10.1016/j.ejca.2012.12.027.

69. Daly BJ. Caring for the critically ill patient with cancer. AACN Adv Crit Care. 2011;22:321–2. https://doi.org/10.1097/NCI.0b013e31822f57b5.

70. Demshar R, Vanek R, Mazanec P. Oncologic emergencies: new decade, new perspectives. AACN Adv Crit Care. 2011;22:337–48. https://doi.org/10.1097/NCI.0b013e318230112b.

71. Azoulay E, Soares M, Darmon M, Benoit D, Pastores S, Afessa B. Intensive care of the cancer patient: recent achievements and remaining challenges. Ann Intensive Care. 2011;1:5. https://doi.org/10.1186/2110-5820-1-5.

72. Wiencek CA, Ferrell BR, Jackson M. The meaning of our work: caring for the critically ill patient with cancer. AACN Adv Crit Care. 2011;22:397–407. https://doi.org/10.1097/NCI.0b013e318232c6ef.

73. Dondorp AM, Iyer SS, Schultz MJ. Critical care in resource-restricted settings. JAMA. 2016;315:753–4. https://doi.org/10.1001/jama.2016.0976.

74. Makamure M, Makamure M, Mendiola W, Renteria D, Repp M, Willden A. A review of critical care nursing and disease outbreak preparedness. Dimens Crit Care Nurs. 2013;32:157–61. https://doi.org/10.1097/DCC.0b013e318299801f.

75. Garnacho-Montero J, Dimopoulos G, Poulakou G, Akova M, Cisneros JM, De Waele J, et al. Task force on management and prevention of Acinetobacter Baumannii infections in the ICU. Intensive Care Med. 2015;41:2057–75. https://doi.org/10.1007/s00134-015-4079-4.

76. Colatrella S, Clair JD. Adapt or perish - a relentless fight for survival: designing superbugs out of the intensive care unit. Crit Care Nurs Q. 2014;37:251–67. https://doi.org/10.1097/CNQ.0000000000000029.

77. Chertow DS, Palmore TN, Masur H. Critical care medicine after the 2014–2015 Ebola outbreak: are we ready if it happens again? Crit Care Med. 2016;44:457–9. https://doi.org/10.1097/CCM.000000000001590.

78. Casalino E, Astocondor E, Sanchez JC, Díaz-Santana DE, Del Aguila C, Carrillo JP. Personal protective equipment for the Ebola virus disease: a comparison of 2 training programs. Am J Infect Control. 2015;43:1281–7. https://doi.org/10.1016/j.ajic.2015.07.007.

79. MacIntyre CR, Chughtai AA, Seale H, Richards GA, Davidson PM. Uncertainty, risk analysis and change for Ebola personal protective equipment guidelines. Int J Nurs Stud. 2015;52:899–903. https://doi.org/10.1016/j.ijnurstu.2014.12.001.

80. York NL, Kane C. Caring for the critically ill patient with tuberculosis. Dimens Crit Care Nurs. 2013;32:6–11. https://doi.org/10.1097/DCC.0b013e3182768045.

81. Johnson SS, Barranta N, Chertow D. Ebola at the National Institutes of Health: perspectives from critical care nurses. AACN Adv Crit Care. 2015;26:262–7. https://doi.org/10.1097/NCI.0000000000000103.

# Erratum to: Venous Thromboembolism Prevention and Prophylaxis

**Matteo Manici, Giacomo Alemanno, and Margherita I. Nuzzaco**

**Erratum to:**
**Chapter 13 in: I. Comisso et al., *Nursing in Critical Care Setting,***
**https://doi.org/10.1007/978-3-319-50559-6**

The author name was misspelled as Magherita I. Nuzzacco and it has now been corrected as Margherita I. Nuzzaco.

The updated online version of the original chapter can be found at
https://doi.org/10.1007/978-3-319-50559-6_13